Pathogenesis of Idiopathic Scoliosis

Masafumi Machida • Stuart L. Weinstein
Jean Dubousset
Editors

Pathogenesis of Idiopathic Scoliosis

Springer

Editors
Masafumi Machida
Department of Spine and Spinal Cord Surgery
Yokohama Brain and Spine Center
Yokohama, Kanagawa, Japan

Stuart L. Weinstein
University of Iowa
Iowa, USA

Jean Dubousset
Academie Nationale de Medecine
Paris, France

ISBN 978-4-431-56539-0 ISBN 978-4-431-56541-3 (eBook)
https://doi.org/10.1007/978-4-431-56541-3

Library of Congress Control Number: 2017964308

Printed on acid-free paper

This Springer imprint is published by Springer Nature
The registered company is Springer Japan KK
The registered company address is: Shiroyama Trust Tower, 4-3-1 Toranomon, Minato-ku, Tokyo 105-6005, Japan

Foreword

I first met Dr Masafumi Machida in 1989, when he came to France with a Cotrel Fellowship program, for a training on CD instrumentation.

Years later, in 2000, one of his research projects on etiopathogenesis of idiopathic scoliosis was selected by the members of the scientific Board of the Fondation Cotrel. Ever since then, I have witnessed his dedication to attending the annual meetings in Paris, sharing his progresses with all the researchers.

As the founder of the Fondation Cotrel for spinal research—Institut de France and as a friend, it is now my pleasure to write a few words for this book dedicated to the pathogenesis of idiopathic scoliosis.

I am pleased to see such a book being published.

I have known most of the authors—if not all of them—for many years. I know of their dedication to fundamental basic science and research as well as clinical work on this topic.

Despite the obvious major improvements of the last four decades for the surgical treatment of scoliosis, the scientific explanation of its occurrence will be a great step forward.

I am sure the readers of this book will find the historic aspect as well as a real update of this problem of high interest.

This book brings up the most recent results as well as some openings for future works, leading one day, hopefully, to the prevention of such disorder.

These works put the stress on the importance of the most early detection possible and the risk of progression, in order to start the proper treatment and get the best result possible. The purpose is to avoid the surgery: even though the techniques have improved, they still ankylose, at more or less extent, the spinal organ.

I want to thank Professor Machida and the authors who have participated into this book for sharing their scientific knowledge, hopes and aims oriented toward a better and comprehensive understanding of the initiation of the disease.

This will, no doubt, benefit to the patients and their families.

Docteur Yves Cotrel

Preface

Idiopathic scoliosis comprises a three-dimensional deformity of the spine with lateral curvature combined with vertebral rotation that develops in the absence of congenital spinal anomaly or neurologic musculoskeletal disorders. First described by Hippocrates, the entity became known as "idiopathic scoliosis", the term probably introduced in the middle of nineteenth century by Bauer, used by Nathan in 1909 and defined by Whitman in 1922.

A number of genetic, biochemical, skeletal and neuromuscular abnormalities have emerged as contributing elements in the pathogenesis of idiopathic scoliosis in humans and experimentally induced scoliosis in animals. These multiple factors, however, may constitute its epiphenomena rather than etiologic causes. More recent studies using magnetic resonance imaging have aimed to investigate the potential contribution of the central nervous system. Developments in diffusion tensor imaging allows the assessment of white matter microstructure such as synchronization of axonal myelination and pruning. Advances in human genome mapping and genetic methodology has made it possible to screen the entire genome of an individual with genetic markers evenly spaced along the chromosomes. Using this technique, called positional cloning or linkage analysis, recent genome-wide association study yielded candidate genes that implicate neuromuscular disease origins. Next-generation genomic technologies may enable the creation of idiopathic scoliosis mutations in the animal model.

A couple of text books dealing with this subject matter are already available: "Pathogenesis of Idiopathic Scoliosis" by Scoliosis Research Society in 1983 and "The Aetiology of Idiopathic Scoliosis" by Gordon Robin in 1990. Since their publication, a large number of articles appeared relative to pathogenesis of idiopathic scoliosis. We have incorporated these new data in preparing the current volume. I have asked my mentors, Dr. Jean Dubousset, to describe the definition of idiopathic scoliosis and Dr. Stuart Weinstein, to summarize its natural history based on his own Iowa experience. Both also served as editors of the remaining chapters, which introduce new concepts and current topics in each area of pathogenies of idiopathic scoliosis.

A majority of investigators now regard idiopathic scoliosis as a multifactorial disease with genetic predisposing factors. In most current studies, observed abnormalities may represent secondary features of the disease, making it difficult to distinguish the primary cause of the disease. We hope future studies will identify various factors directly involved in the causation of this disorder. Only then, we will be able to elaborate on its effective treatment and undertake plans for its eventual eradication.

Yokohama, Japan Masafumi Machida

Contents

Chapter 1
Definition of Adolescent Idiopathic Scoliosis

Jean Dubousset

1.1 Introduction

1.1.1 First Statement

The normal spinal organ must be considered as the skeleton of the trunk. It starts from the head, considered physiologically as the first vertebra. The head is heavy (4–5 kg) and forms a reverse pendulum with the spine when in an upright position. This head vertebra is supported by the cervical part of the spine with its seven vertebrae. Below this are the12 thoracic vertebrae, then the lumbar region with its five vertebrae. The entire pelvis (sacrum plus iliac bones) can be considered as the pelvic vertebra, because the motion of the sacroiliac joint is physiologically below 1.5°, as measured by White and Panjabi [1]. This pelvic vertebra plays the major role of an intercalary bone between the trunk and the lower limbs. The pelvis is mobile upon the two hip joints and the skeleton of the lower limbs, where several segments and mobile joints reach the bones of the feet. The system adapts the weight of the body and its motion to the polygon of support to achieve the "chain of balance" of the human body. The definition for me of the human body balance is " stability within movement"!

1.1.2 Second Statement

This anatomical entity is mobile and strong, straight on the frontal plane, and presents harmonious curves in the lateral plane, such as the cervical lordosis and thoracic kyphosis lumbar lordosis. Pelvic orientation adapts to realize a harmonious chain of balance. The major functions of the spinal organ are to (1) protect the central nervous system and particularly the spinal cord; (2) support the skeleton of the thoracic cage with its respiratory and circulatory organs and, thus, support the upper limbs; and (3) support the abdomen viscera and muscles and all constitutive masses of the body, giving them stability within movement.

J. Dubousset, M.D.
Académie Nationale de Médecine, Paris, France
e-mail: jean.dubousset@wanadoo.fr

M. Machida et al. (eds.), *Pathogenesis of Idiopathic Scoliosis*,
https://doi.org/10.1007/978-4-431-56541-3_1

1.1.3 Third Statement

This mixture of stability and movement allows the spinal organ to play an important role in compensation mechanisms in regard to a variety of inherited or acquired pathological problems or physiological difficulties, especially those correlated with aging. The common factor leading to these phenomena is the necessity for the human to maintain horizontal vision when in an erect posture.

1.2 Scoliosis

The word "scoliosis" comes from the Greek language and means "crooked" or twisting, as applied to a pathway in the middle of a rocky mountain or the visual aspect of the trunk of a tree after difficult growth subsequent to multiples injuries but trying always to recover the vertical axis. It is not surprising that the first description of scoliosis in humans was made by Hippocrates [2] and applied to all kinds of malalignment of the spine. It was a remarkable observation because Hippocrates recognized that many deformities occurred in patients that were otherwise in good health, but also he also recognized the poor prognosis when it was an early onset of the disease.

The first accurate description of scoliosis, especially adolescent idiopathic scoliosis (AIS) was made by Ambroise Paré (1510–1590), who tried to treat patients with the well-known iron brace [3]. It is noticeable that he was probably the first to describe congenital anomalies of the spine as the origin of some deformities. Every orthopedic surgeon remembers the crooked tree symbol of orthopedics given by Nicolas Andry in 1741 [4]. This author favored poor posture to be the initiator of the disease. It took time to differentiate between postural and structural deformities, despite beautiful anatomical descriptions given by many authors during the nineteenth century on both sides of the Atlantic ocean, long before Roentgen's discovery (28 Dec 1895). Before this date, everybody was thinking in terms of three dimensions (3D). Numerous testimonies describe the deformity exactly in 3D, thanks to observation of clinical cases and specimens. These appeared in the publications and beautiful drawings by Shaw (1824), Adams, and Bouvier (1858). Ingenious machines were invented, like that of Schulthess, which was able to give simultaneously the shape of the back, frontal, and sagittal. The cyrtometer of Zander gave the horizontal shape of the trunk at any level. Some works were very suggestive of a 3D approach, long before X-rays were discovered. Samuel Hare of London (1849) gave practical observations on the prevention, causes, and treatment of curvatures of the spine. He used cast molding to beautifully demonstrate, before and after, the reduction of deformity thanks to extended (over 12 months) traction from shoulders and feet. By the end of the nineteenth century, surgeons could distinguish some differences in the etiologies of the spinal deformities called scoliosis, but the basic deformity with lateral inflexion and non-reducible torsion was still called scoliosis, whatever the etiology.

When the era of X-rays began at the beginning of the twentieth century, it was so revolutionary to see the "inside" of the body (the skeleton) on film that the 3D aspect was forgotten. It took time (almost half a century, especially for spinal morphology) to integrate that, in reality, these beautiful X-rays showed only the projection on one plane ("Chinese shadow" as we say in the French language) of the spinal organ, which is built and developed in 3D (Fig. 1.1). When I started my residency in 1960, most of the AIS patients were diagnosed, treated (even with surgery), and monitored only with frontal plane X-rays. Studies with antero-posterior (AP) and sagittal X-rays were more used to study limited congenital, infectious, or traumatic lesions. It took almost another 20 years (1979) before systematic AP and lateral X-rays were used to study AIS patients. Simultaneously, imaging using tomography (or laminography) was developed, but was reserved for exploring a localized region of the spine. Subsequent development of computed tomography (CT) (1973) gave one or a succession of transverse slices of the localized spinal element being studied. Personally, the 3D became evident when preparing the yearly meeting of the French Scoliosis Group in 1972; the topic was "paralytic pelvic obliquity." At the meeting in Feb 1973, I used the term "3D" and explicitly presented drawings showing each one of the three planes, the deformity of the pelvis, and the deformity of the spine (Fig. 1.2). I did the same with drawings at the combined GES/SRS meeting in Lyon (1973) when Pierre Stagnara asked me to present the prognostication and treatment of congenital anomalies of the spine. The concept was easily understood by everybody for

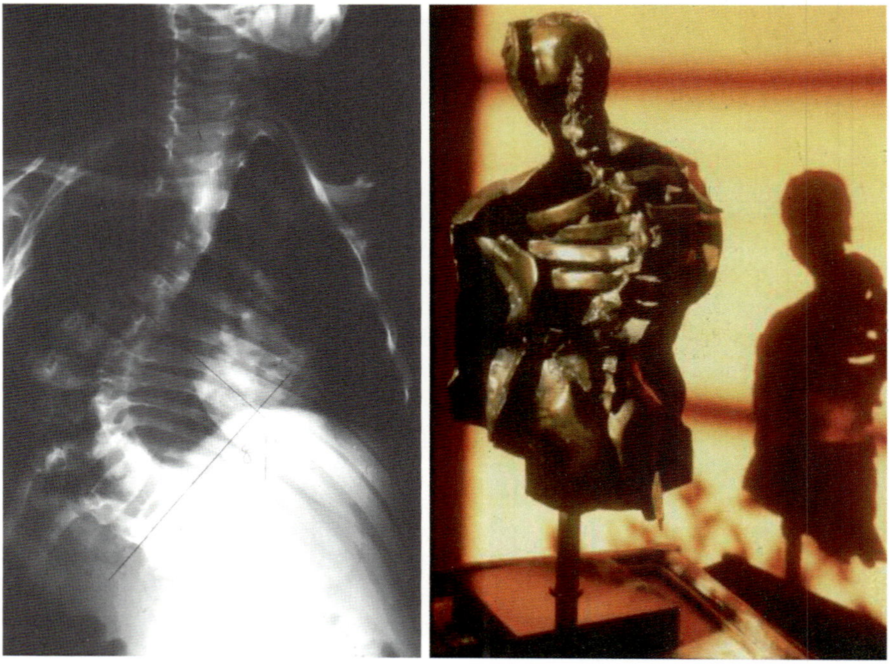

Fig. 1.1 X-rays are shadows from the projection of a 3D object onto one plane

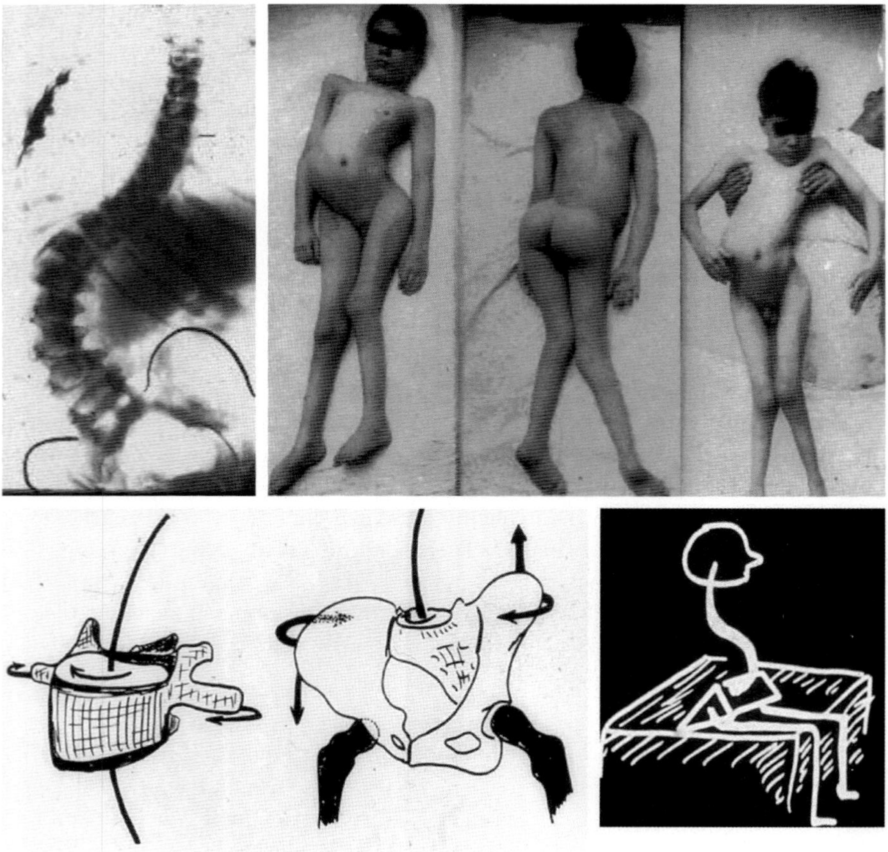

Fig. 1.2 Scoliosis and pelvic obliquity. The entire pelvis is considered as one unique vertebra, displaced in the three dimensions of the space. The clinical picture of such a patient is very demonstrative of such definition, but not so well approached by the X-ray projection

these congenital deformities. However, it was not well understood for AIS because the surgeons were "addicted" to their habitual AP and (sometimes) lateral views (Fig. 1.3a, b). Nevertheless, many spine surgeons realized the problem of the false image of a curve given by X-rays; for example, Sommerville and Roaf in England and Pierre Stagnara in France, who described the "plan d'élection" (plane of maximum deformity). In addition, the beautiful work of René Perdriolle, done between 1976 and 1979, was published at that time in *La Scoliose: son etude tridimensionnelle* [5]. René established the basis for understanding 3D and its implication for the pathogenesis of AIS. In 1977, together with Henry Graf and Jerome Hecquet (a computer engineer), we attempted [6] to reconstruct the spine in 3D, starting from two successive X-rays (AP and lateral). We used a simplified model for the vertebrae: a simple line to represent each vertebra in space first, then the surface of an ideal model, and then the volume of such model. The final step was to modify the same

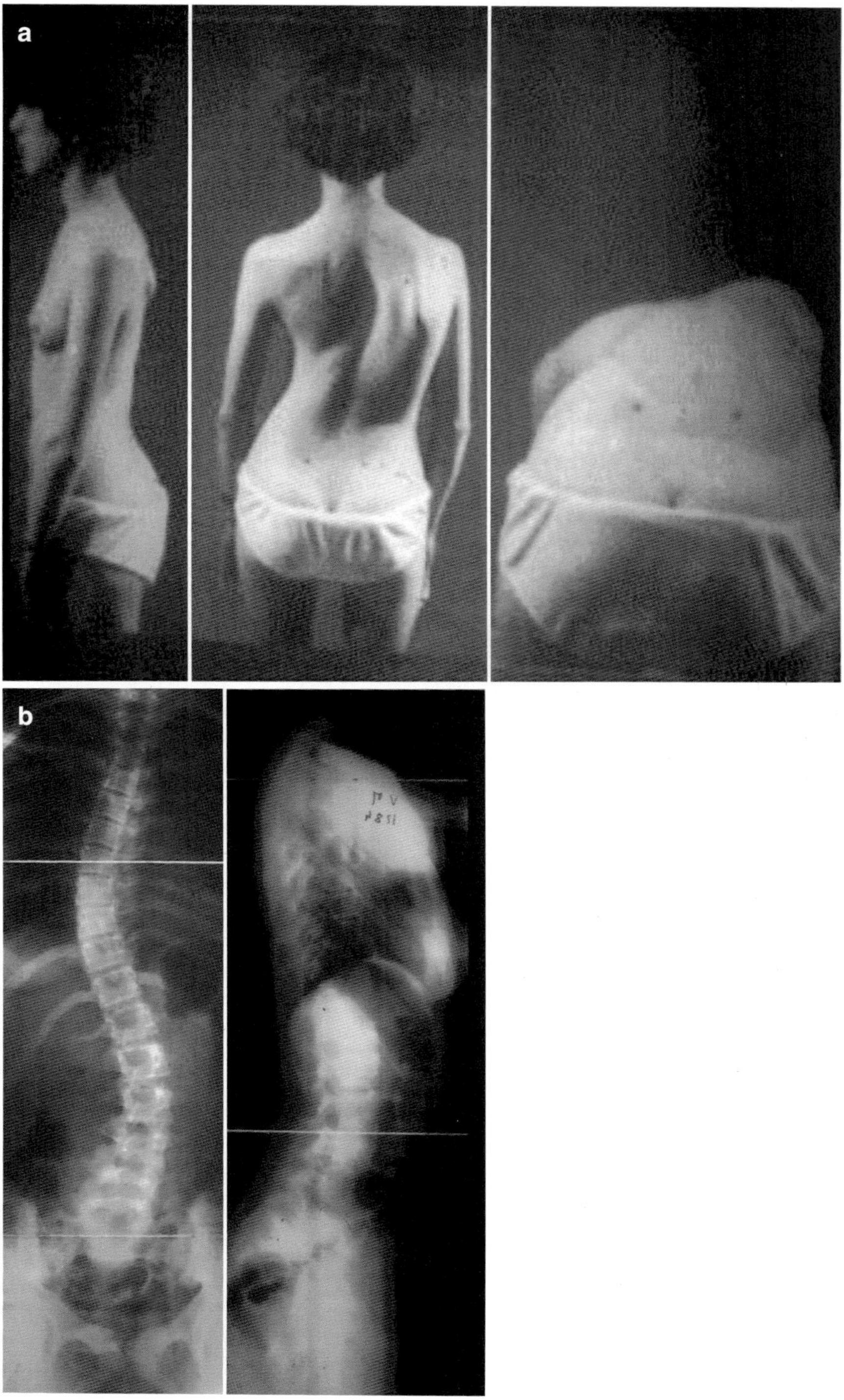

Fig. 1.3 (**a**) Clinical aspect of a right thoracic idiopathic scoliosis. (**b**) Radiological aspect AP and lateral of a right thoracic scoliosis

volume by hand so that the projected reconstruction closely matched the real X-rays (Fig. 1.4). The results were compared with a skeleton specimen of AIS and conformed well to reality, especially the view from the top. We presented this work at the Scoliosis French group meeting in Montreal in 1979, where the main topic was "AIS seen from the lateral." From that time, French doctors became more sensitive to the problem of the sagittal plane. We presented this at the SRS meeting in Chicago in 1980, but none of the orthopedic surgeons were interested; only Al Schultz (a well-known biomechanical engineer) came to me to ask questions. The development in 1990 of 3D CT reconstruction (not acceptable in children because of the excessive amount of radiation needed) demonstrated the value of this 3D concept, but it took a long time to be accepted and used in practice.

Although study of the sagittal plane has entered daily practice, especially because of the development of adult degenerative spine surgery, the horizontal plane remains one of the most forgotten despite beautiful specimens and reconstructions proving clearly that a scoliotic curve cannot be inscribed in one plane, but requires an infinity of successive planes. We inspired the team of Georges Charpak to develop a new imaging device (EOS imaging) [7]. The EOS system uses low doses of radiations and 3D computer surface and volume reconstruction (thanks to joint work from the engineers of ENSAM Paris and LIO Montreal) and has helped to introduce 3D into the daily clinical approach to AIS (Fig. 1.5). All analyses of the deformity, before and after treatment (surgical or not), can be carried out using this technique, as well as simulations of different ways of correction and studies of prediction of progression for early detected cases with mild deformity. For these reconstructions, the most attractive view (but also the less studied up to now) is the view from the top, which address the horizontal plane beautifully and shows the basic deformity of the scoliosis – torsion/rotation (Fig. 1.6).

The most important word in the definition of scoliosis is "curve." What is a curve? It is a segment of the spine that, instead of being normally aligned straight, as seen on the frontal plane of a normal spine, is bent laterally on either the right or left side. Seen on the lateral plane, the normal spine presents physiological curves; when the alignment is bent toward the front it is kyphosis and toward the back it is lordosis. Generally, in a normal posture the spine does not present any axial rotation. During motion, when the spine is bent laterally, a combined axial rotation occurs called coupled. This is normal mobility and returns to normal when the motion is finished. It is why it is important to make the distinction between postural and structural deformity:

- *Postural* means that the deformity is completely reducible in all its components. For example, a discrepancy in the length of limbs creates lateral tilting of the spine with lateral inclination, which is easily seen on an AP standing X-ray, but disappears completely when the discrepancy is compensated for with a lift under one foot.
- *Structural* means that the deformity generally includes lateral inclination, axial (horizontal) rotation, and sagittal displacement in flexion (kyphosis) or extension (lordosis). Most importantly, the deformity cannot be reduced completely in any

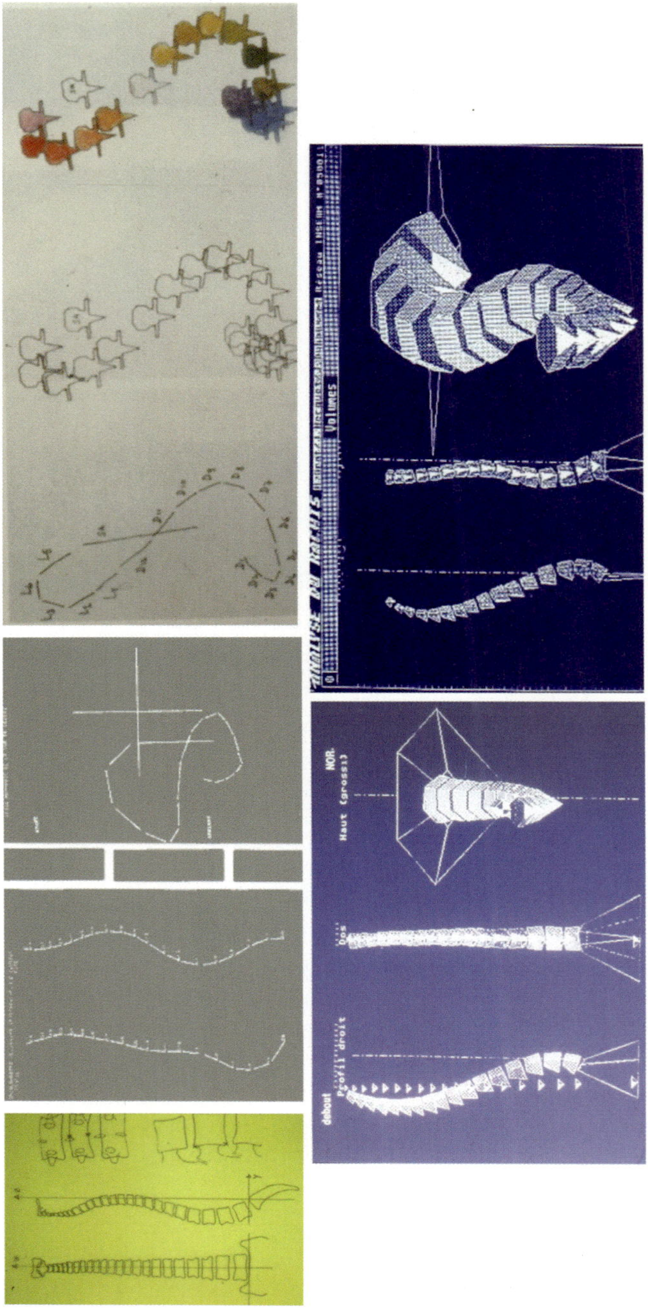

Fig. 1.4 Jerome Hecquet computer reconstruction from two orthogonal X-rays of a scoliotic spine: lines first, then simple surface model, then volume. Notice the view from the top, demonstrating clearly the "piling up" of the vertebrae from feet to head

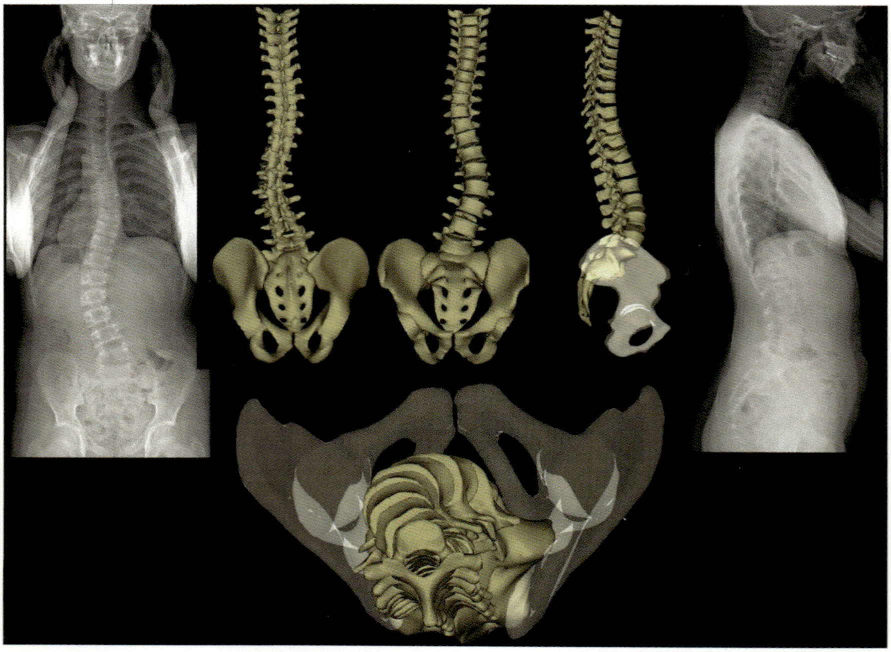

Fig. 1.5 EOS imaging system: 3D computer reconstruction of an idiopathic scoliosis

position or through traction, bending etc. In summary, a structural curve is a segment of the spine with a 3D deformity and a lack of sufficient flexibility to reduce the deformity (Fig. 1.7).

The next step in defining scoliotic deformity of a normally built spine (without congenital anomalies and without evident paralytic or dystrophic components) depends on *the way of installation*; there are two major ways.

The first situation develops during childhood and growth, creating a progressive torsion/rotation/inclination of a normally constructed spine, but in any component (bone tissue, cartilage, discs, ligaments, and muscles – almost any cell!!!). There is progressive structural change and deformation of the tissues of the vertebra, but with continuity between the components during the piling up process that occurs with growth. This lead to the type of idiopathic scoliosis where the bone deformity is primary. I used to teach my students using the term "ascending scoliosis." The end result is a scoliotic spine with a succession of structural and compensatory curvatures to achieve a more or less balanced alignment between head and feet.

The second situation, discogenic cascade, occurs much later, in adulthood or when ageing is more or less advanced. Here, the piling up of the vertebrae is progressively destroyed by primary disc degeneration; bone deformity can occur but is secondary. For my students, I used the term "descending scoliosis." The end result is also a succession of curves, very often linked by zones of rotatory dislocation at the level of a junction.

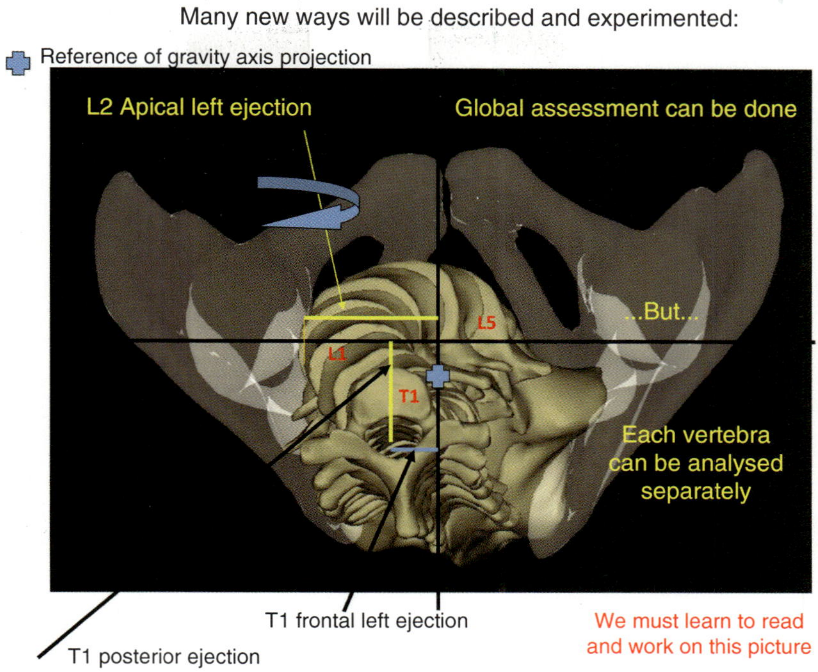

Fig. 1.6 The view from the top allows study of the horizontal plane deformity and the 3D localization of the curves of a scoliotic spine

The distinction between the two groups is important because the method of reduction can differ from one group to the other. With ageing, the scoliotic spine of the first group may develop degenerative changes, creating a mixture of the two pathologies.

Measurement of these deformities can be done by clinical examination and imaging with X-rays or magnetic resonance imaging (MRI).

Clinically, static measurements from the gravity line axis include the center of polygon of support, feet to head or head to feet alignment using a plumb line or force plate, leg length discrepancy, and alignment of the shoulders and pelvis from the front, back, and lateral. With a forward bending of the trunk, measurement of the rib hump (Adams test) is done at the apex by the arithmetical rule (in millimeters or centimeters) and by angulation using a scoliometer. Sophisticated measurements can be done using cyrtometry, which gives the circular shape of the thorax at various levels (upper, middle, and lower thorax). This measurement can be better obtained from the plaster molding used by orthotists before surface topography measurements with a computer. I must mention the optical surface topography device developed by the Russian Institute of Novosibirsk. The device gives stimulating information by approaching the 3D in a better way.

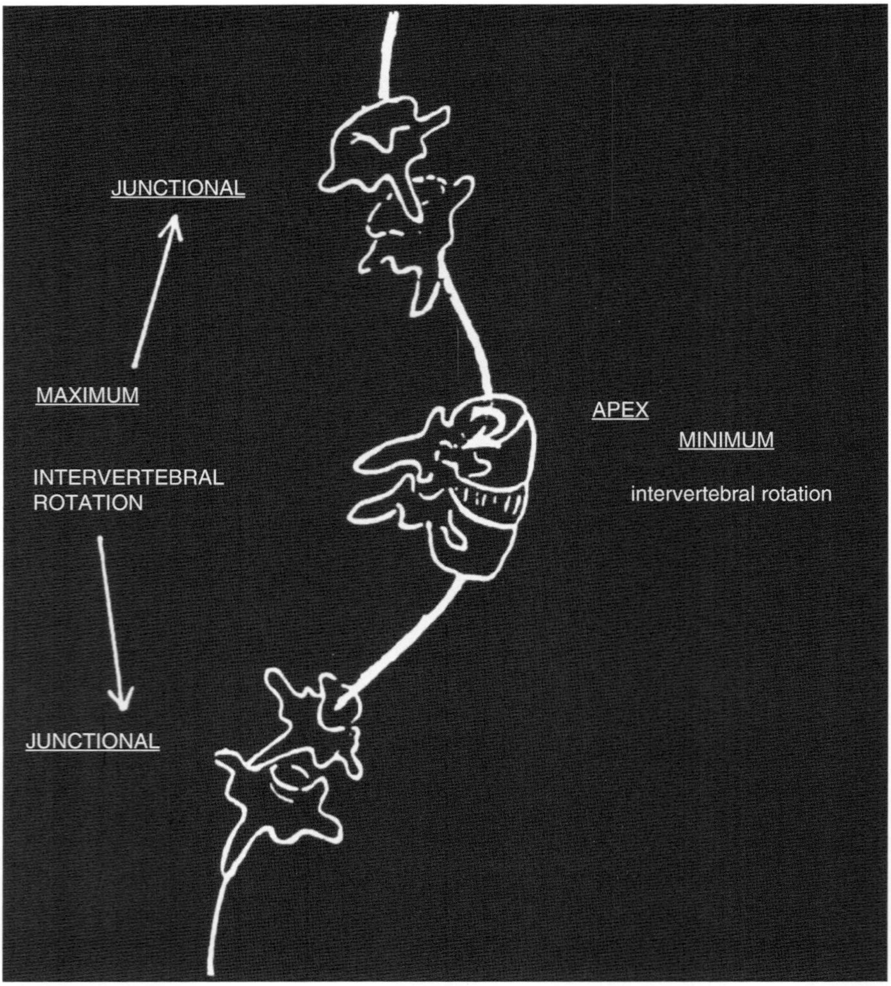

Fig. 1.7 Schematic 3D drawing of a scoliotic spine, demonstrating the structural curve and the junctional zone

Dynamic measures during bending (front, back, lateral, and rotatory) check the relative flexibility or stiffness of the spine so that a differential diagnosis of non-idiopathic etiology can be made.

Imaging is generally carried out using X-ray machines or MRI. Most of the measurements are 2D, resulting from the projection on one plane of the shadow of a 3D skeleton. The most used index is the Cobb angle, obtained on the frontal projection from the crossing of the line parallel to the upper or lower plateau of upper end vertebra of the curve and the line parallel to the lower plateau of the lower end vertebra of the curve. The same Cobb angle is measured on the lateral projection, giving an idea of the projected kyphosis or lordosis. We know that these angles are not true because they do not represent the 3D, but they are used by habit and accepted as reference by the scoliosis community. The rotation in the horizontal or axial plane of the vertebra is measured by the Nash and Moe method (classified as +, ++, +++), coming from the projection of the pedicles relative to the projection of the lateral walls of the vertebral body. More precise and reliable measurement of rotation is obtained with the Perdriolle torsiometer, which measures angles. For example, axial rotation of the vertebra is maximum at the apex of the curve, but intervertebral rotation (with the vertebra immediately adjacent) is minimum. When we reach the superior or inferior end vertebrae of the curve, axial rotation is close to 0° for the neutral vertebra, but intervertebral rotation with the immediately adjacent vertebrae is maximum. When we obtained a 3D reconstruction of the entire curve using 3D CT or the EOS imaging system, we were able to measure the 3D coordinates of the deformity. One of the easiest ways to measure these 3D coordinate is to use the "vertebral vector" described by Tamas Illes [8].

Software can give the real orientation of each vertebra according each coordinate. The view from the top gives an excellent appreciation of these orientations relative to the gravity line (Fig. 1.8). A lot of new research will come from that, probably giving a nice adjunct to the work of Carl-Eric Aubin in Canada, who used "da Vinci" views coming from the plane of maximum deformity of each curve [9]. This 3D aspect is especially useful for addressing thoracic cage deformity, where we can also measure the spinal penetration index [10]. The spinal penetration index measures the invasion of the spine inside the thoracic volume and is a parameter used in assessment of all structural scolioses. CT scan measurements can also be used to check the real size of a pedicle to be implanted with a pedicular screw, or to check the morphology of a post joint modified by early degenerative changes.

1.2.1 Conclusion

A scoliotic spine is defined as a spine with a succession of structural curves (each with a 3D deformity and not completely reducible by any maneuver) where the convexity is turned toward the right side for most of the thoracic curves (compensatory curves are more or less reducible) and turned toward the left side when located below a right-sided curve; they are linked together by junctional zones. Each structural curve must be studied regarding the localization of the apical vertebra (the least tilted from the horizontal) and the end vertebrae above and below (the most tilted on the horizontal), which are part of the junctional zone with either another structural curve or a compensatory curve. The scoliotic spine must be considered part of the entire chain of balance (feet to head) and no longer studied only at C1/S1 or worse T1/S1, as it was for many years; the scoliotic section must be studied simultaneously with the entire spine and the entire skeleton of the body.

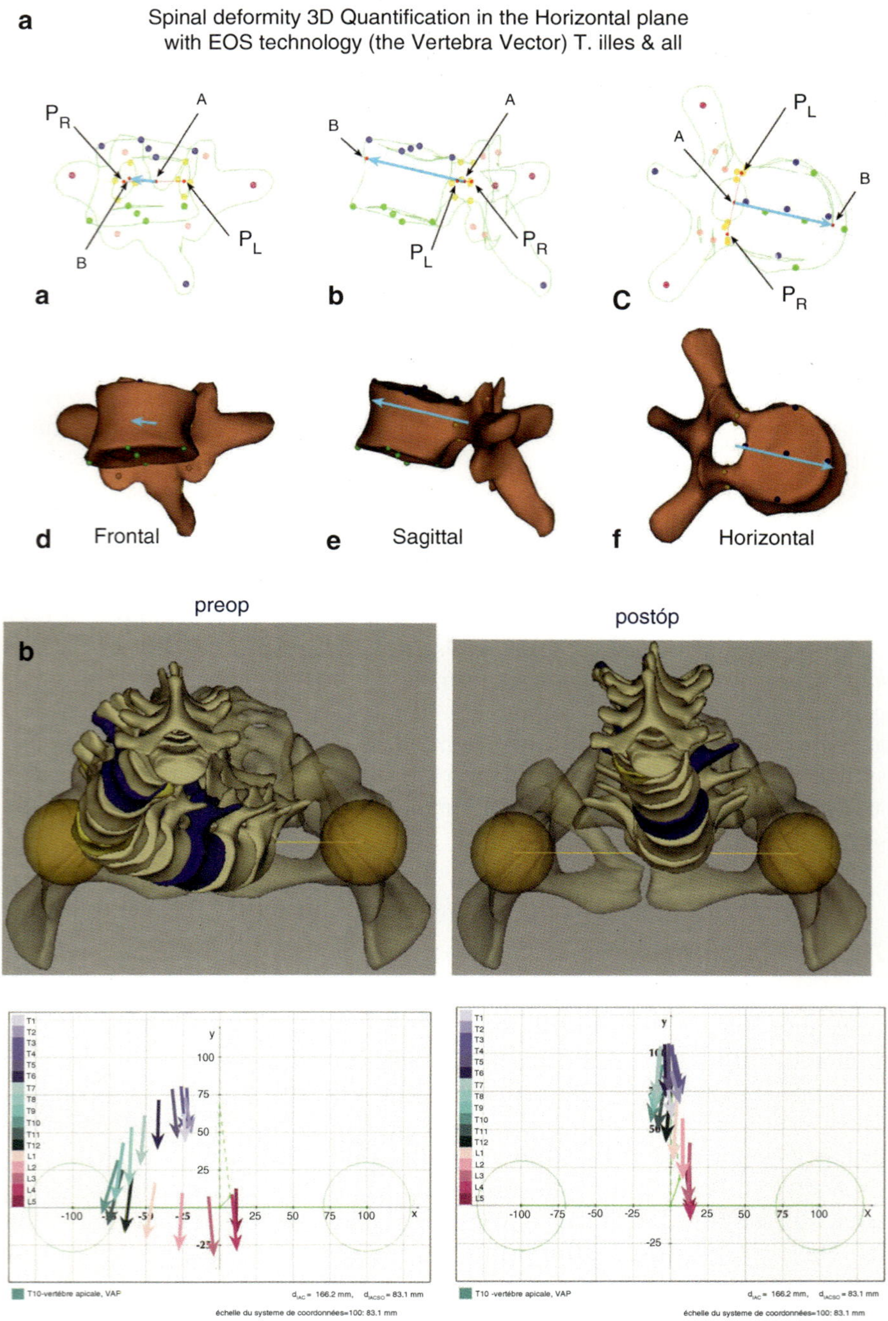

Fig. 1.8 (**a**) The "vertebral vector" give the 3D orientation of each vertebra of the scoliotic spine. (**b**) Example of EOS imaging reconstruction view from the top of a scoliotic spine before and after surgery and the respective vertebral vectors on the horizontal plane

1.3 Adolescent Scoliosis

The definition of "adolescent" lies in the different stages of the development of a growing child, from infancy to adulthood. Adolescence starts when growth has been completed, but is very variable in terms of chronological age. It corresponds to the big hormonal crisis that causes significant changes in stature, sexual characteristics, mood, and personality development.

The determination of the real biological age of a patient is difficult, especially when dealing with adolescents of different ethnic origin. Because so much variation exists between chronological age and biological age, it is accepted in the spine community to use a combination of clinical and radiological signs to assess biological age. Clinical signs of sexual maturation (Tanner) can be used to keep track of the onset of the puberty spurt, with a particular importance and reliability of the onset of pubic hair development for girls and increase in testis size for boys, as pointed out by Ginette Duval-Beaupère [11]. Radiological signs of bone maturation and bone age regard mainly the maturation of the spine (Risser sign, triradiate cartilage of the hip joint, growing cartilage of the elbow and hand.)

When we look at the graphics and curves established to analyze and record the growth in stature (in length) of a child, and measure the velocity of this growth, it is clear that the rate of growth is maximum during the first months of life. Growth then declines to reach a plateau, generally between 5 and 9 years old. A later peak of rapid growth corresponds to the onset of puberty. During this period, the main radiological sign is the triradiate cartilage, which closes before the maximum peak in rate of growth. At this time, the Risser sign is still 0, called by Alain Dimeglio "Risser minus 1." To distinguish between growth of the lower limbs and growth of the spine, measurement of the sitting height, as proposed by Alain Dimeglio, is clinically demonstrative [12]. This peak of rapid growth is reached when the growing cartilages of the elbow are closed; the Risser sign is still 0, but within 6 months it becomes 1. This descending period of the peak of puberal growth continues slowly, with progressive ossification of the iliac crest and the growing cartilages of the hand. The end of this growing stage is reached clinically when sexual signs are completely mature in girls and boys and when ossification of all growing cartilage is obtained, corresponding to the end of growth in height. Remember that the growth of the thorax in size (especially enlargement) continues for about 2 years. Although it is well known that the mean difference between girls and boys is about 2 years in chronological age, each case is different and the study must be done individually. It is here that the beautiful work of Ginette Duval-Beaupère, first on paralytic polio patients then extended to patients with idiopathic scoliosis, demonstrated clearly that the progression of scoliosis deformity was strictly correlated with the puberty growth spurt and with the initiation of clinical signs of puberty.

Because the discovery of a scoliotic deformity very often occurs during the period of adolescent rapid growth, it was called "adolescent scoliosis" or scoliosis discovered after the onset of puberty and before the bony maturation. Others have called it "puberal scoliosis."

The classical classification of structural idiopathic scoliosis is according to the age of discovery of the symptoms. Scoliosis is classified as infantile when discovered during the first 3 years, juvenile when diagnosed in children of 3 to 10 years old, then adolescent when discovered after the age of 10 years.

This terminology is accepted by the majority of orthopedic spine surgeons, including the terminology committee of the Scoliosis Research Society (SRS) and other spine specialists all over the world. It is a useful classification but does not cover the etiopathogenesis of the disease. In my opinion, it is more logical to imagine a kind of continuum of the infantile, juvenile, and adolescent types of idiopathic scoliosis. We are not aware of any longitudinal study giving reliable information about the status of the spine prior to discovery of the deformity in children who develop so-called AIS.

1.4 Idiopathic Scoliosis

Many diseases of congenital, dystrophic, paralytic, infectious, tumor or post-surgical sources can produce spinal deformities with the 3D aspect of scoliosis, but the majority of scoliotic deformities are called idiopathic because no clear etiological factor has been demonstrated. It is the purpose of this book to point out the results of the extensive research done to elucidate the etiology of AIS.

1.5 Classification of Adolescent Idiopathic Scoliosis

Numerous classifications have been proposed for AIS and they are useful for comparison in terms of etiology, epidemiology, and treatment and for discussions between surgeons or doctors. However, they are not so useful for the patient unless they are used by the physician in front of their patient as a check list! The following points should be taken into account:

- Concerning the chronological age of onset (in reality, the age of discovery!): Infantile scoliosis is seen before age 3; juvenile is seen in 4- to 10-year-olds; and adolescent is seen from age 10 to maturity. This helps to predict the worst or mildest cases in function of the remaining growth potential.
  My personal conclusion about the development of idiopathic scoliosis is that the 3D deformity is similar for a growing child whatever his age; only the amount of deformity is variable and depends on the biological age of the patient and the status of evolution of the different etiological disorders.
- Concerning whether the curve is structural or nonstructural: Compensatory curves can be structural or nonstructural and are there to maintain normal body alignment. At first, a compensatory curve is completely flexible and reducible,

but with time and progressive contracture of the surrounding soft tissues, it becomes not reducible and therefore structural, but still compensatory.

- Sometimes physicians speak about the primary curve as the one that appears first; the secondary curve is that seen later during a second look. Very often, these correlate with the magnitude of the deformity as measured with the Cobb angle.
- Ponseti, and Friedman classified AIS into only two types [13] (i.e., with one or two major curves). AIS with only one major curve includes 70% of cases. Curves are divided according to localization. Cervico-thoracic curves are generally convex to the left (apex C7 or T1); thoracic (25%) generally convex to the right (apex between T2 and T11); thoraco-lumbar (19%) most often convex to the right (apex T12 or L1); and lumbar (25%) generally convex to the left (apex between L2 and L4). AIS with two major curves include 30% of cases. The curves are generally of same magnitude (±10%), the most frequent being the double major right thoracic/left lumbar and the double thoracic left upper thoracic (T1/T5) and lower thoracic (T6/T12).
- Concerning the localization of the deformities along the spine's skeleton: We can speak of cervical when the apex of the structural curve is between C1/C7 (I personally have never seen such a localization in idiopathic scoliosis); cervico-thoracic when the apex is located between C7 and T3; thoracic (the most frequent) when the apex is located between T4 and T11; thoraco-lumbar when the apex is located between T11 and L2; lumbar when the apex is located between L2 and L5; and lumbo-sacral when the apex is located at L5 or the L5/S1 junction (in my experience, such cases are often because of a congenital anomaly at that level). Of course, multiple curves can be associated, such as the double major thoracic and lumbar or double thoracic; triple curves upper thoracic, lower thoracic, and thoraco-lumbar; and "serpentine" with four curves upper thoracic, lower thoracic, lumbar, and lumbo-sacral.
- Concerning the junctional zones: A junctional zone is group of three or two vertebrae or even only one disc located at the junction between either two structural curves or structural and compensatory curves. Generally at that level, the axial rotation of the vertebra above the junction is in one direction and the axial rotation of the vertebra below is in the opposite direction, giving a kind of scissoring effect on the disc between. Thus, at that level, the major concern is stability/instability. This concept is evident for the degenerative spine (rotatory dislocation) but potentially exists in AIS. It is not so difficult to recognize when the disc above a vertebra is yawning on one side and the disc below is doing the same but on the other side; this vertebra must be considered unstable.
- Concerning the position of the pelvis: The position of the pelvis is important, especially for the thoracic and lumbar double curves. The "pelvic vertebra concept" was developed in France by Jean Dubousset in 1973 and, under the influence of Christian Salanova and Maurice Bergoin, the importance of the position of the pelvis relative to the convexity or concavity of the thoracic curve became understood. Salanova describes the pelvis as "included" within the lumbar curve when the iliac crest is elevated on the side of the concavity of the lumbar or con-

vexity of the thoracic; subsequently the fusion has to include the lumbar curve. The pelvis is called "excluded" when elevated on the side of the convexity of the lumbar curve or concavity of the thoracic. In such cases, the lumbar spine must be preserved from fusion. Unfortunately, this simple and very practical observation has never crossed the ocean.

Many other well-known classifications have originated from the guidelines for the treatment, especially when instrumentation is used:

- Paul Harrington gave the important definition of a "stable zone" for the level of his lower instrumentation area. The stable zone includes the vertebrae completely within the area delineated by two parallels lines elevated from both right and left posterior joints at the low lumbar and lumbo-sacral area.
- The King and Moe classification [14] was widely used but designed only for thoracic scoliosis based on the radiological view from the frontal plane. The five types of scoliosis curves came from their position relative to a vertical line elevated from the mid-sacrum central line, ignoring the lumbar curves, ignoring the sagittal plane, and ignoring pelvic positioning.
- Currently, the most widely used classification is indisputably that designed by Larry Lenke [15]. This scheme has the advantage that the lateral plane is considered, but it is still 2D because the horizontal plane is ignored. This classification system requires analysis of the upright coronal and sagittal X-rays, along with supine side bending views. The triad classification system consists of a curve type (types 1–6) [1–4, 11, 16], a lumbar spine modifier (A, B, C), and a sagittal thoracic modifier (−, N, +). All three regions of the radiographic coronal and sagittal planes (the proximal thoracic, main thoracic, and thoracolumbar/lumbar) are designated as either the major curve (largest Cobb measurement) or minor curves. The minor curves are separated into structural and nonstructural types. For treatment, the recommendations are that the major and structural minor curves are included in the instrumentation and fusion and the nonstructural minor curves are excluded.
  Despite so many types, this classification has three great advantages: (a) It provides a common language for comparison of similar cases between different origins, surgeons, and treatments. (b) It integrates a kind of check list into the brains of physicians and surgeons, making them think about a more precise anatomo-pathology of the deformity. (c) It establishes a series of guidelines for posterior approach treatment.
- The Montreal team with the support of SRS [9] attempted to design a way to create a 3D classification. However, the way chosen is not easy to understand and even worse to apply. The decision to put each curve in a plane (the plane of maximum deformity) is curious and open for discussion, because it is well known that a scoliotic curve cannot be inscribed in one plane. But, this classification is useful because it is the only study specifically addressing the horizontal plane deformity with the "da Vinci" view from the top. Can this method replace the Cobb angle?

We personally do not use any classification and analyze the scoliotic spine in two ways:

1. Globally, from feet to head, looking simultaneously at the three planes.
2. Clinically, by vision and clinical measurements:
    - Static: frontal from the front, then from the back; sagittal, right then left; and horizontal, first from the top (generally in sitting position) and then with the Adams test seen from the front and seen from the back. Optical topography gives excellent 3D measurements with the modern devices.
    - Dynamic: using classical motion exercises standing or lying in order to assess muscle function of the various segments of the body with or against gravity.
3. Imaging is best obtained with the EOS imaging system for static and some dynamic measurements, but must be supplemented by bending or traction X-rays to address the flexibility and, for instance, prognostication after surgical treatment of the patient's body balance.
4. Locally, each curve and each junction is analyzed with a 3D aspect using all the criteria developed by each researcher and brought out by each classification, remembering that the most important criteria both before and after surgery are balance and motion, not the Cobb angle correction. Alignment and balance should not be confused. The maximum reduction is not always optimum.

1.6 Personal Conclusion

Unicity in the biological development of idiopathic scoliosis:

- According the anatomic structure of the vertebral functional unit (vertebra, disc above, disc below) and spinal arrangement with the chain of balance, emphasizing the important role of the pelvic and cephalic vertebra.
- According the physiological function of the surrounding muscles close to or away from the spine.
- According the maturation of the bone and soft tissues of the spine.
- According the maturation of the central and peripheral nervous system.
- According to the clinical observations of (1) development, progression, stabilization, and reduction of the scoliotic curves in infancy and early childhood; (2) evolution of the juvenile group; and (3) evolution of the adolescent (or puberal) group.

It is logical to think that the phenomenon creating the curves and their arrangement in the spine is unique or universal and that is a mistake to concentrate only on the adolescent idiopathic group, ignoring the younger group. On the contrary, the fact that the group with progressive benign infantile scoliosis (even with a 70° Cobb angle) can be completely corrected either spontaneously or with appropriate non-surgical treatment (cast plus brace) and go through the adolescent spurt without cast or brace, pushes us to support the hypothesis of unicity in the development of idiopathic scoliosis.

Glossary[1]

Adolescent scoliosis: Scoliosis detected between age 10 and maturity.

Adult scoliosis: Scoliosis considered more or less after the end of growth.

Alignment: 3D positioning of the body's elements from head to feet along the gravity line. This can be used for the entire body or for the bone and joint elements of the entire spine.

Apex, apical vertebra: Vertebra located in a curve and farthest away from the gravity line, most horizontal, and generally the most axially rotated in a standing position.

Balance: Stability of the body in 3D when static or within any movement in relation to the gravity line.

Barycentrometry: Measurement of the center of mass of different parts of the body (head, thorax, abdomen, etc.) relative to the gravity line and evaluation of the mass value of the body corresponding to each vertebral level and its location relative to the gravity line axis.

Basement: Lower part of the spine (generally the lumbo-pelvic area), considered the most fixed zone for alignment of the spine. This term can also be used for the polygon of support of the body.

Bending: Image or measurement obtained either clinically or by X-ray of a curvature, bent to the right or left (for the frontal plane) or toward the front or back (for the sagittal plane), to check the flexibility of the curve. It can be passive or active.

Bone age: Skeletal X-ray landmarks demonstrating the maturation of the bony tissues.

Café au lait spot: Brown (varying from light to dark) skin spots anywhere on the body, suggesting neurofibromatosis 1.

Cephalic vertebra: The entire head is considered as one unique heavy (7% body weight) vertebra that plays the role of a reverse pendulum on the chain of balance of the body.

Cervico-thoracic curve: Curve located at the cervico-thoracic junction between C5/T5, with apex generally at C7 or T1.

Chain of balance: 3D positioning of the successive parts of the body from polygon of support to the head, creating a harmonious "piling up" of the different bones and joints of the skeleton, in order to achieve balance in both the static posture of the human and during motion of the entire body.

---

[1] It seems useful to present an extensive glossary of scoliosis terms to help the reader understand better the contents of the different chapters of this book.

Cobb angle: X-ray measurement (in degrees) of a curve from lines tangential to the end vertebrae plateau of the most tilted vertebrae (one superior, one inferior) in opposite directions.

Compensation: Clinical (3D static or dynamic) or radiological evaluation of the realignment or rebalance of part of the spine to approach the gravity line reference.

Compensatory curve: Curve either structural (generally minor) or postural that realigns the spine within the gravity line.

Congenital scoliosis: 3D spinal deformity secondary to vertebral bony malformations.

Cone of Economy: 3D volume occupied by the human body in standing or sitting position requiring a minimum of muscle function to achieve balance.

Crankshaft phenomenon: 3D hyper-rotatory deformity, generally post-operative after early posterior fusion for scoliosis on a growing child, secondary to the continuing anterior growth of the twisted body in front of a posterior solid fusion.

Cuneiform vertebral body: Loss of normal parallel aspect of the upper and lower vertebral plateau.

Curve: Deformity of the spine with mainly lateral deviation from the midline, maximum at its apex where the extremities or end vertebrae come back toward the midline.

Curve measurement: Curve measurement can express curve magnitude in degrees (the Cobb angle is the most used) or the inclination of the curve projected onto the horizontal plane, obtained using a scoliometer. It can be the projection of the curve onto the oblique plane of maximum deformity or the contrary minimum deformity. The best measurements are 3D, where each plane requires specific measurement.

Degenerative scoliosis: Spinal scoliotic deformity secondary to degenerative changes primarily at the disc level, due to aging and occurring either on an already scoliotic spine (known from childhood or adolescence) or on a normal spine.

De novo scoliosis: Scoliotic deformity of an adult normal spine developed during adulthood.

Discogenic cascade: The succession of degenerative changes occurring at the disc level, sometimes limited at first to one level, then extending progressively to a larger part of the spine, especially the thoraco-lumbar, lumbar, or lumbo-sacral area.

Dislocation: Complete loss of continuity in the alignment of vertebral units; (*Subluxation*: Partial loss of continuity, reducible or not).

Double major scoliosis: Spine with two significant structural curves of equal magnitude, generally one thoracic and one lumbar.

Double thoracic scoliosis: Spine with two significant structural curves, both located within the thoracic area.

Election vertebra: Name given by Christian Salanova to the lower end vertebra of an instrumentation, obtaining all the criteria for stability in static or dynamic conditions before operation.

End vertebrae: Ultimate vertebra located at each side of a curve (upper and lower ends).

Erect posture: A human characteristic, defining the position of the entire body or trunk within the gravity axis in a standing or sitting position, with the head aligned vertically above the feet for standing, or above the buttocks when sitting.

Flat back: Loss or severe decrease in normal sagittal alignment for part or all of the spine.

Fractional curve: Part of a curve including one or more levels, realizing a division of the full curve; sometimes useful to plan the map of the instrumentation.

Full curve: Complete curve from upper end to lower end vertebrae.

Gaze: Orientation of the axis of the vision. Horizontal gaze is a characteristic of human beings.

Gibbus: Protrusion on the back, more or less pronounced and acute or rounded, generally secondary to severe kyphotic or kypho-scoliotic deformity

Ginette Duval-Beaupère: French physician who described the law of progression of scoliotic deformity in a growing child, as well as the "incidence angle."

Greulich and Pyle atlas: Radiological tables used to determine bone age.

Hump: Clinical sign demonstrating the asymmetry of paravertebral structures of the back. Generally, a hump represents the axial rotation of vertebral bodies and is associated with posterior bulging of the ribs in the thoracic area. In the lumbar zone, it represents the consequence of the axial rotation of vertebrae.

Hyper-kyphosis: Sagittal alignment of the thoracic spine with a kyphosis angle greater than the normal range.

Hypokyphosis: Sagittal alignment of the thoracic spine where the kyphosis angle is less than the normal value, but where the severity is not yet lordotic.

Hysterical scoliosis: Spinal nonstructural deformity at the initiation, secondary to transient or permanent central neurological problems such as conversion. With time, structural changes may develop.

Idiopathic scoliosis: Scoliosis with unexplained etiology

Iliac epiphysis, apophysis: Epiphysis develops along the wing of an ilium, giving a radiological sign of maturation according to the extent of ossification (Risser sign 1–5).

Ilio lumbar angle: Angle between the horizontal axis of the superior part of both iliac wings and the vertical alignment of L4 and L5 vertebrae. It may be symmetrical right and left, or asymmetrical. If asymmetrical, we speak about "asymmetrical ilio-lumbar basement."

Ilio lumbar asymmetrical basement: See above.

Incidence angle: Anatomical angle from the sagittal alignment (defined by Ginette Duval-Beaupère), created by the junction between one line perpendicular to the middle of the S1 plateau and the line from this center to the center of femoral head (or the middle of the line that centers both femoral heads). It is important to determine the postural sagittal alignment according the formula Pelvic incidence = Pelvic version (tilt) + Sacral slope (angle between vertebral plateau S1 and the horizontal).

Inclination angle: Generally used for the thoracic spine. It is the angle between the horizontal reference plane and the plane across the thoracic cage passing at the maximum of rib cage pro-eminence (rib hump).

Inclinometer: Instrument used to measure the thoracic inclination angle on the back of a patient, bent 90° frontward onto the hip joints; also called a scoliometer.

Infantile scoliosis: Scoliosis, idiopathic type, appearing and discovered between birth and 3 years old

Intermediate vertebra: In a scoliotic curve, the vertebrae located between the apex and the end vertebrae.

Junction, junctional zone: Part of the spine consisting of one unique vertebra, one unique disc, or a group of three vertebrae with their surrounding discs, located between two curves, either structural or compensatory.

Juvenile scoliosis: Scoliosis, idiopathic type, appearing and discovered between 3 years old and the first signs of puberty

King classification: Five types of idiopathic scoliosis determined from the localization of the curves relative to the central sacral line.

Kyphosis: Deformity developed purely in the sagittal plane with a shape or angle greater than found in normal alignment. They are classified into two types: (1) *Angular*, meaning that a sudden change between two adjacent vertebrae occurs in this sagittal alignment, giving an acute sinus open toward the front. (2) *Regular*, meaning mild progressive change in the sagittal alignment, giving an angle greater than normal. If we consider the vertical line (the plumb line) as 0°, vertebrae are bent toward the front in kyphosis, toward the back in lordosis.

Kyphoscoliosis: A kyphotic spine has scoliosis and a true hyperkyphosis. Kyphoscoliosis must be differentiated from (1) a spine looking kyphosis but where this aspect results from a hyper-rotatory deformity of the apical vertebrae (apparent kyphosis). In this case, the apex of scoliosis and the apex of kyphosis are at the same level; (2) a junctional kyphosis where the apex of the kyphosis lies at the junction between two lordotic curves.

Kyphosing scoliosis: Scoliotic spine with marked axial rotation, where the lateral bending of these rotated vertebrae look like kyphosis.

Lenke classification: The most used 2D classification for idiopathic scoliosis, based on six types of primary curves, with adjuncts of a lumbar modifier and a sagittal modifier.

LIV: Lower instrumented vertebra

Lordosis: Negative sagittal alignment of the vertebrae of a curve, relative to the vertical sagittal line (plumb or line tragus/S1, or C7/S1 etc. reference lines) considered as 0°.

Lordoscoliosis: Scoliosis where the sagittal projection is lordotic (different from hypokyphotic).

Lumbar curve: Curve located between T12 and L5, apex generally L2 or L3.

Lumbo-sacral curve: Curve located betweenL3/L4 and pelvis, apex generallyL4/L5 orL5/S1 disc.

Major curve: Structural curve with the largest magnitude on the spinal alignment.

Menarche: Female menstrual regimen.

Min Mehta index: Measure of the rib-vertebra angle difference, concave/convex on the apical vertebra.

Minor curves: Structural or compensatory curves with a magnitude lower than others in the spinal alignment; generally more flexible than the major curves.

Nash and Moe Index: Simple method for measuring the axial rotation of a vertebra (in three grades) by the relation of the axis of the convex pedicle to the lateral border of the body.

Nonstructural curve: Curve without structural characteristics, generally corrects completely or overcorrects in the bending tests.

Occipital axis: Vertical line from the midline of the occiput or occipital crest down to the center of the polygon of support.

Pelvic anteversion: Sagittal tilt frontward of the pelvis from the normal alignment.

Pelvic obliquity: 3D position of the pelvic vertebra relative to the gravity line axis in standing, sitting, or lying posture.

Pelvic retroversion: Sagittal tilt backward of the pelvis from the normal alignment.

Pelvic tilt (or pelvic version): Sagittal tilt from the normal alignment.

Pelvic vertebra: The entire pelvis is considered as one unique vertebra because mobility of the sacroiliac joint is minimal (1.5° according White and Panjabi) playing the role of an intercalary bone in the chain of balance of the body.

Plan d'élection: French expression to define the plane of maximum deformity, corresponding to an oblique plane where the projection of the scoliotic spine on the X-ray film develops a maximum of deformity. It is possible to use the same expression for the plane, still oblique, showing the minimum of deformity (generally, a plane orthogonal to the first one).

Plumb line: Vertical reference line for gravity, given by a string with attached weight at one extremity and presented at a fixed reference point of the body.

Polygon of support: Surface created by the weight-bearing surface of both feet.

Ponseti classification: Early classification for idiopathic scoliosis, based on the number of curves and their localization.

Postural scoliosis: Spinal deformity with only positional (not structural) disorders, generally completely reversible and secondary to extra-vertebral factors.

Predominant: Element more important for function or any other criteria, in any further time.

Primary curve: The spinal curve developed first or earliest; can be associated with other curves called secondary, structural, or postural generally compensatory for the alignment toward the gravity line.

Prone positioning: Lying position on the stomach.

Reduction, reducible: Ability of a curve to reduce its characteristics of magnitude (Cobb angle, axial rotational index, etc.) in any direction or in a selective direction, secondary to various maneuvers such as longitudinal traction, supine or standing side bending, correction in a brace or a cast, or after surgery.

Reverse pendulum: Generally, the fixed part of a pendulum is the upper part and the weight is oscillating at the lower part. A reverse pendulum means that the fixed point is at the bottom (i.e., polygon of support) and the oscillating weight at the upper part (i.e., the head). Describes the biomechanics of the chain of balance in the human.

Risser sign: Radiological ossification of the iliac wing apophysis is divided into five stages from 1 (beginning appearance) to 5 (complete ossification). The Risser sign is used to evaluate growth maturation.

Ring apophysis: Growing radiological marker that is the most reliable index of the maturation of the vertebra, given by the amount of ossification of the periphery of the vertebral plateau growth plate.

Rotational prominence: The prominence seen when looking at the back of the patient when it is in a frontward bend. Generally, a thoracic prominence is caused by the axial rotation of the vertebrae and the subsequent deformity of the ribs (most frequently seen on the right for right thoracic scoliosis). At the lumbar level, prominence is a result of the axial rotation of the vertebrae.

Rotatory dislocation: Anatomical and pathological phenomenon realized by a combined movement in the disc between two vertebrae (or around one vertebra with the two discs above and below) that associates axial rotation in an opposite direction above and below, lateral ejection, and kyphosing deformity between the two vertebrae. It is a localized phenomenon corresponding to junctional kyphosis between two lordotic curves.

Sacral slope: Sagittal angle between superior plateau of S1 and the horizontal.

Scoliometer: Instrument used to measure the angle of slope of the back surface from the horizontal reference at various levels of the back and especially at the apex of the rib hump.

Skeletal age: Bone age

Spinal penetration index: Amount of the invasion of the thoracic cage by the spinal elements measured at one transversal, axial, or horizontal level of the thorax, or in volume relative to the entire thoracic cage.

Stability/instability: Stability is the normal anatomical relationship between two vertebral units or two segments of the spine during motion, whereas instability is the loss of this normal relationship during motion. Instability is called "immediate" when demonstrated, for example, on stress films such as Flex/Ext. Instability is "potential" when not demonstrated on these stress films but can occur suddenly after a minor trauma, progressively with time secondary to gravity, or in response to external repeated stress.

Structural curve: Curve where anatomical changes can be found in the alignment (axial rotation, lateral translation, sagittal displacement) that are not reducible by any external passive manipulation, traction, or supine side-bending films for instance.

Supine positioning: Lying position on the back.

Surface topography: Measurement of the 3D shape of the trunk using various non-invasive devices, generally optical. Gives 3D information about the external deformity of the trunk in frontal sagittal and horizontal planes. Useful for diagnosis, quantification of treatments, and follow up.

Thoraco-lumbar curve: Curve located between T8 and L3, apex generally on T12 or L1.

Torsiometer: Accurate instrument designed by René Perdriolle to measure the degree of axial rotation of the vertebrae by the position of the convex pedicle (more precise measurement than that of Nash and Moe).

Torsion and counter-torsion: 3D movement of a segment of the spine or the whole spine, made by the association of axial rotation with lateral and sagittal deviation of the spinal unit relative to the adjacent unit in one direction (right or left). A scoliotic spine is made by a succession of torsion and counter-torsion segments. Torsion is a 3D combined movement of a part of the spine, where axial rotation in one direction increases from superior end vertebra to apical vertebra and decreases from apical vertebra to inferior end vertebra.

Triradiate cartilage: 3D growing cartilage of the acetabulum. Its complete ossification correlates clearly with Risser 0 or Risser −1 for Dimeglio (12 year bone age in girls, 14 year bone age in boys). When still open, the peak of the growth spurt has not yet been reached.

Vertebral end plate: Inferior and superior plates of the vertebral bodies; cortical bone immediately adjacent to the intervertebral disc.

Vertebral growth plate: Growing cartilage covering the superior and inferior surfaces of the vertebral bodies. These plates give the longitudinal growth in height of the vertebrae.

References

1. White AA, Panjabi MM. Clinical biomechanics of the spine, vol. 1978. New York: Lippincott. p. 264.
2. Fuchs R III, editor. Hippocrates. Munich: Artemis; 1900. p. 249.
3. Paré A. Apparel 23td book Gabriel Bruon ed Paris. 1585.
4. Andry N. L'orthopedia ou l'art de prevenir et de corriger dans les enfants les deformities du corps. Paris. 1741.
5. Perdriolle R. La scoliose: son etude tridimensionnelle. Paris: Maloine; 1979.
6. Graf H, Hecquet J, Dubousset J. Approche tridimensionnelle des déformations rachidiennes. Application à l'étude du pronostic des scolioses infantiles. Rev Chirurg Orthoped. 1983;1983:407–16.
7. Dubousset J, Charpak G, Dorion I, et al. A new 2D and 3D imaging approach to musculo-skeleta physiology and pathology with low dose radiation and standing position: the EOS system. Bull Acad Natl Med. 2005;189(2):287–300.
8. Illés T, Somoskeöy S. A new 2D and 3D imaging approach to musculo-skeleta physiology and pathology with low dose radiation and standing position: the EOS system. Bull Acad Natl Med. 2013;189(2):287–300.
9. Sangole AP, Aubin CE, Labelle H. Three dimensional classification of thoracic scoliotic curves. Spine. 2008;34(1):91–9.
10. Dubousset J, Pomero V, et al. Spinal penetration index, a new quantified 3D deformity for lordoscoliosis. J Orthop Sci. 2003;8(1):41–9.
11. Duval-Beaupère G, Dubousset J, Queneau A, Grossiord A. Pour une theorie unique de l'évolution des scolioses. Press Med. 1970;88:1141–6
12. Dimeglio A, Bonnel F. Le rachis en croissance. Paris: Springer; 1990.
13. Ponseti IV, Friedman B. Prognosis in idiopathic scoliosis. J Bone Joint Surg. 1950;32:381.
14. King HA, Moe JH, et al. The selection of fusion levels in thoracic idiopathic scoliosis. J One Joint Surg Am. 1983;65:1302–13.
15. Lenke LG, Betz RR, Harms J, et al. A new and reliable 3 dimensional classification of adolescent idiopathic scoliosis. J Bone Joint Surg. 2001;26:42–7.
16. Nash CL Jr, Moe JH. A study of vertebral rotation. J Bone Joint Surg. 1969;51:223–9.

Chapter 2
Adolescent Idiopathic Scoliosis: Natural History

Cameron B. Barton and Stuart L. Weinstein

2.1 Introduction

Adolescent idiopathic scoliosis (AIS), or late-onset scoliosis, is a condition in adolescents defined by an abnormal coronal plane spine curvature with rotation, for which no cause can be established [1]. AIS is the most common form of scoliosis and is diagnosed after exclusion of other known causes, including syndromic disorders, neuromuscular disorders, or vertebral malformations. The natural history of AIS has been well studied [2–12]. However, many of the initial natural history studies had shortcomings, including retrospective study design, small cohorts, patients lost to follow-up, and inclusion of patients with differing diagnoses. Thorough understanding of the natural history of disease is paramount in determining appropriate treatment. Appropriate treatment decisions should be critically assessed based on the outcome studies of patients treated by various methods, including both surgical and nonsurgical techniques. Knowledge of disease natural history is crucial in determining whether any treatment modality alters a disease in a positive, negative, or neutral way. This chapter will focus on the natural history of untreated adolescent idiopathic scoliosis.

2.2 Etiopathogenesis

Despite substantial basic science and epidemiological and clinical research, much remains unanswered regarding the etiopathogenesis of AIS [3, 13, 14]. This is in contrast to neuromuscular and congenital forms, which have much better

C. B. Barton, M.D. (✉) • S. L. Weinstein, M.D.
Department of Orthopaedics and Rehabilitation, The University of Iowa Hospitals and Clinics, Iowa City, IA, USA
e-mail: cameron-barton@uiowa.edu

M. Machida et al. (eds.), *Pathogenesis of Idiopathic Scoliosis*,
https://doi.org/10.1007/978-4-431-56541-3_2

understood underlying mechanisms. A variety of hypotheses and concepts have been proposed, with etiologies involving genetics, the central nervous system, biomechanics, metabolic pathways, skeletal spinal growth, bone metabolism, and others [3, 13, 15, 16]. The biomechanical pathology of AIS has been described as either primary or secondary to the spinal curve itself and might contribute to the initiation and/or progression of the spinal curve [3]. The upright growing human spine expresses multiple biological and biomechanical processes. Several of the classical concepts pertaining to these processes include biomechanical and neuromuscular factors [17], axial rotational instability [18], biomechanical modulation of growth as a result of asymmetrical mechanical compression and reduced loading (known as the Hueter-Volkmann effect) [17, 19], asynchronous (uncoupled) spinal neuro-osseous growth and relative anterior spinal overgrowth [20, 21], right thoracic curves in females with AIS (the thoracospinal concept) [22], melatonin signaling pathway dysfunction [23, 24], and dysfunction of platelet calmodulin [25]. Advances in 3D imaging have led to new concepts pertaining to the pathogenesis of AIS, including bipedalism causing intrinsic dorsal (posterior) shear forces with axial rotational instability [26]. These various concepts will be discussed in further detail.

AIS has been shown to have a genetic component, with a meta-analysis revealing concordance for AIS in 36% of dizygotic twins and 73% of monozygotic twins [27]. Large pedigree studies have demonstrated different methods of inheritance, including autosomal dominance, maternal factors, multiple gene inheritance, X-linked dominance, and multifactorial inheritance [13, 28, 29]. One large pedigree study of 101 families, including 778 individuals, found that severe forms of AIS could be attributed to an autosomal dominant major gene diallele model with incomplete sex-dependent penetrance [28]. However, the majority of studies have failed to identify a specific gene locus responsible for AIS, concluding that AIS does not follow the classic Mendelian inheritance model [30–34]. Therefore, recent views of the heritability of AIS favor a complex polygenic model with significant genetic heterogeneity.

One model of complex disease inheritance proposes that different sets of environmental and genetic factors could separately contribute to the progression or initiation of spinal curve (Fig. 2.1) [3, 35]. One study found that other complex diseases such as type 1 diabetes, Crohn's disease, and rheumatoid arthritis had sibling risk ratios similar to those of AIS [36]. Male patients might require a greater number of genetic risk factors to be affected by the condition, as pedigree analyses show that male patients with AIS are more likely to have siblings and children with scoliosis when compared to female patients [37, 38]. Complex polygenic mode of AIS inheritance has involved studying genes related to connective tissue structure, bone metabolism, puberty, melatonin signaling pathways and genes encoding melatonin, estrogen receptors, and axon guidance pathways [39]. Some of these genes were associated with AIS curve severity, but to date no association between these genes and the initiation of AIS has been elucidated [40, 41].

Genome-wide association studies (GWASs) examine a genome-wide set of genetic variants in individuals to determine if any variant is associated with a trait [3]. GWASs usually focus on associations between single nucleotide polymorphisms (SNPs) and traits or diseases such as AIS. Several SNPs associated with AIS

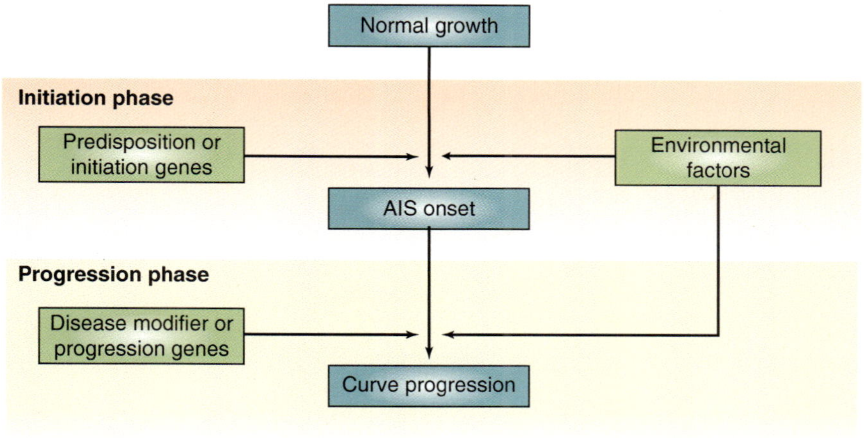

Fig. 2.1 Etiopathogenesis of adolescent idiopathic scoliosis. A general model showing the interaction of environmental and genetic factors to curve onset and progression. AIS, adolescent idiopathic scoliosis. From *Cheng et al.* 2015, Fig. 5, page 7 [3]

have been identified, including ladybird homeobox 1 (LBX1) locus [42, 43], adhesion G protein-coupled receptor G6 (ADGRG6) [44], paired box 1 (PAX1) [45, 46], and fibrillins (FBN1 and FBN2) [47]. Discrepancy has been found regarding association of estrogen receptor protein ESR1 [41, 48, 49]. Overall, these GWAS studies link AIS to possible abnormalities in development, migration, or function of muscle, neural, connective tissue, or hormone receptor proteins [41–50].

The etiopathogenesis of AIS has also been tied to several functional and morphological abnormalities of the central nervous system (Fig. 2.2). Derangements in neurophysiological functions have been found in patients with AIS, including abnormal somatosensory-evoked potentials [51], static and dynamic postural instability [52], abnormal proprioceptive function [52], and vestibular and visuo-oculomotor dysfunction [53]. Patients with AIS have been found to have differences in brain volume ratios and indices via functional MRI, with abnormalities coinciding with functional areas involved in motor control and vestibular and somatosensory systems [54–57]. Studies have also shown that the vestibular apparatus, including semicircular canal abnormalities, may be linked to the etiopathogenesis of AIS, or may alternatively be a compensatory response to in the development of AIS. This could possibly explain the abnormal somatosensory function and poor balance control that may be present in patients with AIS [58, 59].

Abnormal bone growth, metabolism, and remodeling have been suggested in patients with AIS. Neuromorphological abnormalities associated with AIS have included reduced spinal cord to vertebral length ratios [20] and relative anterior spinal overgrowth; supporting a hypothesis that uncoupled neuro-osseous growth may contribute to AIS [20]. Other areas of disproportionate or asymmetric skeletal features reported in AIS have included upper arm length disproportions, periapical

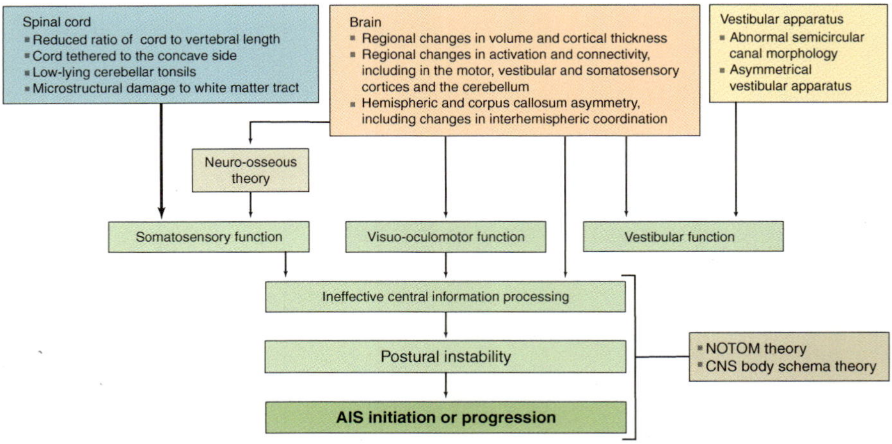

Fig. 2.2 Central nervous system factors involved in AIS. Diagram proposing the possible interactions between central nervous system factors and the initiation or progression of AIS. CNS, central nervous system; NOTOM, neuro-osseous timing of maturation. From *Cheng et al.* 2015, Fig. 6, page 8 [3]

ribs, left-right asymmetry, and abnormalities in iliac height [60, 61]. Osteopenia is suggested to be associated with AIS, as one study shows this diagnosis in 38% of women with AIS [62, 63]. Furthermore, osteopenia can be an important prognostic factor for curve progression in AIS [64]. Other studies have implied that abnormalities that affect bone metabolism could influence development of AIS with associated markers including OST, RANKL, soluble OBR, MATN1, and COMP [3, 65–69]. Specifically, vitamin D deficiency has been linked to osteopenia and osteoporosis, and a recent study found lower vitamin D levels in patients with AIS, with negative correlation to Cobb angle [70].

Abnormal body habitus has also been associated with AIS, with AIS patients having a lower body weight and BMI when compared to controls [71]. One large prospective cohort study found that decreases in leptin, lean mass, and fat mass were associated with an increased risk for scoliosis [72]. Leptin and soluble leptin receptor have been suggested to be responsible for some abnormal phenotypes observed in AIS [73].

Another theory linked to the etiopathogenesis of AIS involves human bipedalism and the three-dimensional biomechanical factors of the spine. Studies have shown that the posterior inclination of the spine is linked to rotational stability [3, 26, 74, 75]. The sagittal profile of males versus females differs, particularly during pubertal growth [32, 76]. Women have a greater posteriorly inclined area of the spine, leading to less rotational stability and possibly contributing to the development or progression of AIS [3, 32, 76].

As mentioned above, the exact factor or combination of factors that lead to the initiation of scoliosis is unknown. However, several other biomechanical theories regarding the initiation of scoliosis have been proposed and include ligamentous and muscular "tethering" of the spine, uncoupled neuro-osseous growth, and anomalies of neuromuscular control [3, 17, 21, 77]. Once scoliosis is initiated, asymmetrical stresses act on a laterally curved spine and associated vertebral growth plates, producing asymmetrical spinal growth [19, 67, 78]. This concept is known as the Hueter-Volkmann principle, where increased compressive loading slows growth and decreased loading accelerates growth [67], thus producing wedging of the vertebrae in the coronal plane.

In summary, the etiopathogenesis of AIS is likely multifactorial. Factors contributing to the initiation or progression of AIS include genetic; CNS; bone metabolism, growth, and remodeling; body composition; and biomechanical contributions.

2.3 Prevalence

The prevalence of AIS in the at-risk population (children age 10 to 16 years of age) is 0.4–3%, with differences noted based on geographic location, ethnicity, and sex [79, 80]. Prevalence ranged from 0.4 to 3.9% in North America, 0.7 to 7.5% in Spain, 0.4 to 2.5% in Asia, and 1.9% for both the Middle East and Australia [79, 80]. High northern latitudes hold a greater prevalence of AIS compared to regions of lower latitude [81]. A study from Hong Kong is currently the largest cohort study evaluating prevalence. It assessed children from 10 years of age until skeletal maturity and found that the prevalence of spinal curves >10° during adolescence was 2.5% [80].

The percentage of individuals with significant curves greater than 20° or those requiring treatment is even smaller. A 2010 meta-analysis, including data from 36 studies on AIS, found that a pooled prevalence of spinal curves greater than or equal to 20° was 0.22% (95% CI: 0.15–0.30%) [79]. Further, the prevalence of individuals who had been treated for scoliosis with surgery or back brace was 0.07% [79]. If these percentages are applied to current population figures, more than 620,000 adolescents in the United States have AIS [82]. An estimated 602,884 visits to private physician officers were made for this condition in 1995 [83]. The number of surgical operations for AIS has been increasing every year. In 2012, over 5000 patients in the United States were surgically treated for AIS, which corresponded with a national bill of $1.1 billion [84].

2.4 Diagnosis

The diagnosis of AIS is often sought after a patient's primary care physician, coach, parent, or other close contact notices body asymmetry. Chest prominences, thoracic prominences, scapular prominences, variance in shoulder height, an asymmetrical waist, or sagittal plane decompensation may be noted. Many screening tests aid in the diagnosis of AIS, including the standard Adams forward bend test, a scoliometer, or formetric screening [69, 80]. For the general practitioner, the Adams forward

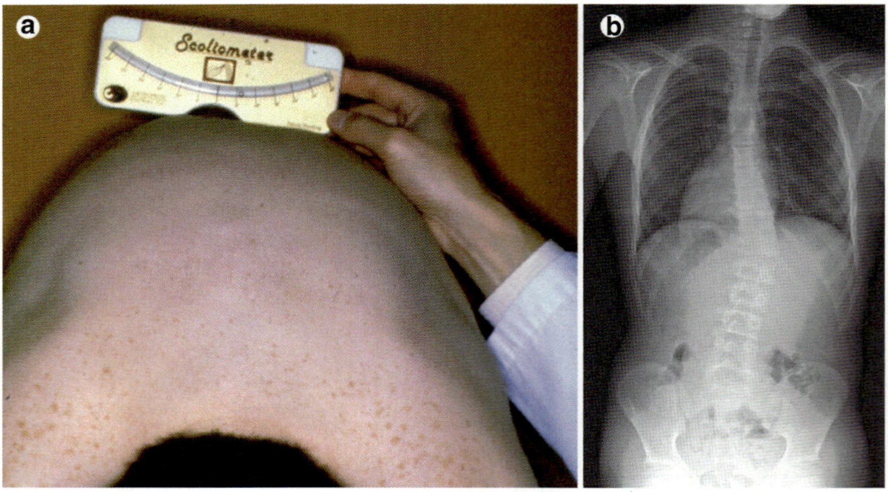

Fig. 2.3 Screening for scoliosis by clinical exam and radiography. (**a**) Scoliometer measurement during Adams forward bend test. (**b**) Long-standing posterior-anterior radiograph of a 13-year-old boy showing a 30° curve and Risser 2. From *Weinstein et al.* 2008, Fig. 1, page 1528 [110]

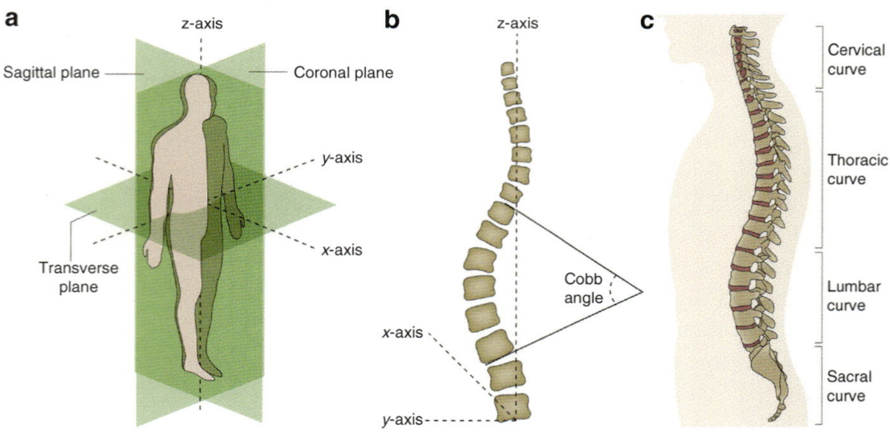

Fig. 2.4 Human spine curvature. (**a**) The three axes and associated planes of the human body. (**b**) Method of measuring the Cobb angle, an angle formed from the most superior vertebral endplate to the most inferior vertebral endplate in the coronal plane. (**c**) The sagittal contours of the spine, including cervical, thoracic, lumbar, and sacral regions. From *Cheng et al.* 2015, Fig. 1, page 2 [3]

bend test and the scoliometer are the most useful (Fig. 2.3). The Adams forward bend test is useful in detecting rotational deformity. While these screening tests are sensitive for detecting body asymmetry, they are not specific for scoliosis and give little information to curve magnitude. The diagnosis of scoliosis can only be confirmed by a coronal spine curvature of at least 10°, measured by the Cobb method (Fig. 2.4 schematic) on a standing PA radiograph of the spine [1, 3]. The human

Table 2.1 Various described classification and subclassification of scoliosis

Pathological	Age of onset	Curve magnitude	Curve level and apex
– *Structural* – *Functional*: no demonstrable spinal column abnormalities	– *Infantile*: 0–3 years of age – *Childhood*: 4–9 years of age – *Adolescent/adolescent idiopathic scoliosis*: 10 years of age until closure of growth plate (most common[a]) – *Adult*: 18 years of age or older – *Early-onset scoliosis*: curve occurs before 10 years of age – *Late-onset scoliosis*: curve occurs after 10 years of age	– Use Cobb method on standard spinal radiographs to obtain the Cobb angle	– Classify as cervical, thoracic, thoracolumbar, or lumbar – May combine with other descriptors (right or left thoracic, lumbar major)
Three-dimensional nature of curve	*Nonsurgical treatment*	*Surgical treatment*	
– *Negrini classification*: based on direction, shift, and phase of curve [130] – *Poncet classification*: based on three distinct patterns of geometric torsion of the major curve [131]	– *Rigo classification*: defines principles of the corrections necessary for effective brace design and fabrication, based on both radiological and clinical curve pattern [132] – *Lehnert-Schroth classification*: includes the "three curve pattern" with the shoulder, thoracic, and lumbopelvic block deviated and rotated against each other in the frontal plane [133]	– *King classification* – *Lenke classification* – *Peking Union Medical College classification*	Defines five curve types [130, 134, 135] Defines six curve types [134] Defines three major curve types and 13 subtypes [135]

[a]Modified from box 1, Cheng et al. 2015 [3]

spine can be described in three planes, but scoliosis is specifically defined by coronal plane curvature (Fig. 2.4). Further classification of scoliosis as AIS requires exclusion of other known etiologies.

Curve magnitude is important when determining diagnosis and prognosis in AIS. Small curves of 10° are found in equal ratios among males and females. Studies have shown that as Cobb angle increases, overall prevalence decreases but female-to-male ratio increases [1, 5, 85, 86]. Fortunately, natural history and epidemiological studies have shown that less than 10% of positively screened patients (curves >10°) require active treatment [87–91].

Idiopathic scoliosis can be subclassified based on various criteria including age of onset, pathological type, curve magnitude, curve level and apex, three-dimensional nature of curve, and surgical vs. nonsurgical treatment types (Table 2.1) [3]. Curve pattern in AIS is important when considering natural history. Four main curve

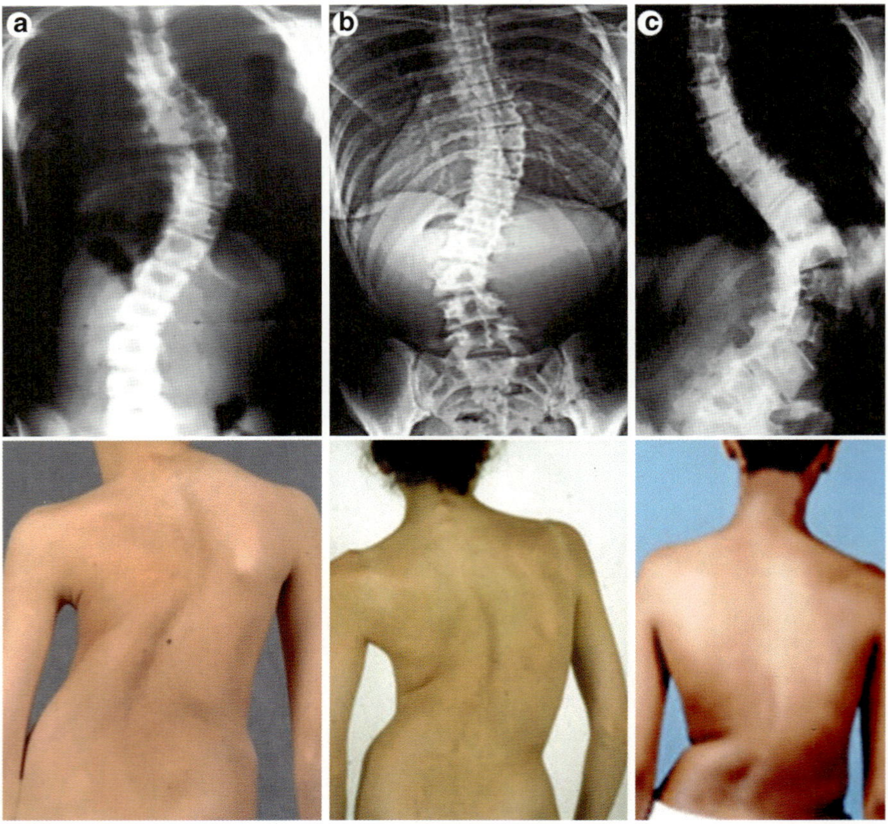

Fig. 2.5 Three curve types based on location of curve. Posterior-anterior standing radiographs of patients (top row) with corresponding clinical photograph (bottom row). (**a**) Right thoracic. (**b**) Thoracolumbar. (**c**) Lumbar. From *Cheng et al.* 2015, Fig. 2, page 4 [3]

patterns have been determined in the literature and include thoracic, lumbar, thoracolumbar, and double major (Fig. 2.5). Other less common curve patterns include cervicothoracic, double thoracic, and thoracic thoracolumbar. These patterns refer to the location of the apical vertebrae. Curve pattern is important to distinguish, as each curve pattern has particular characteristics, predicted course, and associated outcomes.

2.5 Early Studies on Patient Outcomes

Few natural history studies of AIS exist, with early studies portraying a grim prognosis. These studies perpetuated a common misconception that all types of scoliosis inevitably led to disability, cardiopulmonary compromise, and back pain.

Shortcomings of these early studies include retrospective study design, small cohorts, patients lost to follow-up, and inclusion of patients with differing diagnoses. In 1968, Nachemson published one of the first studies regarding patients with untreated scoliosis, not specific to AIS [92]. Their data included a 38-year follow-up of 130 patients. The authors concluded an unfavorable prognosis, including a 100% increase in mortality rate compared to general population, with 16/20 deaths due to cor pulmonale. Further, 37% of patients had constant back pain, 14% complained of cardiopulmonary symptoms, and 30% claimed disability because of their deformity. However, only 45% of patients had idiopathic scoliosis; and the remainder included congenital, paralytic, and scoliosis due to various other causes including tuberculosis, neurofibromatosis, and other miscellaneous diseases. Of note, only 3 out of the 16 deaths due to cor pulmonale were in patients with idiopathic scoliosis, and it is uncertain whether these patients had adolescent-, juvenile-, or infantile-onset forms.

A more recent natural history study of scoliosis patients was published by Pehrsson et al. and included 115 patients with various forms of scoliosis, including 30 with infantile-onset scoliosis, 31 juvenile-onset scoliosis, 52 adolescent-onset scoliosis and scoliosis due to polio [26], rickets [19], and unknown [9, 69]. The average age of death was 54 years (range 16–75), with 60 patients still alive at the time of follow-up. Causes of death included 21 cases of respiratory failure, 17 with cardiovascular disease, and 17 with other causes. Of note, no patient with adolescent-onset scoliosis of unknown etiology (AIS) died from respiratory failure in this study [9].

A 50-year follow-up in 113 patients with scoliosis was reported by Nilsonne and Lundgren [93]. The reported mortality rate in this cohort was twice the rate of the general population, with 60% of deaths due to cardiopulmonary disease. Pertaining to the living patients, half were unable to work, 76% were unmarried, 90% had back symptoms, 30% were on disability pension for back pain or scoliosis, and 17% were on disability without pension. The notable shortcoming of the study was absence of radiographs to ascertain the etiology of scoliosis.

A separate study of patients with scoliosis of mixed etiologies was performed by Fowles and associates in 1978 [5]. They followed 65 patients for an average of 23 years. Ten patients died during the course of the study, and of the remaining, 40% had intermittent back pain, 22% were unemployed, 9% were on disability pensions, and 63% of the women were unmarried. Of note, only 44% of the living patients had a diagnosis of idiopathic scoliosis.

A four-part follow-up of an adolescent idiopathic scoliosis cohort from Ste. Justine in Montreal demonstrated a 45% incidence of current back pain in the non-treated patient group [6, 7]. This information was obtained via questionnaire survey during 14-year follow-up. The authors also concluded that scoliosis patients experienced limitations in specific activities including lifting, walking long distances, sitting or standing for long periods of time, traveling, and socializing outside of the home. They also concluded that patients with scoliosis perceived themselves to be less healthy than other people of the same age. Compared to controls, scoliosis patients also reported more current and intense back pain. This study had many notable shortcomings, including a population-based control group that consisted of patients randomly selected from the telephone directory, but not actually evaluated and screened to exclude the presence of spinal deformity. Further, most of the information was obtained by a telephone survey and questionnaire, and patients were not reevaluated personally or radiographed at follow-up.

Unfortunately, the majority of these early studies portrayed a poor prognosis and implied that all types of scoliosis inevitably led to high mortality rates, disability from back pain, cardiopulmonary compromise, and lower marriage rates. However, as stated previously, these prior studies were not specific to AIS.

The University of Iowa has published one of the longest natural history study series on AIS patients. The first study was performed by Ponseti and Friedman in 1950, and it followed 394 patients with untreated AIS at 2-year follow-up [10]. This particular study showed that overall prognosis can be attributed to curve pattern and age of onset [10]. In 1969, a second follow-up illustrated the importance of collecting specific data during AIS follow-up visits, including radiographic data, pulmonary and back symptoms, living situation, occupation, activities, marriage, and children [4]. In 1976, Weinstein and colleagues continued to follow this cohort with regard to radiographic, clinical, and psychosocial outcomes [11]. Factors related to curvature progression were studied in a second report of the cohort [12]. At an average follow-up of 51 years, this unique cohort was studied again with a comprehensive assessment including clinical exam, radiographs, rating of back pain, pulmonary symptoms, general function, depression, and body image [94]. These studies specific to AIS have shown more favorable outcomes. The most frequently noted long-term sequelae of untreated AIS are curve progression, back pain, cardiopulmonary issues, and psychosocial concerns, all of which will be the remaining focus of this chapter [4, 10–12, 94, 95].

2.6 Curve Progression

2.6.1 Skeletal Maturity

Curve progression in scoliosis varies according to etiology. The natural history of patients with untreated AIS does not necessarily apply to scoliosis of other known etiologies. Outcomes in AIS are tied to curve progression, as progressive curves are thought to eventually lead to pain, diminished pulmonary function, and psychosocial problems. Therefore, surgical and nonsurgical treatment decisions are often centered around probable or actual curve progression. Early work implied that curve progression would stop at skeletal maturity [96]. However, many studies have since shown that many curves may continue to progress throughout life [2, 11, 12, 94, 95, 97].

In the skeletally immature patient, the progression risk is related to specific curve factors and growth potential. Overall, curves that reach 50° are likely to progress into adulthood at a rate of 1° per year, which is largely based on the Iowa long-term studies [4, 10–12, 94, 95]. Assessment of skeletal maturity and associated growth potential through methods such as age of menarche, digital skeletal age, and Risser sign are essential for prognostication [98–101]. Spinal growth is directly tied to specific events of puberty [41, 81, 102, 103, 136]. Curves often progress in early adolescence, known as the curve acceleration phase [99]. The Tanner-Whitehouse-III RUS skeletal maturity assessment method has been shown to correlate well with curve progression in adolescence [99, 100, 137]. Careful assessment of maturity is essential during follow-up of AIS patients, as current maturity stage can predict when a curve may progress more quickly and closer follow-up may be required. Maturity also guides type of treatment, such as scoliosis bracing [104–106].

The majority of data on curve progression was obtained from studies with a predominance of females with thoracic curves. Overall, several factors were found to influence the probability of progression in a skeletally immature patient. Two factors relate to curve characteristics and four factors relate to growth potential.

2.6.1.1 Curve Factors

1. The risk of progression is greater for curves of larger magnitude at detection. Curves greater than or equal to 50° at skeletal maturity tend to progress [12, 88, 94, 102].
2. Curves with thoracic apex tend to progress with a prevalence of progression of 58–100% [12, 88, 94, 102, 107]. Thoracic curves and thoracic component of double major curve progress at a greater rate than lumbar curves and lumbar component of double major curve [94].

2.6.1.2 Growth Factors

1. The younger the patient at time of diagnosis, the greater the risk for progression [2, 12, 88, 102].
2. There is a greater risk for progression before the onset of menarche in girls [41, 81, 102, 103].
3. Amount of skeletal growth remaining. The lower the Risser grade or digital skeletal age, the greater the time before skeletal maturity and therefore the greater the risk for progression [88, 99].

In addition, loss of thoracic kyphosis has also been shown to have some influence on the likelihood of curve progression [108, 109]. The specifics of how the loss of thoracic kyphosis affects curve progression are yet to be determined. Regarding postmaturity curve progression, curves <30° at skeletal maturity, regardless of curve pattern, tend not to progress in adult life. More severe curves, particularly thoracic curves between 50 and 80°, do progress [12, 94, 110].

2.6.2 Curve Location

Location of spinal curve is important to curve progression (Table 2.2). Thoracic curves tend to be the most prone to progression, even after skeletal maturity, with an average progression rate of approximately 0.4–0.5° per year [11, 12, 94, 95]. For

Table 2.2 Cobb angles by curve location and follow-up

		Cobb angles at skeletal maturity[a]	Current Cobb angles
Curve type	Number (%)	Mean (SD) [range]	Mean (SD) [range]
Thoracic	34 (43)	60.48 (26.79) [26–108]	84.50 (30.17) [23–156]
Thoracolumbar	11 (14)	43.63 (8.70) [36–64]	89.54 (32.69) [50–155]
Lumbar	22 (28)	35.05 (13.18) [15–63]	49.41 (26.38) [15–90]
Double major			
Thoracic component	12 (15)	66.00 (21.53) [28–97]	79.08 (21.92) [30–104]
Lumbar component	12 (15)	60.75 (18.06) [26–83]	76.42 (21.88) [32–110]

[a]Modified from Weinstein et al. 2003, Table 2, pg. 561 [94]

patients with thoracic curve patterns, those with curves of less than 30° at maturity did not experience progression and tended to have apical vertebral rotation of less than 20° and Mehta angles of less than 20°.

Fewer thoracolumbar curves have been studied [11, 12, 94, 95]. A progression rate of approximately 0.5° per year has also been reported for thoracolumbar curves >30° [11, 12]. The subset of patients with more severe curves (between >40° and 50°) at skeletal maturity progressed even more on average [2, 12, 94]. Patients with thoracolumbar curves also have a propensity to develop translatory shifts, which may be an important factor in development of back pain [11, 12].

Lumbar curves tend to progress at a slower rate compared to thoracic and thoracolumbar curves [2, 12, 94, 95]. All lumbar curves of >30° at maturity tend to have vertebral rotation of more than 33% and tend to progress. Factors associated with progression include right-sided curves, an apical vertebral rotation of more than 33%, and a high-riding fifth lumbar vertebra [11, 12, 94]. Protective factors against progression include curves <30°, a deeply seated lumbar vertebrae and sacralized fifth lumbar vertebra, and absence of translatory shift development [11, 12]. For double curves, no specific factors other than curve magnitude correlate to curve progression after maturity [2, 11, 12, 94]. The ribs tend to remain level in the thoracic component; therefore, the Mehta angles are typically low. Combined curves revealed no prognostic value in the relationship of the fifth lumbar vertebra to the intercrest line [12]. The magnitude of the thoracic component of the double major curve pattern at maturity tends to be larger than the lumbar component. However, there are selectively greater increases in the lumbar curve magnitude compared to the thoracic curve in order to provide improved patient balance [12, 94]. Further, all patients tend to compensate with time by increases in their secondary curvatures [12].

2.7 Back Pain and Disability

Studies have shown varying data pertaining to the incidence of back pain in patients with AIS. The varying results may be partly attributed to the fact that back pain in the general population has been proven to be highly variable and questionnaire

Table 2.3 Intensity of current back pain (top) and duration of current back pain (bottom)

	Score	Control	Scoliosis	*P* value
Description of pain				
	Overall pain			
None	0	31/48 (65)[a]	21/92 (23)	<0.001
Some	1–5	17/48 (35)	71/92 (77)	
	Intensity			
Little/moderate	1–2	12/17 (24)	48/71 (68)	>0.99
Quite bad/unbearable	3–5	5/17 (29)	23/71 (32)b)	
Duration of pain				
<2 years	2–5	4/17 (24)[a]	6/67 (9)	<0.12
≥2 years	6	13/17 (76)	61/67 (91)	

[a]No./total (%). Modified from Weinstein et al. 2003, Table 7, pg. 561 [94]

dependent [111]. Further, natural history studies of back pain in AIS patients have reported different measures of back pain with categories ranging from overall incidence of pain, pain intensity, pain duration, timing of pain during day, pain in relation to physical activity, pain location, and hospitalizations for pain. Therefore, it has been difficult to compare pain measures across studies. Ascani and coauthors as well as data from the Iowa 40-year follow-up reported similar incidence of back pain between patients with AIS and the general population [2, 11]. The Swedish long-term follow-up studies of AIS, all with follow-up periods of longer than 30 years and all with more than 90% of the patients traced, demonstrated that low-back pain is not a significant problem in these patients [92, 93]. Studies have shown that thoracolumbar and lumbar curves tend to have the highest frequency of back pain and thoracic and double major curves with the lowest frequency [2, 11]. Further, patients with radiographic presence of translatory shifts tended to have slightly greater incidence of back pain than in patients with other patterns [11, 94].

In the Iowa 50-year natural history study's evaluation of pain, it was concluded that both acute and chronic pain were more prevalent in AIS patients compared to controls [94]. Sixty-one percent of AIS patients reported chronic back pain at any level of the spine versus 35% of controls. Current back pain was found in 77% of scoliotic patients versus 37% of controls. However, for both AIS individuals and controls with pain, no significant differences with respect to pain intensity or duration were found (Table 2.3). Of note, only one AIS patient at 50-year follow-up reported using narcotic medications to control pain. To aid in comparison, approximately 50% of adults without scoliosis will experience an episode of back pain in any given year, and 15% will have an episode that lasts for greater than 2 weeks [112].The cause of back pain in the adult scoliosis patient is relatively unknown and does not seem to correlate well with curve severity or presence of osteoarthritis [11, 94]. At skeletal maturity, the Iowa series found only 2% of patients had evidence of osteoarthritis. By 40-year follow-up, 38% of patients had evidence of degenerative joint disease of the spine [11, 12]. The Iowa 50-year follow-up study found 91% of patients showed osteoarthritic changes in the spine, but radiographs continued to be unrelated to the duration or intensity of pain [94]. Patients with scoliosis most commonly complained of back pain at the end of a strenuous day or after unusual activities, with pain generally relieved by rest. The location of the pain is variable and usually unrelated to the location or magnitude of the curve [11, 94]. In general, back pain in scoliosis patients should not be assumed to be caused by the curve itself, and other etiologies of back pain should be sought.

These studies have found that AIS does not cause disability, and most individuals are able to work and perform everyday activities similar to a level of unaffected peers. In an epidemiologic study performed by Horal, it was found that scoliosis cases did not represent a disproportionate number of disability pensions [113]. It is estimated that 1% of patients with scoliosis eventually require surgery specifically for back pain, which is similar to the general population [114]. The natural history of AIS should not be confused with other types of scoliosis and associated pain. Lumbar and thoracolumbar curves may arise de novo in adult life, known as “degenerative” scoliosis [115, 116]. Degenerative scoliosis may cause severe pain and discomfort requiring treatment.

2.8 Pulmonary Function

A direct correlation exists between decreased pulmonary function and increasing curve severity in untreated AIS patients with thoracic curves [94, 117–119]. The only symptom that has been consistently associated with curve magnitude is pulmonary function [94]. A recent study used EOS imaging to reconstruct true coronal, sagittal, and apical deformities in preoperative AIS patients [118]. Deformity was then correlated to PFTs and pulmonary function. The study found that the majority of patients with the large thoracic deformities (defined as 3D coronal cobb >80°, 3D thoracic lordosis >20°, and absolute apical rotation >25°) had moderate to severe impairments in pulmonary function. A Cobb angle of 50° or greater at skeletal maturity is a significant predictor of curve progression and later decreased pulmonary function. Further, vital capacity, FEV1, and Pa02 decrease as the severity of thoracic curves increase. No correlation between curve severity and loss of pulmonary function exists for other curve patterns. Affected patients have a uniform pattern of restrictive lung disease. Patients who smoke are generally affected more severely than non-smokers. Significant limitations of FVC in non-smokers usually do not occur until curve approaches 100–120°. Decrease in pulmonary function may also be caused by thoracic hypokyphosis [118–120]. Therefore, curves of lesser magnitude with significant hypokyphosis may cause significant decrease in pulmonary function. Despite decreases in pulmonary function, pulmonary hypertension and right heart failure are rare occurrences in AIS [2, 8, 11, 13, 94, 121, 122], unlike other forms of scoliosis (i.e., early onset.) Other factors that affect pulmonary function include decreased respiratory muscle strength, magnitude of vertebral rotation, and the degree of thoracic lordosis [117, 123, 124].

2.9 Mortality

As described earlier, initial natural history studies including patients with varying etiologies of scoliosis cited increased mortality rates in scoliosis patients. The Iowa long-term studies found mortality rates in patients specific to AIS are comparable to those of the general population [3, 11, 94]. The Iowa 40-year long-term study showed only one case of cor pulmonale due to scoliosis in a patient with a 142° thoracic curve at final follow-up, as the cause of death in AIS, with an overall mortality rate of 15% [11, 12]. By 50-year follow-up, the number of deaths increased expectedly, but did not differ from actuarial predicted rates for patients born during similar years. Of note, at 50 years, scoliosis could be implicated as a contributing cause of death in three cases [94]. In AIS, increased risk of death from cor pulmonale and right ventricular failure only occurs in patients with high-angle thoracic curves of more than 100° [10, 11, 94].

2.10 Psychosocial Effects

Studies citing psychosocial aspects of untreated AIS are limited. The Iowa 50-year follow-up series showed that 32% of patients felt that scoliosis had limited their life, particularly with regard to buying clothes, decreased physical activity, and increased self-consciousness [94]. However, patients with untreated AIS show psychosocial and depression indices similar to those of controls [7, 94]. The latest follow-up in the Iowa 50-year series utilized several psychosocial indices to better evaluate depression, body satisfaction, and perception of limitations in patients with scoliosis [94]. The Self-Rating Depression Scale, which describes common depressive symptoms and asks users to rate how often he/she experiences each symptom, was used to evaluate scoliosis patients and controls for clinical depression. Scores were found to be similar among the control and scoliosis groups. A Body Satisfaction Scale that included 16 body parts, appearance from multiple sides/angles, and appearance in swimsuit/clothes was also utilized to evaluate overall body satisfaction in the control group compared to the scoliosis group. Overall, the control group was slightly to moderately satisfied with their bodies, and patients in the scoliosis group were slightly dissatisfied to slightly satisfied. Additionally, the study found that current Cobb angle was not highly correlated with the body image scores nor was the degree of apical rotation. The last component of this study asked patients, "Do you feel your back has limited your life, or in any way affected you?" (excluding what had already been outlined previously, including pain, medications, treatments, pulmonary complaints, and apparent deformity). Responses to these open-ended questions were variable, but most outlined self-consciousness, decreased physical capacity, and challenges while shopping for clothes as their main concerns. Overall, 32% of the patients in this study felt limited in some regard due to their scoliosis [94].

2.11 Pregnancy

Controversy exists as to whether curves progress during pregnancy and whether or not women with scoliosis can have normal reproductive experiences. Nachemson and colleagues showed a statistically significant effect on curve progression in patients who experienced multiple pregnancies before the age of 23 [125]. The authors' recommendation was to avoid pregnancy in the early 20s, especially in patients treated with bracing. Further studies by Blount and Mellencamp [126] and Berman et al. [127] demonstrated that scoliosis progressed as a result of pregnancy. This effect was attributed to curve stability [126]. However, one study did not detect any negative effect of pregnancy on scoliosis in a natural history study group [102].

Three hundred and fifty-five patients who had reached skeletal maturity were studied by Betz and associates [128]. These patients were divided into two groups based on pregnancy: patients who had had at least one pregnancy and patients who had never been pregnant. Both groups were comparable pertaining to treatment. Progression of curve more than 5° was observed in 25% of patients in each group, and progression of more than 10° was observed in 10% of patients in each group. Patient's age at time of first pregnancy did not influence risk for progression, and the stability of the curve before pregnancy did not reduce the risk of progression during pregnancy. These authors concluded that pregnancy does not increase the risk for curve progression of a scoliotic curve in a patient whose curve is not severe. Age of patient at time of first pregnancy, number of pregnancies, and curve stability did not affect risk for progression.

A study by Visscher and associates demonstrated that reproductive experiences of scoliotic women do not differ from women without scoliosis [129]. Similarly, another series revealed no specific pregnancy or delivery problems were directly related to scoliosis, except in four patients whose delivery posed difficulties [128]. No cesarean sections were directly related to the mother's scoliosis, and the incidence of cesarean section was half of the national average. The long-term Iowa study mirrored these results [11, 12, 94]. In summary, while controversy exists regarding pregnancy in AIS patients, mild to moderate scoliosis likely has little negative effect on pregnancy or delivery.

2.12 Summary

The natural history of adolescent idiopathic scoliosis is based on a limited number of studies with relatively few patients, which are primarily based on information from female patients with thoracic curves. The conclusions presented in this chapter represent general guidelines. Even in patients with progressive curves, it is difficult to predict whether the natural history of a 30° curve would be to progress to a 40° curve or an 80° curve. In general, curves >50° tend to progress, while curves <30 tend to remain stable.

The majority of patients with AIS live relatively normal lives, are able to have children, and work. Some patients may have increased back pain later in life and may be affected by psychosocial issues, including increased self-consciousness and trouble purchasing clothes. Individualized decisions for each patient must be made by taking into account the probabilities of curve progression based on skeletal maturity, sexual maturity, curve magnitude, curve characteristics, and age. An increased number of children are being referred for orthopedic opinion as a result of increased public awareness, national scoliosis associations, and screening clinics. A thorough knowledge of AIS natural history is necessary for appropriate AIS management decisions and proper patient education.

References

1. Kane WJ. Scoliosis prevalence: a call for a statement of terms. Clin Orthop Relat Res. 1977;126:43–6.
2. Ascani E, Bartolozzi P, Logroscino CA, Marchetti PG, Ponte A, Savini R, et al. Natural history of untreated idiopathic scoliosis after skeletal maturity. Spine. 1986;11:784–9. http://www.ncbi.nlm.nih.gov/pubmed/3810293
3. Cheng JC, Castelein RM, Chu WC, Danielsson AJ, Dobbs MB, Grivas TB, et al. Adolescent idiopathic scoliosis. Nat Rev Dis Prim. 2015;1:15030. http://www.nature.com/articles/nrdp201530
4. Collis DK, Ponseti IV. Long-term follow-up of patients with idiopathic scoliosis not treated surgically. J bone Joint Surg Am. 1969;51(3):425–45.
5. Fowles JV, Drummond DS, L'Ecuyer S, Roy L, Kassab MT. Untreated scoliosis in the adult. Clin Orthop Relat Res. 1978;134:212–7.
6. Goldberg MS, Mayo NE, Poitras B, Scott S, Hanley J. The Ste-Justine Adolescent Idiopathic Scoliosis Cohort Study. Part II: perception of health, self and body image, and participation in physical activities. Spine (Phila PA 1976). 1994;19(14):1562–72.
7. Mayo NE, Goldberg MS, Poitras B, Scott S, Hanley J. The Ste-Justine adolescent idiopathic scoliosis cohort study. Part III: back pain. Spine. 1994;19:1573–81.
8. Pehrsson K, Bake B, Larsson S, Nachemson A. Lung function in adult idiopathic scoliosis: a 20 year follow up. Thorax. 1991;46(7):474–8. http://www.pubmedcentral.nih.gov/articlerender.fcgi?artid=463231%7B&%7Dtool=pmcentrez%7B&%7Drendertype=abstract
9. Pehrsson K, Larsson S, Oden A, Nachemson A. Long-term follow-up of patients with untreated scoliosis. A study of mortality, causes of death, and symptoms. Spine (Phila PA 1976). 1992;17(9):1091–6.
10. Ponseti I, Friedman B. Prognosis in idiopathic scoliosis. J Bone Joint Surg Am. 1950;32:381–95.
11. Weinstein SL, Zavala DC, Ponseti IV. Idiopathic scoliosis: long-term follow-up and prognosis in untreated patients. J Bone Joint Surg Am. 1981;63(5):702–12. http://www.ncbi.nlm.nih.gov/pubmed/6453874
12. Weinstein SL, Ponseti IV. Curve progression in idiopathic scoliosis. J Bone Joint Surg Am. 1983;65(4):447–55. http://www.ncbi.nlm.nih.gov/pubmed/6833318
13. Lowe TG, Edgar M, Margulies JY, Miller NH, Raso VJ, Reinker KA, et al. Etiology of idiopathic scoliosis: current trends in research. J Bone Joint Surg Am. 2000;82A(8):1157–68. http://www.ncbi.nlm.nih.gov/entrez/query.fcgi?cmd=Retrieve&db=PubMed&dopt=Citation&list_uids=10954107
14. Burwell RG. Aetiology of idiopathic scoliosis: current concepts. Pediatr Rehabil. 2003;6:137–70. http://www.ncbi.nlm.nih.gov/pubmed/14713582

15. Wang WJ, Yeung HY, Chu WC-W, Tang NL-S, Lee KM, Qiu Y, et al. Top theories for the etiopathogenesis of adolescent idiopathic scoliosis. J Pediatr Orthop. 2011;31(1 Suppl):S14–27. http://www.ncbi.nlm.nih.gov/pubmed/21173615
16. Burwell RG, Dangerfield PH, Moulton A, Grivas TB, Cheng JC. Whither the etiopathogenesis (and scoliogeny) of adolescent idiopathic scoliosis? Incorporating presentations on scoliogeny at the 2012 IRSSD and SRS meetings. Scoliosis. 2013;8(1):4. http://www.pubmedcentral.nih.gov/articlerender.fcgi?artid=3608974&tool=pmcentrez&rendertype=abstract
17. Veldhuizen G, Wever DJ, Webb PJ. The aetiology of idiopathic scoliosis: biomechanical and neuromuscular factors. Eur Spine J. 2000;9(3):178–84.
18. Wong C. Mechanism of right thoracic adolescent idiopathic scoliosis at risk for progression; a unifying pathway of development by normal growth and imbalance. Scoliosis. 2015;10(1):2. http://www.scoliosisjournal.com/content/10/1/2
19. Stokes IA, Spence H, Aronsson DD, Kilmer N. Mechanical modulation of vertebral body growth. Implications for scoliosis progression. Spine (Phila PA 1976). 1996;21(10):1162–7. http://www.ncbi.nlm.nih.gov/pubmed/8727190
20. Chu WCW, Man GCW, Lam WWM, Yeung BHY, Chau WW, Ng BKW, et al. Morphological and functional electrophysiological evidence of relative spinal cord tethering in adolescent idiopathic scoliosis. Spine (Phila Pa 1976). 2008;33(6):673–80.
21. Porter RW. The pathogenesis of idiopathic scoliosis: Uncoupled neuro-osseous growth? European Spine Journal. 2001;10:473–81.
22. Sevastik J, Burwell RG, Dangerfield PH. A new concept for the etiopathogenesis of the thoracospinal deformity of idiopathic scoliosis: summary of an electronic focus group debate of the IBSE. Eur Spine J. 2003;12:440–50.
23. Azeddine B, Letellier K, Wang DS, Moldovan F, Moreau A. Molecular determinants of melatonin signaling dysfunction in adolescent idiopathic scoliosis. Clin Orthop Relat Res. 2007;462(462):45–52.
24. Moreau A, Wang DS, Forget S, Azeddine B, Angeloni D, Fraschini F, et al. Melatonin signaling dysfunction in adolescent idiopathic scoliosis. Spine (Phila Pa 1976). 2004;29(16):1772–81.
25. Lowe TG, Burwell RG, Dangerfield PH. Platelet calmodulin levels in adolescent idiopathic scoliosis (AIS): can they predict curve progression and severity? Summary of an electronic focus group debate of the IBSE. Eur Spine J. 2004;13:257–65.
26. Castelein RM, Van Die'n JH, Smit TH. The role of dorsal shear forces in the pathogenesis of adolescent idiopathic scoliosis – a hypothesis. Med Hypotheses. 2005;65(3):501–8.
27. Kesling KL, Reinker KA. Scoliosis in twins. A meta-analysis of the literature and report of six cases. Spine (Phila PA 1976). 1997;22(17):2009–14. discussion 2015. http://www.ncbi.nlm.nih.gov/pubmed/9306532
28. Axenovich TI, Zaidman AM, Zorkoltseva IV, Tregubova IL, Borodin PM. Segregation analysis of idiopathic scoliosis: demonstration of a major gene effect. Am J Med Genet. 1999;86(4):389–94.
29. Miller NH. Genetics of familial idiopathic scoliosis. Clin Orthop Relat Res. 2007;462(462):6–10.
30. Baghernajad Salehi L, Mangino M, De Serio S, De Cicco D, Capon F, Semprini S, et al. Assignment of a locus for autosomal dominant idiopathic scoliosis (IS) to human chromosome 17p11. Hum Genet. 2002;111(4–5):401–4.
31. Chan V, Fong GCY, Luk KDK, Yip B, Lee M-K, Wong M-S, et al. A genetic locus for adolescent idiopathic scoliosis linked to chromosome 19p13.3. Am J Hum Genet. 2002;71(2):401–6. http://www.sciencedirect.com/science/article/pii/S0002929707604856
32. Wang W, Wang Z, Liu Z, Zhu Z, Zhu F, Sun X, et al. Are there gender differences in sagittal spinal pelvic inclination before and after the adolescent pubertal growth spurt? Eur Spine J. 2015;24(6):1168–74.
33. Justice CM, Miller NH, Marosy B, Zhang J, Wilson AF. Familial idiopathic scoliosis: evidence of an X-linked susceptibility locus. Spine. 2003;28:589–94. http://www.ncbi.nlm.nih.gov/pubmed/12642767

34. Wise C, Barnes R, Gillum J, Herring J, Bowcock M, Lovett M. Localization of susceptibility to familial idiopathic scoliosis. Spine (Phila PA 1976). 2000;25(18):2372–80.
35. Cheng JC, Tang NL, Yeung HY, Miller N. Genetic association of complex traits: using idiopathic scoliosis as an example. Clin Orthop Relat Res. 2007;462:38–44. http://www.ncbi.nlm.nih.gov/entrez/query.fcgi?cmd=Retrieve&db=PubMed&dopt=Citation&list_uids=17534191
36. Wise CA, Gao X, Shoemaker S, Gordon D, Herring JA. Understanding genetic factors in idiopathic scoliosis, a complex disease of childhood. Curr Genomics. 2008;9(1):51–9. http://www.pubmedcentral.nih.gov/articlerender.fcgi?artid=2674301&tool=pmcentrez&rendertype=abstract
37. Ward K, Ogilvie J, Argyle V, Nelson L, Meade M, Braun J, et al. Polygenic inheritance of adolescent idiopathic scoliosis: a study of extended families in Utah. Am J Med Genet Part A. 2010;152(5):1178–88.
38. Kruse LM, Dobbs MB, Gurnett C. Polygenic threshold model with sex dimorphism in clubfoot inheritance: the carter effect. J Bone Joint Surg Am. 2008;90(12):2688–94. http://www.pubmedcentral.nih.gov/articlerender.fcgi?artid=2663333&tool=pmcentrez&rendertype=abstract
39. Gorman KF, Julien C, Moreau A. The genetic epidemiology of idiopathic scoliosis. Eur Spine J. 2012;21(10):1905–19. http://www.pubmedcentral.nih.gov/articlerender.fcgi?artid=3463687&tool=pmcentrez&rendertype=abstract
40. Yeung HY, Tang NL, Lee KM, Ng BK, Hung VW, Kwok R, Guo X, Qin L, Cheng JC. Genetic association study of insulin-like growth factor-I (IGF-I) gene with curve severity and osteopenia in adolescent idiopathic scoliosis. Stud Heal Technol Inf. 2006;123:18–24.
41. Inoue M, Minami S, Nakata Y, Kitahara H, Otsuka Y, Isobe K, et al. Association between estrogen receptor gene polymorphisms and curve severity of idiopathic scoliosis. Spine (Phila PA 1976). 2002;27(21):2357–62.
42. Takahashi Y, Kou I, Takahashi A, Johnson T, Kono K, Kawakami N, et al. A genome-wide association study identifies common variants near LBX1 associated with adolescent idiopathic scoliosis. Nat Genet. 2011;43:1237–40. https://doi.org/10.1038/ng.974.
43. Londono D, Kou I, Johnson T, Sharma S, Ogura Y, Tsunoda T, et al. A meta-analysis identifies adolescent idiopathic scoliosis association with LBX1 locus in multiple ethnic groups. J Med Genet. 2014;51(6):401–6. http://www.ncbi.nlm.nih.gov/pubmed/24721834
44. Kou I, Takahashi Y, Johnson T, Takahashi A, Guo L, Dai J, et al. Genetic variants in GPR126 are associated with adolescent idiopathic scoliosis. Nat Genet. 2013;45:676–9. http://www.ncbi.nlm.nih.gov/pubmed/23666238
45. Wallin J, Wilting J, Koseki H, Fritsch R, Christ B, Balling R. The role of Pax-1 in axial skeleton development. Development. 1994;120(5):1109–21.
46. Sharma S, Londono D, Eckalbar WL, Gao X, Zhang D, Mauldin K, et al. A PAX1 enhancer locus is associated with susceptibility to idiopathic scoliosis in females. Nat Commun. 2015;6:6452. http://www.pubmedcentral.nih.gov/articlerender.fcgi?artid=4365504&tool=pmcentrez&rendertype=abstract
47. Buchan JG, Alvarado DM, Haller GE, Cruchaga C, Harms MB, Zhang T, et al. Rare variants in FBN1 and FBN2 are associated with severe adolescent idiopathic scoliosis. Hum Mol Genet. 2014;23(19):5271–82.
48. Wu J, Qiu Y, Zhang L, Sun Q, Qiu X, He Y. Association of estrogen receptor gene polymorphisms with susceptibility to adolescent idiopathic scoliosis. Spine (Phila PA 1976). 2006;31(10):1131–6.
49. Tang NL-S, Yeung H-Y, Lee K-M, Hung VW-Y, Cheung CS-K, Ng BK-W, et al. A relook into the association of the estrogen receptor [alpha] gene (PvuII, XbaI) and adolescent idiopathic scoliosis: a study of 540 Chinese cases. Spine (Phila PA 1976). 2006;31(21):2463–8.
50. Sharma S, Gao X, Londono D, Devroy SE, Mauldin KN, Frankel JT, et al. Genome-wide association studies of adolescent idiopathic scoliosis suggest candidate susceptibility genes. Hum Mol Genet. 2011;20(7):1456–66.
51. Chen Z, Qiu Y, Ma W, Qian B, Zhu Z. Comparison of somatosensory evoked potentials between adolescent idiopathic scoliosis and congenital scoliosis without neural axis abnormalities. Spine J. 2014;14(7):1095–8.

52. Lao MLM, Chow DHK, Guo X, Cheng JCY, Holmes AD. Impaired dynamic balance control in adolescents with idiopathic scoliosis and abnormal somatosensory evoked potentials. J Pediatr Orthop. 2008;28(8):846–9.
53. Simoneau M, Lamothe V, Hutin E, Mercier P, Teasdale N, Blouin J. Evidence for cognitive vestibular integration impairment in idiopathic scoliosis patients. BMC Neurosci. 2009;10:102.
54. Domenech J, García-Martí G, Martí-Bonmatí L, Barrios C, Tormos JM, Pascual-Leone A. Abnormal activation of the motor cortical network in idiopathic scoliosis demonstrated by functional MRI. Eur Spine J. 2011;20(7):1069–78.
55. Wang D, Shi L, Chu WCW, Paus T, Cheng JCY, Heng PA. A comparison of morphometric techniques for studying the shape of the corpus callosum in adolescent idiopathic scoliosis. NeuroImage. 2009;45(3):738–48.
56. Joly O, Rousié D, Jissendi P, Rousié M, Frankó E. A new approach to corpus callosum anomalies in idiopathic scoliosis using diffusion tensor magnetic resonance imaging. Eur Spine J. 2014;23(12):2643–9. http://www.ncbi.nlm.nih.gov/pubmed/24986356
57. Shi L, Wang D, Hui SCN, Tong MCF, Cheng JCY, Chu WCW. Volumetric changes in cerebellar regions in adolescent idiopathic scoliosis compared with healthy controls. Spine J. 2013;13(12):1904–11.
58. Shi L, Wang D, Chu WCW, Burwell GR, Wong TT, Heng PA, et al. Automatic MRI segmentation and morphoanatomy analysis of the vestibular system in adolescent idiopathic scoliosis. Neuroimage. 2011;54(Suppl. 1):S180–8.
59. Rousie DL, Deroubaix JP, Joly O, Baudrillard JC, Berthoz A. Abnormal connection between lateral and posterior semicircular canal revealed by a new modeling process: origin and physiological consequences. Ann NY Acad Sci. 2009;1164:455–7.
60. Burwell RG, Aujla RK, Freeman BJC, Dangerfield PH, Cole AA, Kirby AS, et al. Patterns of extra-spinal left-right skeletal asymmetries in adolescent girls with lower spine scoliosis: relative lengthening of the ilium on the curve concavity & of right lower limb segments. Stud Health Technol Inform. 2006;123:57–65.
61. Normelli H, Sevastik J, Akrivos J. The length and ash weight of the ribs of normal and scoliotic persons. Spine (Phila Pa 1976). 1985;10(6):590–2.
62. Cheung CSK, Lee WTK, Tse YK, Lee KM, Guo X, Qin L, et al. Generalized osteopenia in adolescent idiopathic scoliosis—association with abnormal pubertal growth, bone turnover, and calcium intake? Spine (Phila PA 1976). 2006;31(3):330–8.
63. Cheng JC, Qin L, Cheung CS, Sher AH, Lee KM, Ng SW, et al. Generalized low areal and volumetric bone mineral density in adolescent idiopathic scoliosis. J Bone Miner Res Off J Am Soc Bone Miner Res. 2000;15(8):1587–95. http://www.ncbi.nlm.nih.gov/pubmed/10934658
64. Hung VWY, Qin L, Cheung CSK, Lam TP, Ng BKW, Tse YK, et al. Osteopenia: a new prognostic factor of curve progression in adolescent idiopathic scoliosis. J Bone Joint Surg Am. 2005;87(2003):2709–16.
65. Cheng JC, Tang SP, Guo X, Chan CW, Qin L. Osteopenia in adolescent idiopathic scoliosis: a histomorphometric study. Spine (Phila PA 1976). 2001;26(3):E19–23. http://www.ncbi.nlm.nih.gov/pubmed/11224874
66. Kouwenhoven JW, Castelein RM. The pathogenesis of adolescent idiopathic scoliosis: review of the literature. Spine (Phila PA 1976). 2008;33(26):2898–908. http://www.ncbi.nlm.nih.gov/pubmed/19092622
67. Stokes IAF, Aronsson DD, Dimock AN, Cortright V, Beck S. Endochondral growth in growth plates of three species at two anatomical locations modulated by mechanical compression and tension. J Orthop Res. 2006;24(6):1327–34.
68. Valteau B, Grimard G, Londono I, Moldovan F, Villemure I. In vivo dynamic bone growth modulation is less detrimental but as effective as static growth modulation. Bone. 2011;49(5):996–1004.
69. Sabirin J, Bakri R, Buang SN, Abdullah AT, Ortho P, Fellow S, et al. School scoliosis screening programme – a systematic review. Med J Malaysia. 2010;65(4):261–7.

70. Balioglu MB, Aydin C, Kargin D, Albayrak A, Atici Y, Tas SK, et al. Vitamin-D measurement in patients with adolescent idiopathic scoliosis. J Pediatr Orthop B. 2017;26(1):48–52.
71. Shohat M, Shohat T, Nitzan M, Mimouni M, Kedem R, Danon YL. Growth and ethnicity in scoliosis. Acta Orthop Scand. 1988;59(3):310–3. http://www.ncbi.nlm.nih.gov/pubmed/3381663
72. Clark EM, Taylor HJ, Harding I, Hutchinson J, Nelson I, Deanfield JE, et al. Association between components of body composition and scoliosis: a prospective cohort study reporting differences identifiable before the onset of scoliosis. J Bone Miner Res. 2014;29(8):1729–36.
73. Tam EMS, Yu FWP, Hung VWY, Liu Z, Liu KL, Ng BKW, et al. Are volumetric bone mineral density and bone micro-architecture associated with leptin and soluble leptin receptor levels in adolescent idiopathic scoliosis? A case-control study. PLoS One. 2014;9(2):e87939. http://www.pubmedcentral.nih.gov/articlerender.fcgi?artid=3916359&tool=pmcentrez&rendertype=abstract
74. Kouwenhoven J-WM, Smit TH, van der Veen AJ, Kingma I, van Dieën JH, Castelein RM. Effects of dorsal versus ventral shear loads on the rotational stability of the thoracic spine: a biomechanical porcine and human cadaveric study. Spine (Phila Pa 1976). 2007;32(23):2545–50.
75. Janssen MM, J-WM K, TPC S, Viergever M, Bartels LW, Castelein RM, et al. Analysis of preexistent vertebral rotation in the normal infantile, juvenile, and adolescent spine. Spine (Phila PA 1976). 2011;36(13):E486–91.
76. Schlösser TPC, Vincken KL, Rogers K, Castelein RM, Shah SA. Natural sagittal spino-pelvic alignment in boys and girls before, at and after the adolescent growth spurt. Eur Spine J. 2015;24(6):1158–67.
77. Jarvis JG, Ashman RB, Johnston CE, Herring JA. The posterior tether in scoliosis. Clin Orthop Relat Res. 1988;227:126–34. http://www.embase.com/search/results?subaction=viewrecord&from=export&id=L18054628
78. Roaf R. Vertebral growth and its mechanical control. J Bone Joint Surg. 1960;42B(1):40–59. http://www.bjj.boneandjoint.org.uk/content/42-B/1/40.abstract
79. Fong DY, Lee CF, Cheung KM, Cheng JC, Ng BK, Lam TP, et al. A meta-analysis of the clinical effectiveness of school scoliosis screening. Spine (Phila PA 1976). 2010;35(10):1061–71. http://search.ebscohost.com/login.aspx?direct=true&db=cin20&AN=2010641169&site=ehost-live
80. Luk KDK, Lee CF, Cheung KMC, Cheng JCY, Ng BKW, Lam TP, et al. Clinical effectiveness of school screening for adolescent idiopathic scoliosis: a large population-based retrospective cohort study. Spine (Phila PA 1976). 2010;35(17):1607–14. http://www.ncbi.nlm.nih.gov/pubmed/20453727
81. Grivas TB, Vasiliadis E, Mouzakis V, Mihas C, Koufopoulos G. Association between adolescent idiopathic scoliosis prevalence and age at menarche in different geographic latitudes. Scoliosis. 2006;1:9.
82. US Census Bureau. Census 2010. Suitland, MD: US Census Bureau; 2010. http://quickfacts.census.gov/qfd/states/13/13135.html
83. Schappert SM, Nelson C. National Ambulatory Medical Care Survey: 1995–96 summary. Vital Heal Stat. 1999;13(142):i122.
84. Vigneswaran HT, Grabel ZJ, Eberson CP, Palumbo MA, Daniels AH. Surgical treatment of adolescent idiopathic scoliosis in the United States from 1997 to 2012: an analysis of 20,346 patients. J Neurosurg Pediatr. 2015;16(3):322–8. http://www.ncbi.nlm.nih.gov/pubmed/26114991
85. Burwell RG, James N, Johnson F, Webb JK, Wilson Y. Standardised trunk asymmetry scores. A study of back contour in healthy school children. J Bone Joint Surg Br. 1983;65(4):452–63. http://journals.lww.com/pedorthopaedics/Abstract/1984/03000/Standardised_Trunk_Asymmetry_Scores__A_Study_of.75.aspx
86. Brooks HL, Azen SP, Gerberg E, Brooks R, Chan L. Scoliosis: a prospective epidemiological study. J Bone Joint Surg Am. 1975;57(7):968–72. http://www.ncbi.nlm.nih.gov/pubmed/1194304

87. Brooks HL, Azen SP, Gerberg E, Brooks R, Chan L. Scoliosis: a prospective epidemiological study. J Bone Joint Surg Am. 1975;57(7):968–72. http://www.ncbi.nlm.nih.gov/entrez/query.fcgi?cmd=Retrieve&db=PubMed&dopt=Citation&list_uids=1194304
88. Lonstein JE, Carlson JM. The prediction of curve progression in untreated idiopathic scoliosis during growth. J Bone Joint Surg Am. 1984;66(7):1061–71.
89. Montgomery F, Willner S. The natural history of idiopathic scoliosis – incidence of treatment in 15 cohorts of children born between 1963 and 1977. Spine (Phila PA 1976). 1997;22(7):772–4.
90. Rogala EJ, Drummond DS, Gurr J. Scoliosis: incidence and natural history. A prospective epidemiological study. J Bone Joint Surg Am. 1978;60(2):173–6.
91. Willner S, Udén A. A prospective prevalence study of scoliosis in Southern Sweden. Acta Orthop Scand. 1982;53(2):233–7.
92. Nachemson A. A long term follow-up study of non-treated scoliosis. Acta Orthop Scand. 1968;39(4):466–76.
93. Nilsonne U, Lundgren K. Long-term prognosis in idiopathic scoliosis. Acta Orthop Scand. 1968;39(4):456–65.
94. Weinstein SL, Dolan LA, Spratt KF, Peterson KK, Spoonamore MJ, Ponseti IV. Health and function of patients with untreated idiopathic scoliosis: a 50-year natural history study. JAMA. 2003;289(5):559–67. http://eutils.ncbi.nlm.nih.gov/entrez/eutils/elink.fcgi?dbfrom=pubmed&id=12578488&retmode=ref&cmd=prlinks%5Cnpapers2://publication/uuid/A3B2B968-56B2-43D1-9E86-54B3EDA1B140
95. Edgar MA. The natural history of unfused scoliosis. Orthopedics. 1987;10(6):931–9. http://www.scopus.com/inward/record.url?eid=2-s2.0-0023181938&partnerID=tZOtx3y1
96. Risser JC, Ferguson AB. Scoliosis: its prognosis. J Bone Joint Surg. 1936;18(3):667–70. http://jbjs.org/content/18/3/667.abstract
97. Weinstein SL. Idiopathic scoliosis: natural history. Spine (Phila PA 1976). 1986;11(8):780–3. http://www.scopus.com/inward/record.url?eid=2-s2.0-0023038198&partnerID=tZOtx3y1
98. Risser JC, Brand RA. The iliac apophysis: an invaluable sign in the management of scoliosis. Clin Orthopaed Relat Res. 2010;2010:646–53.
99. Sanders JO, Khoury JG, Kishan S, Browne RH, Mooney JF, Arnold KD, et al. Predicting scoliosis progression from skeletal maturity: a simplified classification during adolescence. J Bone Joint Surg Am. 2008;90(3):540–53. http://content.wkhealth.com/linkback/openurl?sid=WKPTLP:landingpage&an=00004623-200803000-00011
100. Sanders JO. Maturity assessment and curve progression in girls with idiopathic scoliosis. J Bone Joint Surg. 2007;89(1):64. http://jbjs.org/cgi/doi/10.2106/JBJS.F.00067
101. Tanner J. Assessment of skeletal maturity and prediction of adult height (TW3 method). 3rd ed. London: W.B. Saunders; 2001.
102. Bunnell WP. The natural history of idiopathic scoliosis before skeletal maturity. Spine (Phila PA 1976). 1986;11(8):773–6. http://journals.lww.com/spinejournal/Fulltext/1986/10000/The_Natural_History_of_Idiopathic_Scoliosis_Before.3.aspx
103. Lonstein JE, Winter RB. The Milwaukee brace for the treatment of adolescent idiopathic scoliosis. A review of one thousand and twenty patients. J Bone Joint Surg Am. 1994;76(8):1207–21.
104. Dolan L, Haggerty K, Weinstein S. Evaluation of TLSOS in the bracing in adolescent idiopathic scoliosis trial (BrAIST). Scoliosis. 2013;8(Suppl 1):O48. http://scoliosisjournal.biomedcentral.com/articles/10.1186/1748-7161-8-S1-O48
105. Weinstein S, Dolan L, Wright J, Dobbs M. Effects of bracing in adolescents with idiopathic scoliosis. N Engl J Med. 2013;369(16):1512–21.
106. Weinstein S, Dolan L. The evidence base for the prognosis and treatment of adolescent idiopathic scoliosis: the 2015 Orthopaedic Research and Education Foundation Clinical Research Award. J Bone Joint Surg Am. 2015;18(97):1899–903.
107. Picault C, DeMauroy J, Mouilleseaux B, Diana G. Natural history of idiopathic scoliosis in girls and boys. Spine (Phila Pa 1976). 1986;11:777–8.

108. Deacon P, Flood BM, Dickson R. Idiopathic scoliosis in three dimensions. A radiographic and morphometric analysis. J Bone Joint Surg Br. 1984;66(4):509–12.
109. Shufflebarger HL, King WF. Composite measurement of scoliosis: a new method of analysis of the deformity. Spine (Phila PA 1976). 1986;12:228–32.
110. Weinstein S, Dolan L, Cheng J, Danielsson A, Morcuende J. Adolescent idiopathic scoliosis. Lancet. 2008;3(371(9623)):1527–37. http://www.thelancet.com/pdfs/journals/lancet/PIIS0140-6736(08)60658-3.pdf
111. Frymoyer JW, Newberg A, Pope MH. Spine radiographs in patients with low-back pain: an epidemiological study in men. J Bone Joint Surg Ser A. 1984;66(7):1048–55.
112. Deyo RA, Mirza SK, Martin BI. Back pain prevalence and visit rates: estimates from U.S. national surveys, 2002. Spine (Phila PA 1976). 2006;31(23):2724–7. http://www.ncbi.nlm.nih.gov/pubmed/17077742%5Cn. http://www.uptodate.com/contents/evaluation-of-low-back-pain-in-adults/abstract/7
113. Horal J. The clinical appearance of low back disorders in the city of Gothenburg, Sweden. Comparisons of incapacitated probands with matched controls. Acta Orthop Scand. 1969;118:1–109.
114. Nachemson A. Adult scoliosis and back pain. Spine (Phila PA 1976). 1979;4(6):513–7.
115. Robin GC, Span Y, Steinberg R, Makin M, Menczel J. Scoliosis in the elderly: a follow-up study. Spine. 1982;7:355–9.
116. Kostuik JP, Bentivoglio J. The incidence of low back pain in adult scoliosis. Acta Orthop Belg. 1981;47(4–5):548–59.
117. Kafer ER. Respiratory and cardiovascular functions in scoliosis. Clin Respir Physiol. 1977;13(2):299–321. http://www.embase.com/search/results?subaction=viewrecord&from=export&id=L8055079%5Cn. http://sfx.library.uu.nl/utrecht?sid=EMBASE&issn=02727587&id=doi:&atitle=Respiratory+and+cardiovascular+functions+in+scoliosis&stitle=CLIN.+RESPIR.+PHYSIOL.&title=Clinica
118. Yaszay B, Bastrom TP, Bartley CE, Parent S, Newton PO. The effects of the three-dimensional deformity of adolescent idiopathic scoliosis on pulmonary function. Eur Spine J. 2017;26:1658–64.
119. Newton P, Faro F, Gollogly S, Betz R, Lenke L, Lowe T. Results of preoperative pulmonary function testing of adolescents with idiopathic scoliosis. A study of six hundred and thirty-one patients. J Bone Joint Surg Am. 2005;87:1937–46.
120. Winter RB, Lovell WW, Moe JH. Excessive thoracic lordosis and loss of pulmonary function in patients with idiopathic scoliosis. J Bone Joint Surg Am. 1975;57(7):972–7.
121. Branthwaite MA. Cardiorespiratory consequences of unfused idiopathic scoliosis. Br J Dis Chest. 1986;80(C):360–9.
122. Pehrsson K, Danielsson A, Nachemson A. Pulmonary function in adolescent idiopathic scoliosis: a 25 year follow up after surgery or start of brace treatment. Thorax. 2001;56(5):388–93. http://www.pubmedcentral.nih.gov/articlerender.fcgi?artid=1746049&tool=pmcentrez&rendertype=abstract
123. Kearon C, Viviani GR, Kirkley A, Killian KJ. Factors determining pulmonary function in adolescent idiopathic thoracic scoliosis. Am Rev Respir Dis. 1993;148(2):288–94.
124. Lin MC, Liaw MY, Chen WJ, Cheng PT, AMK W, Chiou WK. Pulmonary function and spinal characteristics: their relationships in persons with idiopathic and postpoliomyelitic scoliosis. Arch Phys Med Rehabil. 2001;82(3):335–41.
125. Danielsson a J, Nachemson a L. Childbearing, curve progression, and sexual function in women 22 years after treatment for adolescent idiopathic scoliosis: a case-control study. Spine (Phila PA 1976). 2001;26(13):1449–56.
126. Blount W, Mellencamp D. The effect of pregnancy on idiopathic scoliosis. J Bone Joint Surg Am. 1980;62(7):1083–7.
127. Berman A, Cohen D, Schwentker E. The effects of pregnancy on idiopathic scoliosis. A preliminary report on eight cases and a review of the literature. Spine (Phila PA 1976). 1982;7(1):76–7.

128. Betz RR, Bunnell WP, Lambrecht-Mulier E, MacEwen GD. Scoliosis and pregnancy. J Bone Joint Surg Am. 1987;69(1):90–6. http://www.ncbi.nlm.nih.gov/pubmed/22070615
129. Visscher W, Lonstein JE, Hoffman DA, Mandel JS, Harris BS. Reproductive outcomes in scoliosis patients. Spine (Phila PA 1976). 1988;13(10):1096–8.
130. Negrini S, Negrini A, Atanasio S, Santambrogio GC. Three-dimensional easy morphological (3-DEMO) classification of scoliosis, part I. Scoliosis. 2006;1(1):20. http://scoliosisjournal.biomedcentral.com/articles/10.1186/1748-7161-1-20
131. Poncet P, Dansereau J, Labelle H. Geometric torsion in idiopathic scoliosis: three-dimensional analysis and proposal for a new classification. Spine (Phila PA 1976). 2001;26:2235–43.
132. Rigo MD, Villagrasa M, Gallo D. A specific scoliosis classification correlating with brace treatment: description and reliability. Scoliosis. 2010;5(1):1–11.
133. Weiss H. The method of Katharina Schroth – history, principles and current development. Scoliosis. 2011;6:17.
134. Lenke LG, Betz RR, Harms J, Bridwell KH, Clements DH, Lowe TG, et al. Adolescent idiopathic scoliosis. A new classification to determine extent of spinal arthrodesis. J Bone Joint Surg. 2001;83(8):1169–81. http://jbjs.org/content/83/8/1169.abstract
135. Qiu G, Zhang J, Wang Y, Xu H, Zhang J, Weng X, et al. A new operative classification of idiopathic scoliosis: a peking union medical college method. Spine (Phila PA 1976). 2005;30(12):1419–26.
136. Greulich W, Pyle S. Radiographic atlas of skeletal development of the hand and wrist. 2nd ed. Stanford, CA: Stanford University Press; 1959.
137. Tanner J. Growth and endocrinology of the adolescent. In: Ll G, editor. Edocrine and genetic diseases of childhood. 2nd ed. Philadelphia, PA: W.B. Saunders; 1974. 14 p.

Chapter 3
The Genetic Architecture of Adolescent Idiopathic Scoliosis

Anas M. Khanshour and Carol A. Wise

3.1 Introduction

Art and literature dating back to the beginnings of modern history have depicted the human struggle with scoliosis. The word itself is derived from the Greek "skoliosis" or "crooked," attributed to Galen in the first-century Greece [1]. Today scoliosis is clinically defined as a rotational deformity of the spine with lateral deviation from the vertical of at least 10°. This measurement is known as the "Cobb angle" and is taken from standing spinal radiographs (Fig. 3.1). Although scoliosis is a common deformity in many congenital disorders, about 80% of the time, it appears to be an isolated, or "idiopathic," problem in an otherwise healthy child. Thus, a diagnosis of idiopathic scoliosis (IS) is reached only after excluding the various common causes of scoliosis. The differential diagnosis of IS includes developmental neurologic conditions, such as spinal cord anomalies (tethered cord, syringomyelia) or spina

A. M. Khanshour
Sarah M. and Charles E. Seay Center for Musculoskeletal Research, Texas Scottish Rite Hospital for Children, Dallas, TX, USA

Department of Integrative Biomedical Sciences, Texas A&M University, College Station, TX, USA

C. A. Wise (✉)
Sarah M. and Charles E. Seay Center for Musculoskeletal Research, Texas Scottish Rite Hospital for Children, Dallas, TX, USA

McDermott Center for Human Growth and Development, University of Texas Southwestern Medical Center, Dallas, TX, USA

Department of Pediatrics, University of Texas Southwestern Medical Center, Dallas, TX, USA

Department of Orthopaedic Surgery, University of Texas Southwestern Medical Center, Dallas, TX, USA
e-mail: Carol.Wise@tsrh.org

M. Machida et al. (eds.), *Pathogenesis of Idiopathic Scoliosis*,
https://doi.org/10.1007/978-4-431-56541-3_3

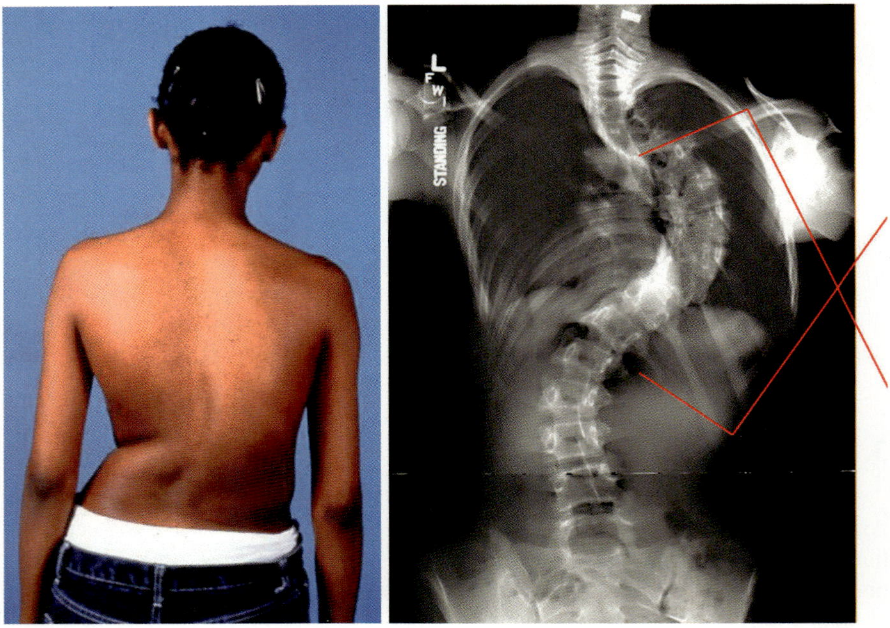

Fig. 3.1 Patient with AIS. Curvature of the spine to the right with shoulder imbalance is evident in the picture on the left. Standing posteroanterior spinal radiograph reveals severe thoracic curvature measuring >70° by the Cobb angle method

bifida, neuromuscular diseases, and disorders of connective tissue, such as Ehlers-Danlos or Marfan syndrome caused by leg length discrepancy or vertebral segmentation anomalies that may be excluded by physical examination and radiography [2, 3]. Clinical examination, imaging, and genetic testing aid to ruling out these possibilities. Idiopathic scoliosis is described further by age at onset: "infantile" (0–3 years of age), "juvenile" (JIS; 4–8 years of age), or "adolescent" (AIS; 10 years and older). Many prefer a simpler classification of "late onset" (6 years of age or older) and "early onset" (up to 6 years of age), as it is more descriptive of the natural history of early spinal growth. However the two systems have led to some semantic confusion [4]. Here we use the traditional terminology and focus on AIS, by far the most common form of idiopathic scoliosis.

Adolescent idiopathic scoliosis is coincident with the prepubertal growth spurt and affects ~2% of the pediatric population or about 29 million children worldwide (Fig. 3.2). Most AIS patients have nonprogressive curves; that is to say, the deformity will not worsen appreciably. About 0.4% of these children, however, will require active treatment to control progression, usually by bracing or surgery [3]. If left untreated, the natural history of progressive AIS is a possible chest wall compromise with concomitant lung restriction, pain, deformity, and possible spinal osteoarthritis [1, 3]. Risk factors for progression in an affected child are well-documented. Female patients and skeletally immature patients who present with

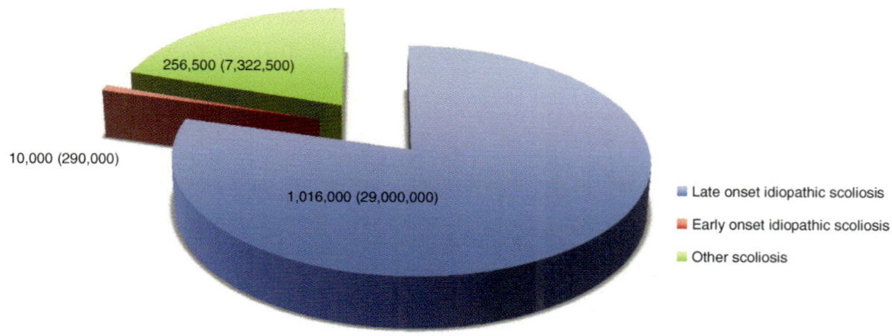

Fig. 3.2 Scoliosis populations. Pie chart depicts the type of scoliosis (idiopathic shown in blue and brown, congenital shown in green) and proportion of each. The estimated numbers of scoliosis patients are given for the USA, with worldwide estimates in parentheses

large curves have a greater risk of progression, but additional predictive markers are highly sought [3]. Certain curve patterns, e.g., in the thoracic region, are also more likely to progress in severity and therefore must be monitored carefully. The potential for a rapid, progressive deformity is significant enough that many professional health organizations recommend school screening programs, although their efficacy remains controversial [5]. The child who has AIS and is at risk of progression typically will be treated by bracing, with the goal of slowing or halting progression of the deformity. Although there is some evidence that bracing can be effective [3, 6], some deformities will continue to worsen, warranting surgery. Today surgery typically involves fixation with instrumentation and spinal fusion [2]. Although outcomes and safety in AIS treatment have benefited from recent advances in surgical and bracing techniques, the methods conceptually have remained the same for decades [3, 6].

As described in this chapter, although AIS is genetically heterogeneous, it bears several distinct features. For one, the location of a spinal deformity in AIS patients (unlike infantile IS or syndromic scoliosis) is remarkably consistent, usually involving vertebrae in the thoracic region [7]. In fact curve patterns in AIS appear to mirror spinal growth at this particular developmental stage in humans, which is known to be at its most rapid, particularly in the thoracic region [8]. Remarkably, greater than ninety percent of thoracic curves are right-sided [2]. Girls are much more likely to have a progressive deformity, leading some to the notion that AIS is a "female disease." It is important to emphasize, however, that males comprise ~12–17% of progressive cases [9]. Perhaps the most notorious of these was King Richard III of England, described by his acquaintance Thomas More as having "….croke backed, his left shoulder much higher than his right….," a description borne out as scoliosis by his recently unearthed skeleton [10].

Less invasive interventions to halt or prevent a scoliotic deformity altogether are clearly desirable. However until recently, etiologic understanding of the disease has lagged despite decades of clinical research. The reasons for this center on the complexity of the problem: the architecture of the spine itself (is AIS a problem of muscle, nerve, bone, or connective tissues?), the complex genetic underpinnings of AIS as described below, and the lack of genetically defined animal models that faithfully recapitulate the AIS phenotype. A recent breakthrough in both genomic technologies and animal modeling are fortunately proving to be powerful tools for deconstructing the causes of AIS in human patients. As outlined in this chapter, recent genetic discoveries have yielded new insights into AIS disease mechanisms. Here we describe the genetic underpinnings of AIS and the progress in understanding AIS pathogenesis derived from gene discovery research. We also discuss emerging genetic investigations of AIS and the prospects for future molecular interventions.

3.2 Epidemiology and Inheritance: How Common and "Genetic" Is AIS?

The prevalence of AIS is similar across all the major ancestral groups (summarized in Table 3.1), although some early studies found otherwise, likely reflecting differences in disease definition or diagnostic screening methods (e.g., physical examination [11–16] versus radiography [17]). Intra- and interobserver error of 5° is generally accepted for measuring the Cobb angle; hence, small curves are more likely to be false positives. If the standard scoliosis definition (>10° Cobb angle

Table 3.1 Published prevalence and heritability estimates for AIS

Country [12]	Populations	Age group (years)	Minimum Cobb angle (degrees)	Prevalence	Inheritance (heritability)	Reference
USA	Black, white	>14	>10[a]	Black: 2.1% White: 1.9%		11
Canada		12–14	>5 >10	4.5% 2.0%		12
Sweden			≥10	Girls: 3.2% Boys: 0.5%		13
England		10–14	≥10	2.8%		16
Japan		Junior high school	≥15	Girls: 1.77% Boys: 0.25%		14
Greece		9–14	≥ 10	1.7%		15
USA	Boston (various ethnicities)	Families			Multifactorial	22
USA	Utah	Families	>10		Mixed polygenic/ recessive (96%)	23
China	Chinese females	Families	≥20		Mixed polygenic/ recessive (87.5 ± 11.1%)	21

[a]Measured from chest X-rays

method from standing lateral radiographs) is applied, most studies report the prevalence of AIS in the range of 2–3% of school-age children. Consequently, AIS does not generally cluster within any particular geographic region, nor is it evident that any population or ethnic group has been spared from AIS. Indeed, there is increasing evidence for genetic risk factors shared between ancestral groups as described later in this chapter.

Genetic influences in AIS have been postulated for almost a century [18]. Twin studies have consistently shown higher concordance in monozygotes compared to dizygotes, pointing to heritable factors [19, 20]. (Lack of full concordance in identical (monozygotic) twins reminds us of complex issues that are still poorly understood for genetic disorders, including reduced penetrance and possible environmental and/or epigenetic effects.) AIS sibling risk and heritability estimates also support significant genetic contributions. One study of AIS compared 415 Chinese index patients and found a sibling recurrence risk of 17.7% and estimated a heritability of 87.5% [21]. It is interesting to note that these results closely mirror an original recurrence risk estimate from a study of Caucasian cases 50 years prior [22]. A separate study of 100 US Intermountain West probands with severe scoliosis (defined as requiring surgical correction) found an even higher recurrence risk of 33% in first-degree female relatives. The latter study also suggested that the location of the scoliotic deformity on the spine may be more heritable than its pattern or severity [23]. At the population level, AIS inheritance is consistent with several to many mutations contributing greater than 80% of disease risk [21–23]. However, Mendelian (single gene) inheritance patterns including autosomal dominant, recessive, and X-linked dominant are also described in AIS families [18, 24]. Accordingly both family- and population-based methods have been used in AIS gene discovery as described later in this chapter. Considering a multi- or polygenic inheritance model, the preponderance of progressive AIS in females suggests that genetic loading may be greatest in affected males. In other words, males may require more risk mutations, or mutations with greater effect sizes, before they manifest disease. This phenomenon is known as the Carter effect [25], and recent data support this model in AIS inheritance [26]. Recent evidence supports a model of sex-specific gene regulation leading to sexual dimorphism in AIS, as has been described for other diseases such as liver cancer [27, 28].

As with other complex disorders, there is considerable uncertainty in predicting an individual genetic risk of developing AIS. For families with history of presumed AIS, care must be given to ensure that there is no underlying syndrome or known Mendelian disorder. Otherwise, it is appropriate to advise patients with familial AIS that their recurrence risk is increased, but that quantifying the absolute risk is difficult [29].

3.3 AIS: A Disease of Bone, Muscle, Nerve, or Cartilage?

Neuropathologic mechanisms have long been proposed for AIS due to the association of scoliosis with neurologic/neuromuscular diseases. In laboratory animals, experimental models of scoliosis have been produced by surgically created small brain lesions. One of the better-described methods involves removal of the pineal gland from chickens, fish, or bipedal rats, reportedly yielding scoliosis that resembles AIS [30–32]. Several investigations of AIS patients have suggested coexisting deficits in an oculo-vestibular (visual/hearing) and proprioceptive function [33–37]. How primary alterations in the nervous system can effect spinal curvature is not altogether obvious but presumably involves cross talk with muscle/bone/connective tissue. Indeed we now understand that sensory innervation may affect bone homeostasis; for example, nerve-specific knockout of the axon guidance gene *Sema3A* produces low bone mass phenotypes in animal models [38]. It is interesting that several studies have found decreased bone mass in girls with AIS [39, 40]. One study found that osteopenia of the femoral neck was a prognostic indicator of curve progression, with an odds ratio of 2.3 [41]. Whether such a mechanism of nerve/bone cross talk functions in skeletal growth and AIS will be important to consider in future hypothesis-driven studies. Other morphologic studies of AIS spinal structures have revealed some disarrangement of fibers of the ligamentum flavum in AIS patients compared to controls [42]; a separate study found decreased glycosaminoglycan content in the intervertebral discs of AIS patients [43]. Histochemical analyses of paraspinous muscles surrounding the scoliotic curve have shown relative hypertrophy and increased electromyographic signaling of type I fibers on the convexity of the curve in AIS patients. This was explained as most likely a compensatory response to curve progression [43, 44]. Although calcification of the cartilage end plate and the adjacent disc occurred in AIS patients is probably a secondary response to altered loading in the patients, the development of cartilage tissues may be highly significant to the progression of the scoliotic curve [45]. The most definitive evidence for tissue of origin in AIS comes from a conditional gene targeting study in the mouse. As described in more detail below, loss of *GPR126* in cartilage altered normal spinal column development and produced a scoliotic phenotype [46]. However, although these data suggest an important role for disc chondrogenesis in AIS, insufficient evidence exists for a primary role for other tissues.

3.4 Identifying AIS Genes in Humans: Mapping Susceptibility Loci

Until recently, AIS research has lacked adequate animal models for defining disease mechanisms. Consequently, most etiological research has focused on human patients. AIS research in humans, consistent with most disease gene discovery efforts, has benefited from hypothesis-free, genome-wide methods that map the location of genetic risk factors in the genome relative to fixed markers [47]. One method, linkage inheritance mapping, relies on identifying candidate mutations that co-segregate with disease in families. Another method, association mapping, identifies polymorphic loci that are shared more frequently in unrelated AIS cases (i.e., populations) compared to control individuals. Here we describe both approaches with their resulting studies of AIS.

3.4.1 Family-Based Studies

Linkage analysis has been powerful for mapping Mendelian traits and has aided mapping candidate regions for common disease. The method relies on demonstrating co-segregation of the disease with genetic markers of known chromosomal location. Although a significant linkage with a disease may be found, further recognition of causal mutations is still difficult in a large genomic region. Therefore, linkage analysis typically is followed by sequencing to identify the candidate mutations involved. Sequencing can be done in two ways: (1) targeted sequencing where a subset of genes or regions of the genome are isolated and sequenced and (2) exome sequencing which is similar to the targeted sequencing but including all the coding regions of the genome. Table 3.2 lists five familial risk loci that were mapped by traditional linkage methods, as given in Online Mendelian Inheritance in Man (OMIM). Three loci, OS1, OS2, and OS5 (OMIM numbers 181,800, 607,354, and 612,239), were mapped to chromosomes 19p13.3, 17p11, and 17q25-qter by linkage mapping in single East Asian (Han Chinese), European (Italian), and European (British) families [48–50]. Two additional loci IS3 (OMIM 608765) and IS4 (OMIM 612238) were each identified in family-based studies using independent cohorts and methods. IS3 was originally mapped to chromosome 8q12 by linkage mapping in a cohort of 52 families analyzed by model-free methods [51]. In similar fashion, IS4 was mapped to 9q31–q34 in a family with dominantly inherited AIS; moreover, a suggestive linkage to this region was previously reported in a study of 202 affected sibling pair families [50, 52]. Consequently, the IS4 locus is potentially the first and only independently replicated AIS linkage. One candidate gene, *CHD7* encoding the chromodomain *h*elicase *D*NA binding protein *7* transcription factor, has been proposed for the IS3 locus [51]. Loss-of-function *CHD7* mutations are well described in the CHARGE syndrome of multiple developmental anomalies that can include scoliosis [53, 54]. A more recent genome-wide linkage analysis in three large IS families reported a perfect marker disease co-segregation in two regions at 3q12.1 and 5q13.3 only in one family, whereas intrafamilial genetic heterogeneity was observed in the other two families [55] (Table 3.2). Further exome sequencing revealed a rare missense variant in the 5q13.3 centriolar protein gene *POC5* that co-segregated with the disease in the original extended family [56]. Another study using exome sequencing of a multigenerational family with familial AIS concluded that rare variants in the *HSPG2* gene potentially contribute to the AIS phenotype [57]. The lack of overlap in genes and loci identified by these studies suggests considerable genetic heterogeneity in familial AIS [55]. Consequently, further genome-wide sequencing-based studies are warranted to discover other AIS causal mutation.

Table 3.2 Susceptibility loci in AIS

Locus	Region	Marker	Mapping method	LOD score	*p*-Value (odds ratio)	Candidate gene	Reference
IS1	19p13.3	D19S216	Genome-wide linkage in seven families	3.63	–	–	48
IS2	17p11.2	D17S799	Genome-wide linkage in extended family	3.20	–	–	49
IS3	8q12.1	D8S1136 rs1038351	Targeted linkage association across *CHD7*	2.77	0.0002 (GRR = 3.1)	*CHD7*	51
IS4	9q31.2-34.2	D9S2157	Genome-wide linkage in extended family	3.64	0.0005	–	50
		D9S915	Genome-wide linkage in affected sibling pair families[a]	–		–	52
IS5	17q25.3	AAT095	Genome-wide linkage in two families	4.08	–	–	50
–	5q13.3 3q12.1	D5S2003 D3S2462	Genome-wide linkage	3.01	–	–	55
–	3p26.3	rs10510181	GWAS[b]	–	8×10^{-7} (1.37)	*CHL1*	58
–	10q24.31	rs11190870	GWAS[b]	–	1.24×10^{-19} (1.56)	*LBX1*	59
–	17q24.3	rs12946942	GWAS[b]	–	6×10^{-12} (1.56)	*SOX9*	60
–	6q24.1	rs6570507	GWAS[b]	–	1.27×10^{-14} (1.27)	*GPR126*	61
–	20p11.22	rs6137473	GWAS[b]	–	2.15×10^{-10} (1.30)	*PAX1*	28
–	9p22.2	rs3904778	GWAS	–	2.46×10^{-13} (1.21)	*BNC2*	77
–	10q24.32	rs678741	GWAS	–	9.68×10^{-37} (1.44)	*LBX1AS1*	62
–	18q21.33	rs4940576	GWAS	–	2.22×10^{-12} (1.23)	*BCL-2*	62
–	2q36.1	rs13398147	GWAS	–	7.59×10^{-13} (1.28)	*PAX3/EPHA4*	62
–	1p36.32	rs241215	GWAS	–	2.95×10^{-9} (0.83)	*AJAP1*	62

Regions in the human genome providing statistically significant evidence of harboring an AIS risk factor are denoted by their OMIM locus number (column 1) where applicable

The markers shown are those that provided most significant evidence in the region

[a]This analysis used nonparametric methods; all other linkage analyses used parametric, two-point methods

[b]Listed in Catalog of Published Genome-Wide Association Studies

3.4.2 Population-Based Studies

Genome-wide association studies (GWAS) typically involve genotyping case and control DNA samples for a high density of common single nucleotide polymorphisms (SNPs) (≥350,000) that span the genome. Subsequent statistical comparisons of genotyped SNP allele frequencies between cases and controls can pinpoint regions or even single genes that are commonly associated with disease. GWAS are proving effective for mapping common susceptibility loci in large cohorts of AIS. The Catalog of Published Genome-Wide Association Studies (http://www.genome.gov/gwastudies/) currently lists five studies (Table 3.2). The first GWAS of AIS utilized 419 families of various ethnicities, in a trio design that is robust to the effects of a population substructure. This mostly non-Hispanic white cohort yielded the strongest signals near the *CHL1* gene encoding close homolog of L1, a cell adhesion protein involved in axon guidance [58]. The second study of 1033 East Asian (Japanese) cases and 1473 matched controls yielded the strongest signals on chromosome 10q24.31 near the *LBX1* gene. *LBX1* encodes the ladybird homeobox 1 protein involved in muscle and nerve specification [59]. This association was subsequently replicated in independent East Asian cohorts, and a larger combined analysis from multiple ethnic groups (i.e., mostly East Asian and non-Hispanic white) has provided further evidence for this susceptibility locus (Table 3.2). Thus, *LBX1* is the first identified major AIS susceptibility locus. In the third study, including 12,000 Japanese subjects where cases were limited to severely affected AIS patients, a novel susceptibility locus near the *SOX9* gene was reported and followed by replication studies in Japanese and Chinese populations [60]. The fourth study, an expanded East Asian study, yielded significant association with SNPs on chromosome 6q24.1 in the *GPR126* gene encoding G protein-coupled receptor 126. It is interesting that SNPs in *GPR126* also have been associated with sitting height in humans [61]. The fifth study using 3102 individuals identified significant associations with a locus on chromosome 20p11.22 that is distal to *PAX1*. Further investigation revealed that this association is specific to females making it the first sex-specific AIS locus. *PAX1* encodes paired box 1 which is a transcription factor involved in spine development. This association was also found in independent North American, Japanese, and East Asian female cohorts [28].

More recently, two additional studies were published but not yet included in the Catalog of Published Genome-Wide Association Studies. A study of 2109 East Asian cases (Japanese) and 11,140 controls identifies a new AIS susceptibility locus on chromosome 9p22.2 ($p = 2.46 \times 10^{-13}$) in the *BNC2* gene. This associated locus could potentially regulate the *BNC2* transcriptional activity. A second recent study identified three new susceptibility loci on chromosomes 2, 18, and 1 near *PAX3/EPHA4*, *BCL2*, and *AJAP1*, respectively, and refined a previously reported region near the *LBX1* gene associated with AIS in East Asian (Han Chinese) girls using 4317 cases and 6016 controls [62].

3.4.3 Population-Based Studies of Rare Mutations

The "Common Disease, Rare Variant (CDRV)" hypothesis suggests that multiple rare DNA sequence variations, each with relatively high penetrance, may collectively contribute genetic susceptibility to common diseases. The CDRV hypothesis is now supported by many sequencing and re-sequencing studies of human genic variation [63, 64].

The contribution of rare variants in unrelated AIS populations was recently tested in cohorts of unrelated AIS cases and controls by whole exome sequencing and gene-based association [65]. Gene-based association "burden" is a test that collapses many rare variants in a genomic region or pathway into single risk score so-called burden testing. One study of 91 AIS cases and 337 controls showed fibrillin-1 (*FBN1*) and *FBN2* as the most significant associated genes with AIS with further supporting evidence in a larger cohort [65]. Another study of 391 severe AIS cases and 843 controls of European ancestry examined the burden of rare variants by gene class or pathway and found rare mutation in extracellular matrix (ECM) genes in AIS ($p = 6 \times 10^{-9}$). In particular, novel coding variants in musculoskeletal collagen genes increased AIS risk by >2-fold, with those in *COL11A2* being most strongly associated [66]. This suggests that rare variants may contribute to AIS.

3.4.4 Chromosomal Breakpoint Mapping

Many chromosomal alterations with phenotypes that include scoliosis have been reported, although most do not appear to recapitulate idiopathic forms, i.e., without obvious vertebral anomalies or coexisting diagnoses. One family segregating a pericentric inversion of chromosome 8 with AIS has been reported [67]. Using methods of chromosomal breakpoint mapping, Bashiardes et al. found that one end of this inversion disrupted the 8q11.2 gene encoding gamma-1-syntrophin (*SNTG1*), while the other end of the inversion occurred in a gene-free region of 8p23. Subsequent analysis of the *SNTG1* gene in 152 additional AIS patients revealed an apparent mutation in DNA samples from three unrelated patients. These changes were not detected in screens of 480 healthy control individuals. These results suggested that rare mutations in *SNTG1* could occur in a small percentage of AIS patients and left open the possibility that other nearby genes could be important in AIS. While chromosomal breakpoint mapping is still a powerful method for pinpointing disease genes, the majority of AIS cases are cytogenetically normal and not amenable to study by this method.

3.5 Candidate Genes and AIS Etiology

What have genetic mapping and association studies revealed about AIS biology? It is important to emphasize that, at this stage, candidate genes have been implicated by statistical association, rather than by direct demonstrations of causality. Nevertheless, AIS candidate genes (Table 3.2) underscore potentially important disease pathways as illustrated during somite development shown in Fig. 3.3.

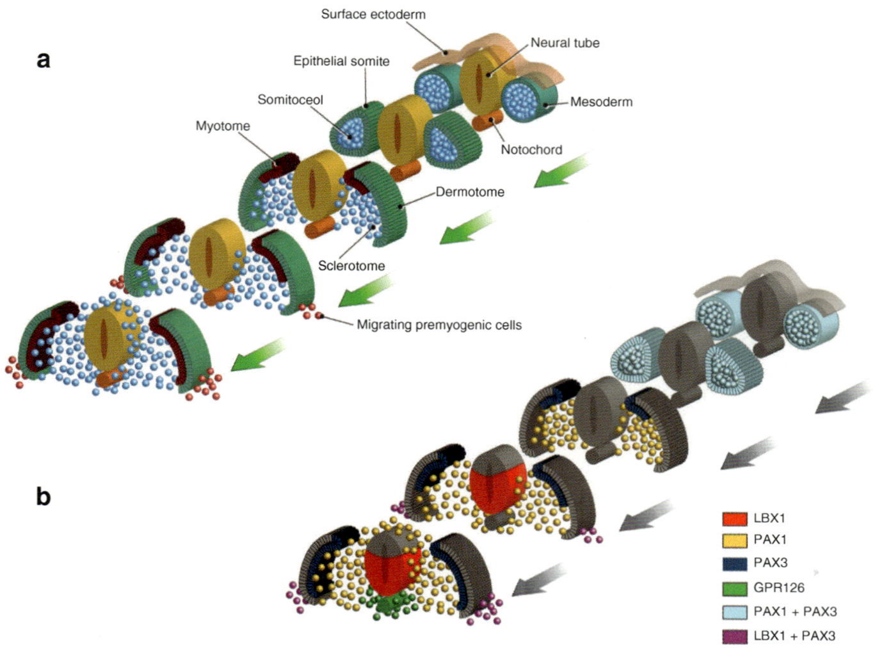

Fig. 3.3 A schematic of somite development. (**a**) The maturation into lineage-specific cellular compartments in somite development; (**b**) AIS candidate genes involved in somite development

3.5.1 LBX1

LBX1 is the vertebrate ortholog of ladybird late (lbl) homeobox gene originally discovered in the fruit fly *Drosophila melanogaster* [68, 69]. In the fly, lbl participates in segmentation and cell specification of heart and muscle precursors. Targeted inactivation in the mouse has shown that this gene is necessary for lateral migration of muscle precursors into the limbs [70]. Further, loss of *LBX1* causes loss of dorsal association neurons, cells of the dorsal spinal cord that relay somatosensory information, and disruption of dorsal horn innervation by nociceptive afferent neurons along with an increase in dorsal commissural neurons [71, 72].

3.5.2 GPR126

GPR126, regulated by *SOX9*, is a member of the adhesion G protein-coupled receptor (GPCR) family that functions in cell adhesion and migration [73]. In zebrafish, gpr126 is required for Schwann cell myelination, an effect that could be overcome by elevating cAMP levels with forskolin. Originally characterized as an orphan receptor, these data suggested that *GPR126* signals through G proteins [74]. *GPR126* studies in other vertebrates reveal a potential role in bone, cartilage, and nerve development. Mouse Gpr126$^{-/-}$ null mutants fail to grow and also have severe neurologic deficits, displaying hypomyelinating peripheral neuropathy [75–77]. More recently, a novel genetic mouse model showing many of the hallmarks of AIS was provided by genetically deleting Gpr126 in cartilage. The loss of Gpr126 results in apoptosis in axial cartilage prior to onset of AIS, emphasizing its critical role during postembryonic cartilage development by regulating morphogenesis of the annulus fibrosis, chondrocyte survival, and the expression of Gal3st4 in cartilage tissues [46].

In humans common variants in this gene are also associated with overall height and trunk length as noted, implying that a *GPR126* signaling pathway somehow regulates appropriate truncal growth in three dimensions.

3.5.3 BNC2

BNC2 is a highly conserved gene that belongs to the group of *C2H2* zinc finger proteins. In humans, this gene is most highly expressed in the uterus and spinal cord, and expression is also evident in bone and cartilage. As reported by Ogura et al. 2015 [78], AIS susceptibility alleles may confer a gain of function and increase *BNC2* expression. *BNC2* overexpression produces body curvature in developing zebrafish in a gene-dosage-dependent manner. Thus increased *BNC2* expression is proposed in the etiology of AIS [78].

3.5.4 PAX1 *and* PAX3

The paired box (PAX) family, highly conserved developmental control genes, encodes transcription factors with a role in pattern formation during vertebrate embryogenesis [79]. *PAX3* regulates both myogenesis and neurogenesis in the neural tube [80–82]. The neural tube/notochord complex has a key role during the development of vertebral muscle [83]. It was reported that mutations in *PAX3* can lead to muscular and neural tube defects, as well as malformation of the vertebral column [84, 85]. Abnormality of the paravertebral muscles has been proposed as the cause of AIS [86]. *PAX1* is expressed during the development of the skeleton, thymus, and parathyroid glands [87, 88] and is required for normal development of ventral vertebral structures [89]. In mice, *PAX1* is expressed in paraspinal muscles, and to a lesser extent in spinal cord, at time points well after the initial patterning of the axial skeleton has been completed. This suggests a later developmental role for *PAX1*, possibly in the growth or maintenance of these tissues [28].

3.5.5 SOX9

SOX9 gene encodes a transcription factor that involved in cartilage formation [90]. In adult mice, *SOX9* was reported to regulate the *GPR126* gene and control the homeostasis of connective tissues such as the growth plate, the articular cartilage, and the intervertebral disk [91]. Recently the *SOX5/6/9* trio proteins were shown to act cooperatively genome-wide, through super-enhancers (SEs), to implement the growth plate chondrocyte differentiation program [92]. Furthermore, mutations in *SOX9* cause campomelic dysplasia, a skeletal dysplasia characterized by bowed, long bones, small scapula, tracheobronchial narrowing, sex reversal, and kyphoscoliosis [93].

3.5.6 Other Genes

Neurologic mechanisms are also suggested by the *CHL1* gene that was highlighted in the first AIS GWAS [58]. *CHL1* encodes an immunoglobulin-class neural cell adhesion protein that participates in commissural axon guidance, i.e., axon crossing at the midline of the corticospinal tract. Deficiencies in commissural axon guidance mechanisms are known to cause scoliosis, as evidenced by the Mendelian disorder *h*orizontal *g*aze *p*alsy with *p*rogressive *s*coliosis (HGPPS, MIM #607313). This disease is caused by recessively inherited mutations in the *ROBO3* gene encoding a transmembrane receptor controlling axon guidance in the same functional and molecular class as *CHL1* [60]. Remarkably, HGPPS patients exhibit only severe scoliosis and absent horizontal eye movement clinically. Imaging studies in these patients confirm that motor and sensory axonal projections do not properly cross within the corticospinal tract of the hindbrain, consistent with their clinical presentation secondary to lesions in ROBO3-mediated axon guidance. *BCL-2* gene encodes an integral outer mitochondrial membrane protein known to have a key role in apoptosis [94]. In *BCL-2* knockout mice, endochondral ossification was accelerated owing to the premature loss of terminal hypertrophic chondrocytes in the growth plate [95]. Differential growth kinetics in the bilateral growth plate of the vertebrae has been suggested in AIS patients as indicated by differences in cellular activity between the convex and concave side of the curve [62]. Further targeted studies of *BCL-2* are necessary to test this hypothesis.

3.6 AIS Candidate Genes from Model Systems

Etiologic studies of AIS have suffered from the lack of an appropriate animal model. However, thanks to modern genome editing and high-throughput forward genetic screens, the field has seen recent breakthroughs in animal modeling.

3.6.1 PTK7

PTK7 is an evolutionarily conserved atypical receptor tyrosine kinase that has been implicated in vertebrate *Wnt* signal transduction [96, 97]. The critical regulators of early spinal development included in the network of Notch, Wnt/β-catenin, and fibroblast growth factor might be involved in IS pathogenesis through disrupting the traveling wave of gene expression along the embryonic axis. Recently, a study reported that zygotic mutation in *PTK7* in zebrafish, that is, a mutant zygote in a normal maternal background, produced an AIS phenotype [98]. Furthermore, the study also identified a novel sequence variant within a single AIS patient that disrupted *PTK7* function, consistent with a role for dysregulated Wnt signaling activity in disease pathogenesis.

3.6.2 KIF6

Another zebrafish study utilized large-scale forward mutagenesis coupled with whole-genome sequencing to produce models of spinal deformity, one of which resembled human AIS, identified in the kinesin family member 6 (*kif6*) gene [99]. Although *kif6* is poorly characterized and its specific cellular functions are still unknown, this zebrafish model clearly implicates its role in spinal development and stability.

3.7 Quantitative Analyses: Do Genetic Factors Influence Disease Course?

Genetic factors exert quantitative effects on various complex traits, such as plasma levels of HDL cholesterol or blood pressure [100, 101]. Quantitative effects are central issues in AIS as well, i.e., what is the risk of severe scoliosis, and how fast will it progress, in a given patient? Genetic risk factors are hypothesized, but identifying them first requires objective, standardized outcome measures. "Severity" is typically measured as the Cobb angle of the major curve, but what constitutes "mild," "moderate," or "severe" deformity? This measure varies between first diagnosis and skeletal maturity, so time is also a covariate to consider. Severity at the time of surgical intervention is necessarily a surrogate final endpoint in many patients. Happily, existing statistical models are developed that can consider AIS curve measurement/surgical intervention endpoints. The rate of AIS curve progression is more easily measured as an increase in the Cobb angle over time. Survival analysis methods with longitudinal data may facilitate the identification of input variables predicts differing times to "severe" curvature [102]. In these methods, input variables may include, for example, SNP genotypes, gender, ethnicity, and initial measures of age, curve magnitude, curve pattern, and Risser sign, with the outcome variable being curve magnitude at a later time point. In this way it may be possible to identify combinations of genotypes and phenotypes that classify progressive AIS. In fact a genetic test predicting the likelihood of curve non-progression in AIS is commercially available [103]. At present the true efficacy of this test and its applicability to general AIS populations are unclear.

3.8 AIS Genetics: Ongoing and Future Research

As noted, genetic discoveries to date explain a small fraction of the trait variance for AIS. In other words, the great majority of genetic risk responsible for AIS awaits discovery. It is clear that genomic methods will continue to bear new insights into AIS etiology. Systems for modeling the disease in animals are needed, not only to understand the physiologic origins of disease but also as vehicles for therapeutic testing.

3.8.1 Genomic Studies

GWAS with sufficient power to detect new AIS risk loci are clearly warranted, but challenging to design. Several tactics may help in this regard: (1) increasing sample size by recruiting larger cohorts, (2) utilizing more informative genotyping platforms, and (3) reducing genetic heterogeneity in the screened cohorts. The first goal, recruiting larger cohorts, is largely an effort to overcome the "signal-to-noise" problem posed by genetic heterogeneity. Research consortia that can combine large datasets productively are key. The first such group, the International Consortium for Scoliosis Genetics (ICSG), formed in 2012 for this purpose and subsequently produced the first AIS large-scale genetic meta-analysis, a study of the chromosome 10 *LBX1* locus in multiple cohorts [104]. Ongoing consortium efforts also will include genome-wide meta-analysis of existing datasets and organizational efforts to support the creation of much larger cohorts, on the order of >10,000 patients. We can anticipate that large consortium-driven cohorts will also enable studies of underrepresented ethnic/ancestral groups. Fortunately, genotyping platforms continue to improve in both chemistry and in density and content of markers [105]. The ultimate genotyping platform, whole-genome sequencing, should be more feasible in the near future due to decreasing costs and improved data storage capability. An alternative "hybrid" approach has been developed that involves inferring genotypes from lower-coverage, whole-genome sequencing [106]. This method is proving superior to standard GWAS of common variants for providing information for less common variants that may confer larger effects on disease [107, 108]. Well-powered genetic studies in richly phenotyped cohorts should yield better AIS classification schemes. Consequently prospective, detailed, and standardized phenotyping of existing cohorts is a key goal in the AIS research community represented by ICSG.

As described in this chapter, most AIS genetic research has centered on discovery of common risk factors. Rare variants are expected also to contribute significantly to the overall disease burden [109–111]. Such mutations are predicted to be important in AIS as well. Extended families with AIS are certain to prove useful in this endeavor, but appropriate validation in additional cohorts will be warranted [55, 112]. It is worth noting that rare variants may contribute considerable risk to individual patients and may prove to be valuable in disease prediction [113].

Many different diseases and syndromes, including cancer, neurological disorders, diabetes, cardiovascular disease, and obesity, are clearly associated with mutations outside of protein-coding genes; i.e., within enhancer or noncoding RNAs [114]. These elements regulate gene expression by facilitating or inhibiting chromatin decompaction, transcription initiation, and the release of RNA polymerase II (Pol II) into productive elongation, as well as by maintaining the three-dimensional architecture of the nucleus [115]. Many of the AIS-associated loci identified by GWAS occur in noncoding regions near or within genes, and recent genomic studies have demonstrated possible functional links between enhancers of *LBX1* and *PAX1* and AIS susceptibility [28, 116]. Clearly the functional annotation of candidate mutations in regulatory regions will be important for mechanistic understanding of AIS.

3.8.2 Epigenetics

Another contribution to the genetic architecture of AIS in fact may be epigenetic, that is, alterations to the genome that do not involve changes in the DNA sequence itself. Two mechanisms, DNA methylation and histone modifications, are primarily associated with epigenetic consequences. Variations in either phenomenon are expected to alter gene expression and may consequently confer specific phenotypes. For example, DNA methylation patterns are known to vary between males and females, leading to sex-specific imprinting of impacted genes. Two relevant diseases caused by effects on imprinting are Angelman/Prader Willi and maternal uniparental disomy chromosome 14, both of which can involve progressive scoliosis [117]. As these disorders may be caused by alterations in sex-specific methylation, it is reasonable to speculate that other epigenetic changes could figure in AIS.

3.8.3 Disease Modeling in Animals

The path from gene discovery to molecular intervention is unpredictable. As described above, proof of concept that zebrafish can model AIS was established with targeted mutagenesis of PTK7 [98]. It is worth noting that ease of drug screening is proving useful in zebrafish models of other disorders such as Duchenne's muscular dystrophy [118]. Thus forward and reverse genetics, that is, from zebrafish screens to humans and vice versa, may prove quite powerful in the next few years of AIS gene discovery and analysis. Likewise conditional mouse mutants that recapitulate AIS, for example, as described for *GPR126* [46] (Fig. 3.4), will be

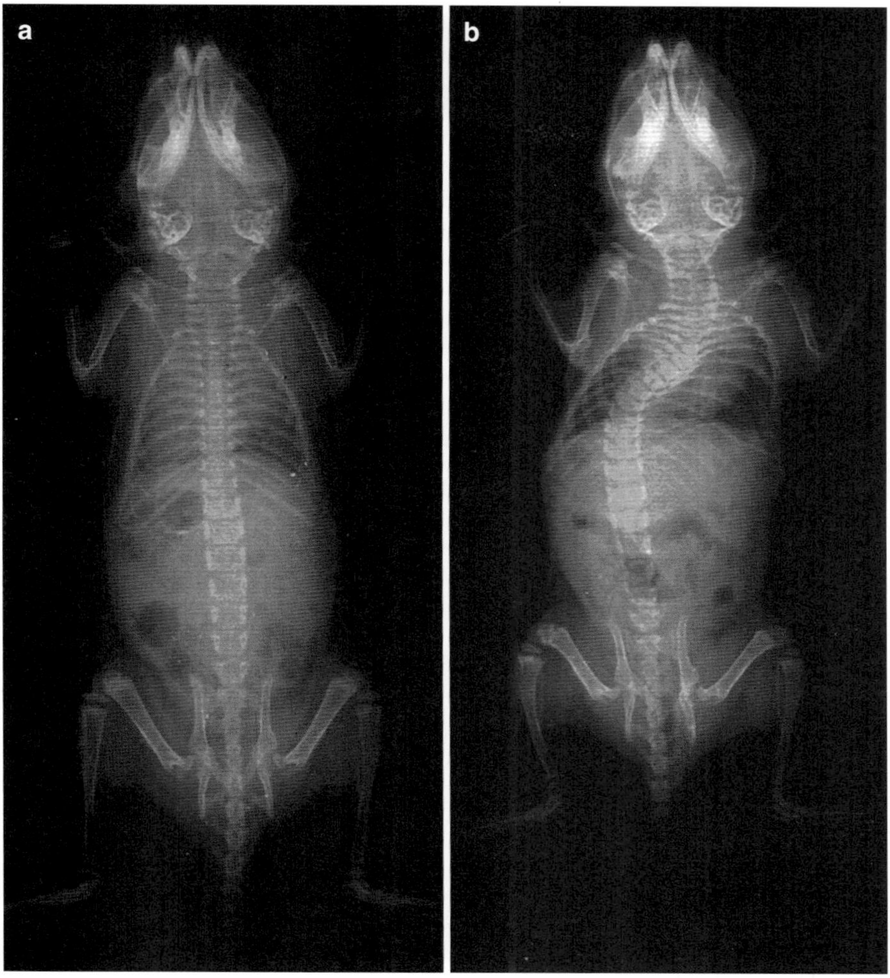

Fig. 3.4 Conditional loss of Gpr126 in chondrocyte lineages results in scoliosis in mice as shown by dorsal X-ray images in P20 wild type (**a**) and mutant (**b**)

critically important resource for mechanistic studies of AIS, including spatial-temporal effects in its pathogenesis.

Theories explaining AIS as a phenomenon of bone, muscle, nerve, connective tissue, or even brain abound, but direct evidence has been lacking. As described in this chapter, breakthroughs in developing animal models for AIS, particularly the mouse, will be completely enabling for testing the spatiotemporal development of the disease. Also, appropriate model systems will facilitate the functional validation and interpretation of prior genetic findings.

3.9 Summary

Adolescent idiopathic scoliosis is one of the most common diagnoses in pediatric orthopedic practice. Despite centuries of treatment and decades of study, the underlying pathogenesis of AIS has been poorly understood due largely to a lack of naturally occurring, genetically defined model systems. Consequently, progress in the field has been driven mostly by genetic studies in human populations. However, recent breakthroughs have yielded animal models of AIS that present exciting opportunity for hypothesis testing. These discoveries and tools set the stage for defining the mechanism in AIS pathogenesis and for the prospect of testing pharmaceutical interventions.

Acknowledgments We thank Drs. Courtney Karner and Ryan Gray for kindly contributing images of genetically engineered mice. We thank Stuart Almond from the Media Department at Texas Scottish Rite Hospital for Children and Benjamin Dupree for helping in Fig. 3.3. We also thank patients, other individuals, and families who have participated in the studies described here.

References

1. Tachdjian MO. Scoliosis. In: Herring J, editor. Tachdjian's pediatric orthopaedics. 4th ed. Philadelphia, PA: WB Saunders; 2008.
2. Herring JA. Tachdjian's pediatric orthopaedics. Philadelphia, PA: WB Saunders; 2008.
3. Hresko MT. Clinical practice. Idiopathic scoliosis in adolescents. N Engl J Med. 2013;368(9):834–41. https://doi.org/10.1056/NEJMcp1209063.
4. Akbarnia BA. Management themes in early onset scoliosis. J Bone Joint Surg Am. 2007;89(Suppl 1):42–54. https://doi.org/10.2106/JBJS.F.01256.
5. Richards BS, Vitale MG. Screening for idiopathic scoliosis in adolescents. An information statement. J Bone Joint Surg Am. 2008;90(1):195–8. https://doi.org/10.2106/jbjs.g.01276.
6. Katz DE, Herring JA, Browne RH, Kelly DM, Birch JG. Brace wear control of curve progression in adolescent idiopathic scoliosis. J Bone Joint Surg Am. 2010;92(6):1343–52. https://doi.org/10.2106/JBJS.I.01142.
7. Lonstein JE, Carlson JM. The prediction of curve progression in untreated idiopathic scoliosis during growth. J Bone Joint Surg Am. 1984;66(7):1061–71.
8. Akbarnia GMB. Idiopathic scoliosis: infantile and juvenile. In: Thompson BAAMYGH, editor. The growing spine: management of spinal disorders in young children. New York, NY: Springer-Verlag; 2011. p. 199–212.
9. Karol LAM, Johnston CE II, Browne RH, Madison M. Progression of the curve in boys who have idiopathic scoliosis. J Bone Joint Surg. 1993;75-A(12):1804–10.
10. http://www.richardiii.net/2_4_0_riii_appearance.php#description.
11. Shands AR Jr, Eisberg HB. The incidence of scoliosis in the state of Delaware; a study of 50,000 minifilms of the chest made during a survey for tuberculosis. J Bone Joint Surg Am. 1955;37-A(6):1243–9.
12. Rogala EJDD, Gurr J. Scoliosis: incidence and naturel history A prospective epidemiological study. J Bone Joint Surg Am. 1978;60(2):173–6.
13. Willner S, Uden A. A prospective prevalence study of scoliosis in Southern Sweden. Acta Orthop Scand. 1982;53(2):233–7.
14. Ohtsuka Y, Yamagata M, Arai S, Kitahara H, Minami S. School screening for scoliosis by the Chiba University Medical School screening program. Results of 1.24 million students over an 8-year period. Spine (Phila Pa 1976). 1988;13(11):1251–7.

15. Soucacos PN, Soucacos PK, Zacharis KC, Beris AE, Xenakis TA. School-screening for scoliosis. A prospective epidemiological study in northwestern and central Greece. J Bone Joint Surg Am. 1997;79(10):1498–503.
16. Dickson RA. Scoliosis in the community. Br Med J. 1983;286(6365):615–8.
17. Horton WA. Common Skeletal deformities. In: Rimoin DL, JMC REP, Korf BR, editors. Emery and Rimoin's principles and practice of medical genetics. 4th ed. London: Churchill Livingstone; 2002. p. 4236–44.
18. Sharma S, Wise C. Current understanding of genetic factors in idiopathic scoliosis. In: Dunwoodie KA, editor. The genetics and development of scoliosis. New York, NY: Springer; 2010. p. 167–90.
19. Kesling KL, Reinker KA. Scoliosis in twins: a meta-analysis of the literature and report of six cases. Spine. 1997;22(17):2009–15.
20. Andersen MO, Thomsen K, Kyvik KO. Adolescent idiopathic scoliosis in twins: a population-based survey. Spine (Phila Pa 1976). 2007;32(8):927–30. https://doi.org/10.1097/01.brs.0000259865.08984.00.
21. Tang NL, Yeung HY, Hung VW, Di Liao C, Lam TP, Yeung HM, et al. Genetic epidemiology and heritability of AIS: A study of 415 Chinese female patients. J Orthop Res. 2012;30(9):1464–9. https://doi.org/10.1002/jor.22090.
22. Riseborough EJ, Wynne-Davies R. A genetic survey of idiopathic scoliosis in Boston, MA. J Bone Joint Surg Am. 1973;55(5):974–82.
23. Ward K, Ogilvie J, Argyle V, Nelson L, Meade M, Braun J, et al. Polygenic inheritance of adolescent idiopathic scoliosis: a study of extended families in Utah. Am J Med Genet A. 2010;152A(5):1178–88. https://doi.org/10.1002/ajmg.a.33145.
24. Raggio CL, Giampietro PF, Dobrin S, Zhao C, Dorshorst D, Ghebranious N, et al. A novel locus for adolescent idiopathic scoliosis on chromosome 12p. J Orthop Res. 2009;27(10):1366–72. https://doi.org/10.1002/jor.20885.
25. Carter CO, Evans KA. Inheritance of congenital pyloric stenosis. J Med Genet. 1969;6(3):233–54.
26. Kruse LM, Buchan JG, Gurnett CA, Dobbs MB. Polygenic threshold model with sex dimorphism in adolescent idiopathic scoliosis: the Carter effect. J Bone Joint Surg Am. 2012;94(16):1485–91. https://doi.org/10.2106/JBJS.K.01450.
27. Li Z, Tuteja G, Schug J, Kaestner KH. Foxa1 and Foxa2 are essential for sexual dimorphism in liver cancer. Cell. 2012;148(1–2):72–83. https://doi.org/10.1016/j.cell.2011.11.026.
28. Sharma S, Londono D, Eckalbar WL, Gao X, Zhang D, Mauldin K, et al. A PAX1 enhancer locus is associated with susceptibility to idiopathic scoliosis in females. Nat Commun. 2015;6:6452. https://doi.org/10.1038/ncomms7452.
29. Pyeritz RE. Common disorders of connective tissue. In: King RA, Motulsky AG, editors. Genetic basis of common diseases. Oxford: Oxford University Press; 2002. p. 638–45.
30. Machida M, Dubousset J, Imamura Y, Iwaya T, Yamada T, Kimura J. An experimental study in chickens for the pathogenesis of idiopathic scoliosis. Spine (Phila Pa 1976). 1993;18(12):1609–15.
31. Machida M, Miyashita Y, Murai I, Dubousset J, Yamada T, Kimura J. Role of serotonin for scoliotic deformity in pinealectomized chicken. Spine (Phila Pa 1976). 1997;22(12):1297–301.
32. Fjelldal PG, Grotmol S, Kryvi H, Gjerdet NR, Taranger GL, Hansen T, et al. Pinealectomy induces malformation of the spine and reduces the mechanical strength of the vertebrae in Atlantic salmon, Salmo salar. J Pineal Res. 2004;36(2):132–9.
33. Guo X, Chau WW, Hui-Chan CW, Cheung CS, Tsang WW, Cheng JC. Balance control in adolescents with idiopathic scoliosis and disturbed somatosensory function. Spine. 2006;31(14):E437–40. https://doi.org/10.1097/01.brs.0000222048.47010.bf. 00007632-200606150-00029 [pii]
34. Lonstein JE. Adolescent idiopathic scoliosis. Lancet. 1994;344(8934):1407–12. doi:S0140-6736(94)90572-X [pii]
35. Mallau S, Bollini G, Jouve JL, Assaiante C. Locomotor skills and balance strategies in adolescents idiopathic scoliosis. Spine. 2007;32(1):E14–22. https://doi.org/10.1097/01.brs.0000251069.58498.eb. 00007632-200701010-00026 [pii]

36. Rousie D, Hache JC, Pellerin P, Deroubaix JP, Van Tichelen P, Berthoz A. Oculomotor, postural, and perceptual asymmetries associated with a common cause. Craniofacial asymmetries and asymmetries in vestibular organ anatomy. Ann N Y Acad Sci. 1999;871:439–46.
37. Wiener-Vacher SR, Mazda K. Asymmetric otolith vestibulo-ocular responses in children with idiopathic scoliosis. J Pediatr. 1998;132(6):1028–32. doi:S0022347698002704 [pii]
38. Fukuda T, Takeda S, Xu R, Ochi H, Sunamura S, Sato T, et al. Sema3A regulates bone-mass accrual through sensory innervations. Nature. 2013;497(7450):490–3. https://doi.org/10.1038/nature12115.
39. Cheng JC, Guo X, Sher AH. Persistent osteopenia in adolescent idiopathic scoliosis. A longitudinal follow up study. Spine (Phila Pa 1976). 1999;24(12):1218–22.
40. Lee WT, Cheung CS, Tse YK, Guo X, Qin L, Lam TP, et al. Association of osteopenia with curve severity in adolescent idiopathic scoliosis: a study of 919 girls. Osteoporosis Int. 2005;16(12):1924–32. https://doi.org/10.1007/s00198-005-1964-7.
41. Hung VW, Qin L, Cheung CS, Lam TP, Ng BK, Tse YK, et al. Osteopenia: a new prognostic factor of curve progression in adolescent idiopathic scoliosis. J Bone Joint Surg Am. 2005;87(12):2709–16. https://doi.org/10.2106/JBJS.D.02782.
42. Hadley-Miller N, Mims B, Milewicz DM. The potential role of the elastic fiber system in adolescent idiopathic scoliosis. J Bone Joint Surg Am. 1994;76(8):1193–206.
43. Lowe TG, Edgar M, Margulies JY, Miller NH, Raso VJ, Reinker KA, et al. Etiology of idiopathic scoliosis: current trends in research. J Bone Joint Surg Am. 2000;82-A(8):1157–68.
44. Lonstein JE. Adolescent Idiopathic scoliosis. Lancet. 1994;344:1407–12.
45. Roberts S, Menage J, Eisenstein SM. The cartilage end-plate and intervertebral disc in scoliosis: calcification and other sequelae. J Orthop Res. 1993;11(5):747–57. https://doi.org/10.1002/jor.1100110517.
46. Karner CM, Long F, Solnica-Krezel L, Monk KR, Gray RS. Gpr126/Adgrg6 deletion in cartilage models idiopathic scoliosis and pectus excavatum in mice. Hum Mol Genet. 2015;24(15):4365–73. https://doi.org/10.1093/hmg/ddv170.
47. Altshuler D, Daly MJ, Lander ES. Genetic mapping in human disease. Science. 2008;322(5903):881–8. https://doi.org/10.1126/science.1156409.
48. Chan V, Fong GC, Luk KD, Yip B, Lee MK, Wong MS, et al. A genetic locus for adolescent idiopathic scoliosis linked to chromosome 19p13.3. Am J Hum Genet. 2002;71(2):401–6. https://doi.org/10.1086/341607.
49. Salehi LB, Mangino M, De Serio S, De Cicco D, Capon F, Semprini S, et al. Assignment of a locus for autosomal dominant idiopathic scoliosis (IS) to human chromosome 17p11. Hum Genet. 2002;111(4–5):401–4. https://doi.org/10.1007/s00439-002-0785-4.
50. Ocaka L, Zhao C, Reed JA, Ebenezer ND, Brice G, Morley T, et al. Assignment of two loci for autosomal dominant adolescent idiopathic scoliosis to chromosomes 9q31.2-q34.2 and 17q25.3-qtel. J Med Genet. 2008;45(2):87–92. https://doi.org/10.1136/jmg.2007.051896.
51. Gao X, Gordon D, Zhang D, Browne R, Helms C, Gillum J, et al. CHD7 gene polymorphisms are associated with susceptibility to idiopathic scoliosis. Am J Hum Genet. 2007;80(5):957–65. https://doi.org/10.1086/513571.
52. Miller NH, Justice CM, Marosy B, Doheny KF, Pugh E, Zhang J, et al. Identification of candidate regions for familial idiopathic scoliosis. Spine (Phila Pa 1976). 2005;30(10):1181–7. doi:00007632-200505150-00013 [pii]
53. Vissers LE, van Ravenswaaij CM, Admiraal R, Hurst JA, de Vries BB, Janssen IM, et al. Mutations in a new member of the chromodomain gene family cause CHARGE syndrome. Nat Genet. 2004;36(9):955–7. https://doi.org/10.1038/ng1407. ng1407 [pii]
54. Doyle C, Blake K. Scoliosis in CHARGE: a prospective survey and two case reports. Am J Med Genet A. 2005;133A(3):340–3. https://doi.org/10.1002/ajmg.a.30564.
55. Edery P, Margaritte-Jeannin P, Biot B, Labalme A, Bernard JC, Chastang J, et al. New disease gene location and high genetic heterogeneity in idiopathic scoliosis. Eur J Hum Genet. 2011;19(8):865–9. https://doi.org/10.1038/ejhg.2011.31.

56. Patten SA, Margaritte-Jeannin P, Bernard JC, Alix E, Labalme A, Besson A, et al. Functional variants of POC5 identified in patients with idiopathic scoliosis. J Clin Invest. 2015;125(3):1124–8. https://doi.org/10.1172/JCI77262.
57. Baschal EE, Wethey CI, Swindle K, Baschal RM, Gowan K, Tang NL, et al. Exome sequencing identifies a rare HSPG2 variant associated with familial idiopathic scoliosis. G3. 2015;5(2):167–74. https://doi.org/10.1534/g3.114.015669.
58. Sharma S, Gao X, Londono D, Devroy SE, Mauldin KN, Frankel JT, et al. Genome-wide association studies of adolescent idiopathic scoliosis suggest candidate susceptibility genes. Hum Mol Genet. 2011;20(7):1456–66. https://doi.org/10.1093/hmg/ddq571.
59. Takahashi Y, Kou I, Takahashi A, Johnson TA, Kono K, Kawakami N, et al. A genome-wide association study identifies common variants near LBX1 associated with adolescent idiopathic scoliosis. Nat Genet. 2011;43(12):1237–40. https://doi.org/10.1038/ng.974.
60. Miyake A, Kou I, Takahashi Y, Johnson TA, Ogura Y, Dai J, et al. Identification of a susceptibility locus for severe adolescent idiopathic scoliosis on chromosome 17q24.3. PLoS One. 2013;8(9):e72802. https://doi.org/10.1371/journal.pone.0072802.
61. Kou I, Takahashi Y, Johnson TA, Takahashi A, Guo L, Dai J, et al. Genetic variants in GPR126 are associated with adolescent idiopathic scoliosis. Nat Genet. 2013. https://doi.org/10.1038/ng.2639.
62. Zhu Z, Tang NL, Xu L, Qin X, Mao S, Song Y, et al. Genome-wide association study identifies new susceptibility loci for adolescent idiopathic scoliosis in Chinese girls. Nat Commun. 2015;6:8355. https://doi.org/10.1038/ncomms9355.
63. Schork NJ, Murray SS, Frazer KA, Topol EJ. Common vs. rare allele hypotheses for complex diseases. Curr Opin Genet Dev. 2009;19(3):212–9. https://doi.org/10.1016/j.gde.2009.04.010.
64. Moutsianas L, Agarwala V, Fuchsberger C, Flannick J, Rivas MA, Gaulton KJ, et al. The power of gene-based rare variant methods to detect disease-associated variation and test hypotheses about complex disease. PLoS Genet. 2015;11(4):e1005165. https://doi.org/10.1371/journal.pgen.1005165.
65. Buchan JG, Alvarado DM, Haller GE, Cruchaga C, Harms MB, Zhang T, et al. Rare variants in FBN1 and FBN2 are associated with severe adolescent idiopathic scoliosis. Hum Mol Genet. 2014;23(19):5271–82. https://doi.org/10.1093/hmg/ddu224.
66. Haller G, Alvarado D, McCall K, Yang P, Cruchaga C, Harms M, et al. A polygenic burden of rare variants across extracellular matrix genes among individuals with adolescent idiopathic scoliosis. Hum Mol Genet. 2016;25(1):202–9. https://doi.org/10.1093/hmg/ddv463.
67. Bashiardes S, Veile R, Allen M, Wise CA, Dobbs M, Morcuende JA, et al. SNTG1, the gene encoding gamma1-syntrophin: a candidate gene for idiopathic scoliosis. Hum Genet. 2004;115(1):81–9. https://doi.org/10.1007/s00439-004-1121-y.
68. Jagla K, Frasch M, Jagla T, Dretzen G, Bellard F, Bellard M. ladybird, a new component of the cardiogenic pathway in Drosophila required for diversification of heart precursors. Development. 1997;124(18):3471–9.
69. Jagla K, Jagla T, Heitzler P, Dretzen G, Bellard F, Bellard M. ladybird, a tandem of homeobox genes that maintain late wingless expression in terminal and dorsal epidermis of the Drosophila embryo. Development. 1997;124(1):91–100.
70. Gross MK, Moran-Rivard L, Velasquez T, Nakatsu MN, Jagla K, Goulding M. Lbx1 is required for muscle precursor migration along a lateral pathway into the limb. Development. 2000;127(2):413–24.
71. Gross MK, Dottori M, Goulding M. Lbx1 specifies somatosensory association interneurons in the dorsal spinal cord. Neuron. 2002;34(4):535–49.
72. Muller T, Brohmann H, Pierani A, Heppenstall PA, Lewin GR, Jessell TM, et al. The homeodomain factor lbx1 distinguishes two major programs of neuronal differentiation in the dorsal spinal cord. Neuron. 2002;34(4):551–62.
73. Langenhan T, Aust G, Hamann J. Sticky signaling—adhesion class g protein-coupled receptors take the stage. Sci Signal. 2013;6(276):re3. https://doi.org/10.1126/scisignal.2003825.

74. Monk KR, Naylor SG, Glenn TD, Mercurio S, Perlin JR, Dominguez C, et al. A G protein-coupled receptor is essential for Schwann cells to initiate myelination. Science. 2009;325(5946):1402–5. https://doi.org/10.1126/science.1173474.
75. Monk KR, Oshima K, Jors S, Heller S, Talbot WS. Gpr126 is essential for peripheral nerve development and myelination in mammals. Development. 2011;138(13):2673–80. https://doi.org/10.1242/dev.062224.
76. Waller-Evans H, Promel S, Langenhan T, Dixon J, Zahn D, Colledge WH, et al. The orphan adhesion-GPCR GPR126 is required for embryonic development in the mouse. PLoS One. 2010;5(11):e14047. https://doi.org/10.1371/journal.pone.0014047.
77. Geng FS, Abbas L, Baxendale S, Holdsworth CJ, Swanson AG, Slanchev K, et al. Semicircular canal morphogenesis in the zebrafish inner ear requires the function of gpr126 (lauscher), an adhesion class G protein-coupled receptor gene. Development. 2013;140(21):4362–74. https://doi.org/10.1242/dev.098061.
78. Ogura Y, Kou I, Miura S, Takahashi A, Xu L, Takeda K, et al. A functional SNP in BNC2 is associated with adolescent idiopathic scoliosis. Am J Hum Genet. 2015;97(2):337–42. https://doi.org/10.1016/j.ajhg.2015.06.012.
79. Chi N, Epstein JA. Getting your Pax straight: Pax proteins in development and disease. Trends Genet. 2002;18(1):41–7.
80. Schubert FR, Tremblay P, Mansouri A, Faisst AM, Kammandel B, Lumsden A, et al. Early mesodermal phenotypes in splotch suggest a role for Pax3 in the formation of epithelial somites. Dev Dynam. 2001;222(3):506–21. https://doi.org/10.1002/dvdy.1211.
81. Buckingham M, Relaix F. The role of Pax genes in the development of tissues and organs: Pax3 and Pax7 regulate muscle progenitor cell functions. Annu Rev Cell Dev Biol. 2007;23:645–73. https://doi.org/10.1146/annurev.cellbio.23.090506.123438.
82. Young AP, Wagers AJ. Pax3 induces differentiation of juvenile skeletal muscle stem cells without transcriptional upregulation of canonical myogenic regulatory factors. J Cell Sci. 2010;123(Pt 15):2632–9. https://doi.org/10.1242/jcs.061606.
83. Rong PM, Teillet MA, Ziller C, Le Douarin NM. The neural tube/notochord complex is necessary for vertebral but not limb and body wall striated muscle differentiation. Development. 1992;115(3):657–72.
84. Xiao Y, Zhang L, He K, Gao X, Yang L, He L, et al. Characterization of a novel missense mutation on murine Pax3 through ENU mutagenesis. Yi Chuan Xue Bao. 2011;38(8):333–9. https://doi.org/10.1016/j.jgg.2011.06.005.
85. Farin HF, Mansouri A, Petry M, Kispert A. T-box protein Tbx18 interacts with the paired box protein Pax3 in the development of the paraxial mesoderm. J Biol Chem. 2008;283(37):25372–80. https://doi.org/10.1074/jbc.M802723200.
86. Kouwenhoven JW, Castelein RM. The pathogenesis of adolescent idiopathic scoliosis: review of the literature. Spine. 2008;33(26):2898–908. https://doi.org/10.1097/BRS.0b013e3181891751.
87. Schnittger S, Rao VV, Deutsch U, Gruss P Balling R Hansmann I. Pax1, a member of the paired box-containing class of developmental control genes, is mapped to human chromosome 20p11.2 by in situ hybridization (ISH and FISH). Genomics 1992;14(3):740-4.
88. Wallin J, Eibel H, Neubuser A, Wilting J, Koseki H, Balling R. Pax1 is expressed during development of the thymus epithelium and is required for normal T-cell maturation. Development. 1996;122(1):23–30.
89. Wallin J, Wilting J, Koseki H, Fritsch R, Christ B, Balling R. The role of Pax-1 in axial skeleton development. Development. 1994;120(5):1109–21.
90. Dy P, Wang W, Bhattaram P, Wang Q, Wang L, Ballock RT, et al. Sox9 directs hypertrophic maturation and blocks osteoblast differentiation of growth plate chondrocytes. Dev Cell. 2012;22(3):597–609. https://doi.org/10.1016/j.devcel.2011.12.024.
91. Henry SP, Liang S, Akdemir KC, de Crombrugghe B. The postnatal role of Sox9 in cartilage. J Bone Miner Res. 2012;27(12):2511–25. https://doi.org/10.1002/jbmr.1696.
92. Liu CF, Lefebvre V. The transcription factors SOX9 and SOX5/SOX6 cooperate genome-wide through super-enhancers to drive chondrogenesis. Nucleic Acids Res. 2015;43(17):8183–203. https://doi.org/10.1093/nar/gkv688.

93. Lekovic GP, Rekate HL, Dickman CA, Pearson M. Congenital cervical instability in a patient with campomelic dysplasia. Childs Nerv Syst. 2006;22(9):1212–4. https://doi.org/10.1007/s00381-006-0071-1.
94. Siddiqui WA, Ahad A, Ahsan H. The mystery of BCL2 family: Bcl-2 proteins and apoptosis: an update. Arch Toxicol. 2015;89(3):289–317. https://doi.org/10.1007/s00204-014-1448-7.
95. Boot-Handford RP, Michaelidis TM, Hillarby MC, Zambelli A, Denton J, Hoyland JA, et al. The bcl-2 knockout mouse exhibits marked changes in osteoblast phenotype and collagen deposition in bone as well as a mild growth plate phenotype. Int J Exp Pathol. 1998;79(5):329–35.
96. Peradziryi H, Kaplan NA, Podleschny M, Liu X, Wehner P, Borchers A, et al. PTK7/Otk interacts with Wnts and inhibits canonical Wnt signalling. EMBO J. 2011;30(18):3729–40. https://doi.org/10.1038/emboj.2011.236.
97. Hayes M, Naito M, Daulat A, Angers S, Ciruna B. Ptk7 promotes non-canonical Wnt/PCP-mediated morphogenesis and inhibits Wnt/beta-catenin-dependent cell fate decisions during vertebrate development. Development. 2013;140(8):1807–18. https://doi.org/10.1242/dev.090183.
98. Hayes M, Gao X, Yu LX, Paria N, Henkelman RM, Wise CA, et al. ptk7 mutant zebrafish models of congenital and idiopathic scoliosis implicate dysregulated Wnt signalling in disease. Nat Commun. 2014;5:4777. https://doi.org/10.1038/ncomms5777.
99. Buchan JG, Gray RS, Gansner JM, Alvarado DM, Burgert L, Gitlin JD, et al. Kinesin family member 6 (kif6) is necessary for spine development in zebrafish. Dev Dynam. 2014;243(12):1646–57. https://doi.org/10.1002/dvdy.24208.
100. Cohen JC, Kiss RS, Pertsemlidis A, Marcel YL, McPherson R, Hobbs HH. Multiple rare alleles contribute to low plasma levels of HDL cholesterol. Science. 2004;305(5685):869–72. https://doi.org/10.1126/science.1099870.
101. Ji W, Foo JN, O'Roak BJ, Zhao H, Larson MG, Simon DB, et al. Rare independent mutations in renal salt handling genes contribute to blood pressure variation. Nat Genet. 2008;40(5):592–9. https://doi.org/10.1038/ng.118.
102. Londono D, Chen KM, Musolf A, Wang R, Shen T, Brandon J, et al. A novel method for analyzing genetic association with longitudinal phenotypes. Stat Appl Genet Mol Biol. 2013;12(2):241–61. https://doi.org/10.1515/sagmb-2012-0070.
103. Ward K, Ogilvie JW, Singleton MV, Chettier R, Engler G, Nelson LM. Validation of DNA-based prognostic testing to predict spinal curve progression in adolescent idiopathic scoliosis. Spine (Phila Pa 1976). 2010;35(25):E1455–64. https://doi.org/10.1097/BRS.0b013e3181ed2de1.
104. Londono D, Kou I, Johnson TA, Sharma S, Ogura Y, Tsunoda T, et al. A meta-analysis identifies adolescent idiopathic scoliosis association with LBX1 locus in multiple ethnic groups. J Med Genet. 2014;51(6):401–6. https://doi.org/10.1136/jmedgenet-2013-102067.
105. Jiang L, Willner D, Danoy P, Xu H, Brown MA. Comparison of the performance of two commercial genome-wide association study genotyping platforms in Han Chinese samples. G3 (Bethesda). 2013;3(1):23–9. https://doi.org/10.1534/g3.112.004069.
106. Pasaniuc B, Rohland N, McLaren PJ, Garimella K, Zaitlen N, Li H, et al. Extremely low-coverage sequencing and imputation increases power for genome-wide association studies. Nat Genet. 2012;44(6):631–5. https://doi.org/10.1038/ng.2283.
107. Morrison AC, Voorman A, Johnson AD, Liu X, Yu J, Li A, et al. Whole-genome sequence-based analysis of high-density lipoprotein cholesterol. Nat Genet. 2013;45(8):899–901. https://doi.org/10.1038/ng.2671.
108. Jonsson T, Atwal JK, Steinberg S, Snaedal J, Jonsson PV, Bjornsson S, et al. A mutation in APP protects against Alzheimer's disease and age-related cognitive decline. Nature. 2012;488(7409):96–9. https://doi.org/10.1038/nature11283.
109. Ng SB, Turner EH, Robertson PD, Flygare SD, Bigham AW, Lee C, et al. Targeted capture and massively parallel sequencing of 12 human exomes. Nature. 2009;461(7261):272–6. https://doi.org/10.1038/nature08250.
110. Iyengar SK, Elston RC. The genetic basis of complex traits: rare variants or "common gene, common disease"? Methods Mol Biol. 2007;376:71–84. https://doi.org/10.1007/978-1-59745-389-9_6.

111. Gibson G. Rare and common variants: twenty arguments. Nat Rev Genet. 2011;13(2):135–45. https://doi.org/10.1038/nrg3118.
112. Asimit J, Zeggini E. Rare variant association analysis methods for complex traits. Annu Rev Genet. 2010;44:293–308. https://doi.org/10.1146/annurev-genet-102209-163421.
113. Antonarakis SE, Chakravarti A, Cohen JC, Hardy J. Mendelian disorders and multifactorial traits: the big divide or one for all? Nat Rev Genet. 2010;11(5):380–4. https://doi.org/10.1038/nrg2793.
114. Lee TI, Young RA. Transcriptional regulation and its misregulation in disease. Cell. 2013;152(6):1237–51. https://doi.org/10.1016/j.cell.2013.02.014.
115. Danko CG, Hyland SL, Core LJ, Martins AL, Waters CT, Lee HW, et al. Identification of active transcriptional regulatory elements from GRO-seq data. Nat Methods. 2015;12(5):433–8. https://doi.org/10.1038/nmeth.3329.
116. Guo L, Yamashita H, Kou I, Takimoto A, Meguro-Horike M, Horike S, et al. Functional investigation of a non-coding variant associated with adolescent idiopathic scoliosis in zebrafish: elevated expression of the ladybird homeobox gene causes body axis deformation. PLoS Genet. 2016;12(1):e1005802. https://doi.org/10.1371/journal.pgen.1005802.
117. Temple IK, Cockwell A, Hassold T, Pettay D, Jacobs P. Maternal uniparental disomy for chromosome 14. J Med Genet. 1991;28(8):511–4.
118. Kawahara G, Karpf JA, Myers JA, Alexander MS, Guyon JR, Kunkel LM. Drug screening in a zebrafish model of Duchenne muscular dystrophy. Proc Natl Acad Sci U S A. 2011;108(13):5331–6. https://doi.org/10.1073/pnas.1102116108.

Chapter 4
Biomechanics of Adolescent Idiopathic Scoliosis

Wafa Skalli and Claudio Vergari

4.1 Introduction

From a biomechanical point of view, the spine is a slender mechanical structure consisting in a construct of quite stiff components (the vertebrae) connected to each other by more deformable components: the intervertebral disc, cartilage at the facet joints and a set of ligaments. The biomechanical role of this complex system is both to withstand the loads to maintain a stable erect posture and to allow multidirectional mobility and stability in any position. Another major role is to prevent excessive intervertebral motion that would affect spinal cord or nerves. The very characteristic shape and mechanical properties of vertebrae and connective tissues at the different intervertebral levels play an essential role, but the spine is only a part of a global neuro-musculoskeletal system involving:

- The head, or cephalic vertebra, weighting 4–5 kg [1].
- The pelvis (called the pelvic vertebra by Jean Dubousset) which is the base of the construct. This base is mobile to allow for postural regulation through pelvic tilt and resulting sacral plate inclination.
- The thorax, with series of ribs to stiffen and strengthen the thoracic spine and protect the vital components (lungs and heart) in the ribcage construct. Specific costovertebral and costotransverse joints allow rib cage mobility for respiration.
- The muscular system, which has an essential role for skeletal mobilization and stabilization.
- The central nervous system allowing regulation of muscle activation and control according to information provided by a wide range of proprioceptive sensors, including those related to vision, to vestibular system, to ligamentous system, and to skin.

W. Skalli, Ph.D. (✉) • C. Vergari, Ph.D.
Arts et Metiers ParisTech, Institut de Biomecanique Humaine Georges Charpak, Paris, France
e-mail: Wafa.skalli@ensam.eu

M. Machida et al. (eds.), *Pathogenesis of Idiopathic Scoliosis*,
https://doi.org/10.1007/978-4-431-56541-3_4

This neuro-musculoskeletal system is particularly complex, and disorders in one of the components may lead to a biomechanical cascade. In the erect position, this system allows keeping subject's balance under gravity loads, with the head upon the pelvis and the eyes in a horizontal plane.

Scoliosis is associated with three-dimensional changes of the whole spine, including lateral and axial deviations and rotations [2]. Local changes occur as well, such as vertebral rotation and wedging, particularly at the apical level. Perdriolle described the continuous torsion within the scoliotic curve with vertebra and disc deformation in the axial plane, resulting in hypokyphosis for the thoracic curve and the so-called specific rotation at its upper extremity [3].

In the growing spine subjected to gravity loads, these changes determine local hyper-pressure that can affect bone growth and disc material properties [4] which can in turn alter the spine's mechanical behavior and induce curve progression. Also muscle forces can become asymmetric for posture regulation. However such biomechanical cascade is not yet fully understood: the aim of the biomechanical engineer is to develop both quantitative methods and models that provide a better understanding of the mechanical behavior, for an improved diagnosis and strategy of treatment. In structural mechanics, the mechanical behavior of a structure is its response to applied loads, in terms of displacements, deformation, and mechanical stress. Such response depends on the geometry, on the material properties of the constitutive components, and on the nature of the applied loads. In biomechanics, the mechanobiology of living tissues also plays a role because both their geometry and properties may change due to remodeling, either because of growth process or according to abnormal internal stress and strain.

This chapter on clinical biomechanics of adolescent idiopathic scoliosis will describe some recent advances on 3D geometric and mechanical modeling of the spinal construct, which provide a novel insight on the scoliotic spine with various clinical implications. First geometric modeling and 3D analysis will be presented; then a brief reminder of the biomechanical characteristics of vertebrae and discs will be provided. Finally biomechanical models will be considered, together with their use for AIS analysis.

Scoliosis is associated with three-dimensional global and local changes of the spine including lateral and axial deviations and rotations. However, for a long time, the routine imaging assessment for AIS analysis was a single frontal X-ray (and this is still the case in many hospitals). The most used clinical parameter for diagnosis and decision making (brace or surgical treatment) is the Cobb angle, which is measured between the limits of a given curve and it quantifies the curve magnitude in a quasi-coronal plane. Nonnegligible biases are related to X-ray projections, as illustrated in Fig. 4.1: when a virtual scoliotic spine is rotated around a vertical axis, the projected angle may differ greatly from the real one. In severe scoliosis, apparent values of Cobb angle may change by more than 15° just due to the different point of view for the projection.

As scoliosis is a disorder that develops in three dimensions, three-dimensional analysis is essential. Lateral X-rays provide information on lordosis and kyphosis, again with projection bias. Axial rotation of the apical vertebra is also a parameter

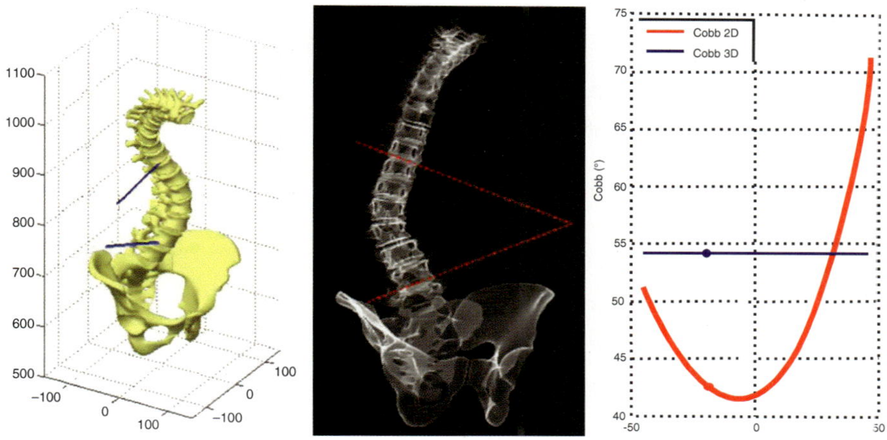

Fig. 4.1 When the spine is rotated along a vertical axis, the 3D Cobb angle (in *blue*) does not change, while 2D angle based on frontal plane projection (in *red*) varies greatly

of primary interest. Its semiquantitative assessment can be performed on the frontal X-ray based on pedicles' projection asymmetry.

CT scan provides useful data for 3D analysis; however, the major issue lies in the high radiation dose [5]. Moreover, as the exam is in supine position, it does not allow taking into account the effect of gravity in functional standing position, and the quantitative analysis of rotations is biased due to the orientation of the CT images [6]. MRI is a noninvasive technology of particular interest for quantitative soft tissue analysis, such as intervertebral discs and muscles. However it is also generally performed in supine position. Moreover, bone signal is much less informative than in CT scan imaging; thus getting 3D reconstruction is still a time-consuming and challenging task. The cost of the MRI exam also is a limitation for use in clinical routine.

Low-dose biplanar X-ray represents a new imaging technique that allows a head to feet exploration of the skeleton, together with accurate model-based 3D reconstruction, thus providing a new insight in scoliosis quantitative analysis. The system itself and the modeling methods are widely described elsewhere [7–10], and they are briefly explained hereafter.

4.1.1 Principles of 3D Reconstruction from Biplanar X-rays

The 3D reconstruction method aims at getting the external *surface shape* of a given bone or structure (e.g., a vertebra) and its *position* in space. First, an a priori model is considered; then a smart deformation of this model is applied in order to make its theoretical biplanar X-rays as close as possible to the real patient's pair of X-rays. This method assumes an a priori knowledge of the bones under consideration to build a

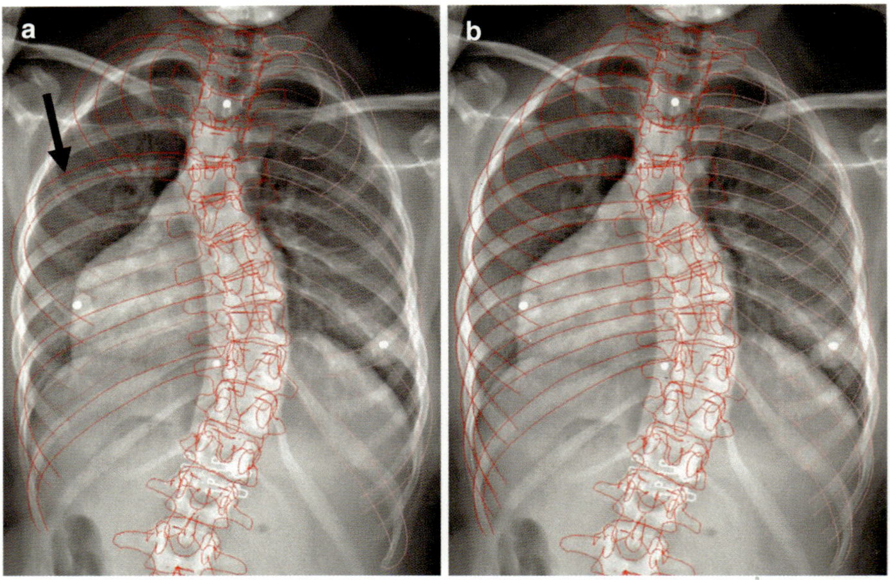

Fig. 4.2 Example of model retroprojection on the real X-rays: (**a**) the virtual contours (in *red*) of the initial virtual model does not perfectly match the real contours, (**b**) final model after adjustments

reference object (such as vertebra, pelvis, or rib or global spine, ribcage, or trunk). This reference object is modeled first using a combination of simple geometric primitives (such as spheres, segments, ellipses) and their associated descriptive parameters (such as radius, length, orientation angle). The 3D reconstruction is then performed in two steps: first a set of landmarks are identified from the X-rays, allowing for quantitative assessment of a set of parameters. Using databases of such objects, together with statistical relationships and template transformation techniques, an initial model estimate is computed and projected to be superimposed on the real X-rays. In a second step, adjustments are performed allowing for matching between virtual and real X-rays, thus yielding the subject-specific accurate model (Fig. 4.2). The process is currently robust, and uncertainty in various situations has been assessed [11–15]. Very active work is in progress for full automatization of the 3D reconstruction process using mathematical modeling and image processing.

4.1.2 *Clinical Relevance of 3D Reconstruction from Biplanar X-rays*

Once the 3D reconstruction is completed, automatic computation of a wide set of 3D parameters can be performed, such as unbiased values of Cobb angle, lordosis, kyphosis, incidence, pelvic tilt, and sacral slope. Particularly, access to horizontal

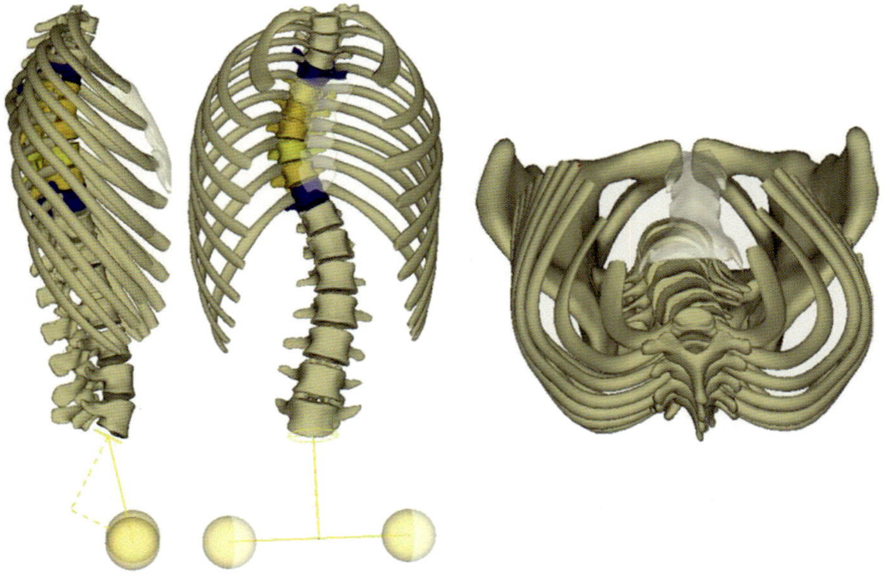

Fig. 4.3 Frontal, lateral, and top view of the 3D model after three-dimensional reconstruction from biplanar X-rays. The spheres represent the femoral heads

plane provides essential information: vertebral axial rotations can be computed and, more qualitatively, the top view of the 3D reconstruction allows to visualize both the spine malalignment and the global torsion within the deformed spine (Fig. 4.3). The simplified vector-based visualization proposed by Illes et al. [16] helps in this global qualitative view.

The very high potential of such quantification and transverse plane analysis is related to the possibility to quantify a geometric phenotype of AIS spine, taking into account deformity in the transverse plane. Datasets of 3D reconstructions were collected for asymptomatic spines, spines with severe scoliosis requiring orthopedic or surgical treatment, and mild scoliosis. The main curve of a severe scoliotic spine can be characterized by several parameters, in complement to the Cobb angle; hypokyphosis at the apical level, when considered in its local plane; axial rotation of the apical vertebra; intervertebral rotations at the junction (which means that the junctional vertebra is rotated with regard to the adjacent one); and torsion index [17], describing the continuous torsion within the curve. Indeed vertebral rotation increases from a junction to the apex and then decreases from the apex to the other junction.

It appeared that seeds of such pattern were also found in mild scoliosis, independently from the main curve location [18]. A specific mathematical method was then used to assess, for each mild scoliotic curve at a very early stage, its "similarity" either to severe or to asymptomatic curves. A severity index quantified this similarity. The validation of this severity index required a long follow-up from the first exam when it was calculated to the end of growth or decision of treatment by brace.

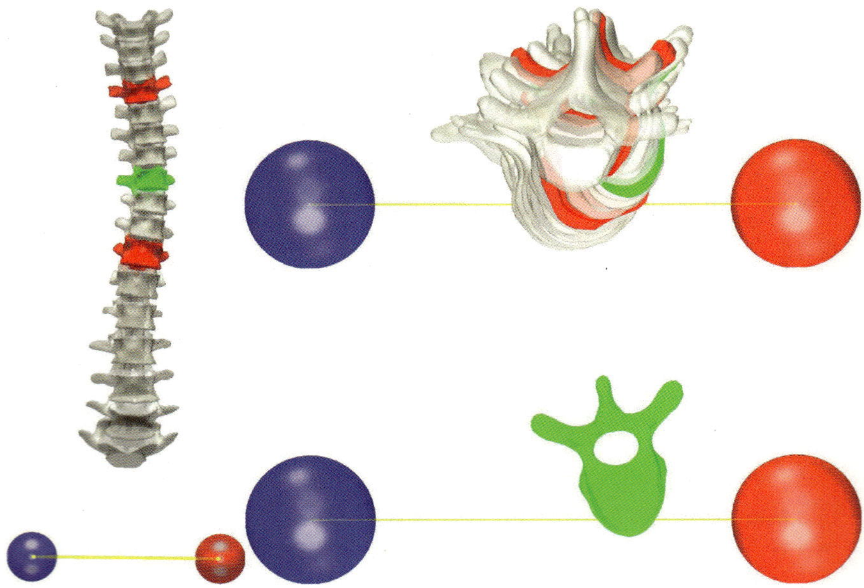

Fig. 4.4 Three-dimensional reconstruction of a scoliotic spine with a Cobb angle of 17° and an axial rotation of the apical vertebra of 13°. Left panel shows a front view, with the junctional vertebrae colored in red and the apical vertebra in green. Top right panel shows a top view of the whole spine, while bottom right panel shows a top view of the apical vertebra, to appreciate its rotation. Red and blue spheres represent the left and right condyles, respectively

On the first 65 patients that were followed until progression status was known, the severity index, set in double blind at the first exam, was in agreement with the real final outcome in more than 80% of the cases [19]. Among the cases where the spine was predicted as progressive, 89% indeed progressed. Figure 4.4 shows a mild scoliosis (17° Cobb angle), for which the top view clearly shows the initiation of the torsion responsible for the scoliosis progression.

3D reconstruction is also essential to quantitatively assess the brace effect. In preliminary studies considering various braces [20, 21], the lordosis reduction was observed in the majority of the cases, which may be unfavorable for sagittal posture. Quantification of the correction in the horizontal plane showed that horizontal plane parameters were corrected only in 30% of the cases and could even be worsened in some cases. Further investigation of the effects of given braces, such as in [22], together with extensive longitudinal studies, should progressively allow better understanding of those parameters that are essential to correct for a successful outcome.

Various studies also propose quantitative analysis of surgery effects [23], which is particularly important to get a better understanding of the mechanisms of correction and to follow the evolution of the levels that remain free after surgery. When the 3D reconstruction is performed both for the spine and the thorax, complementary parameters can be calculated such as the ribcage volume and the spinal penetration index [23, 24]. Research is in progress to assess relationship between ribcage volume and pulmonary function [25].

Another essential issue is the head to feet 3D analysis of the skeleton. Recent research have focused on the position of the head with regard to the hip axis (HA), defined as the vertical line passing through the center point between the femoral heads. Two anatomic landmarks detected on X-rays are close to the head's center of gravity, namely, the center of both acoustic meatus (CAM) and the summit of odontoid (OD). Sixty-nine asymptomatic volunteers younger than 40 years old and forty-four asymptomatic volunteers older than 49 years (up to 76 years old) were considered [26]. The orientation of the lines joining CAM to HA and OD to HA appeared quasi-invariant with a mean angle of 3° with regard to the hip axis and a standard deviation of 2°. Alterations of spine alignment were observed in approximatively one third of the older subjects; however mechanisms of compensation appeared to maintain the head upon the pelvis (mainly from increase of pelvic tilt and cervical lordosis). Recent investigations on 52 AIS patients pre and 3–6 months post brace demonstrated similar quasi-invariance of CAM-HA and OD-HA axes (unpublished data), while in an investigation of CAM-HA on adult patients with severe spine deformities, such invariance was not always preserved [27]. This head to feet analysis with longitudinal follow-up of AIS patients should provide new insights in the mechanisms of progression of a scoliosis curve and the associated mechanisms of compensation.

This global analysis raises the issue of adaptation of the subject to keep an erect posture when a local disorder appears, and maintaining the head upon the pelvis is associated to maintaining the body center of gravity within the support polygon delimitated by the feet. Recent approaches allow getting an accurate body envelope from EOS biplanar X-rays [28, 29]. When associated to improved density models, assessment of the location of the global center of gravity can be obtained only from biplanar X-rays, without requiring an additional force plate [30]. Such new investigation allows large-scale transversal and longitudinal barycentremetry studies, i.e., location of the 3D center of mass of each body segment (Fig. 4.5), which should provide a new insight in the compensation mechanisms that occur in AIS with the progression of the disease.

In synthesis, recent advances in 3D reconstruction from biplanar X-rays allowed drastic progress in the investigation means for AIS patients. Large-scale multicentric studies are still to come, allowing for extensive analysis. While such pooling of multicentric data is facilitated by the fact that the images are already in a digital format, adhering to a common patient positioning during acquisition is essential. We strongly recommend the free-standing position as described by Faro et al. [31] following the SRS recommendation, or a slight modification to place the fingers on the zygomatic arch in order to let full visibility to the cervical spine. Such large-scale analysis should yield new paradigms in investigating scoliosis development understanding, together with improved diagnosis and more focused and efficient treatments. However, geometry is not the only element, and further analysis using

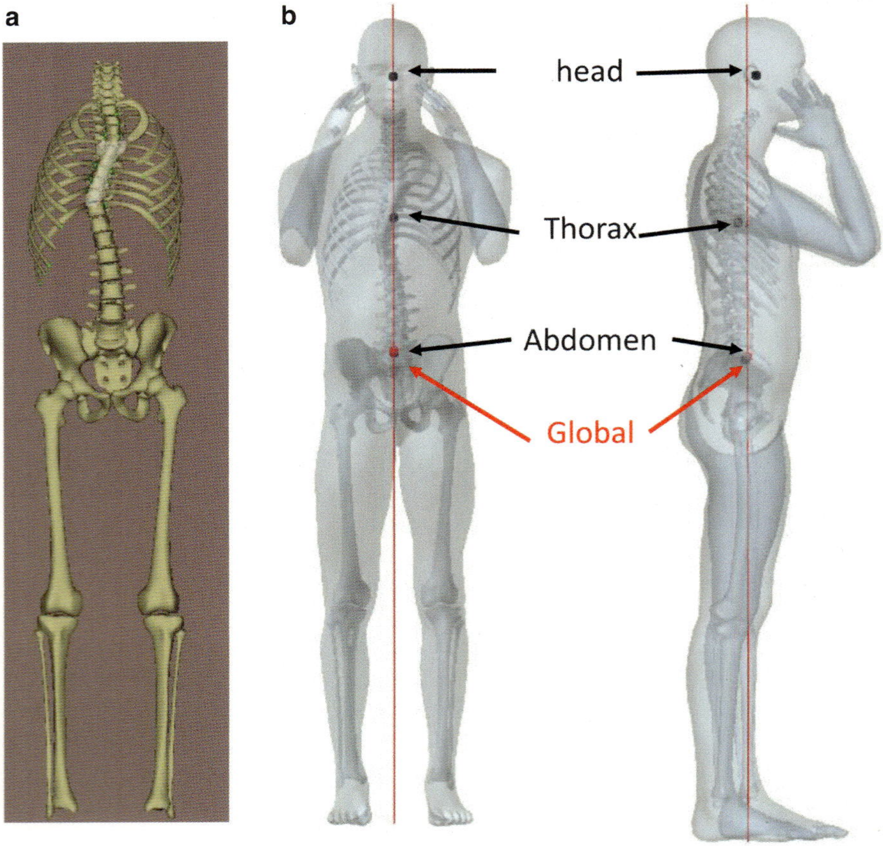

Fig. 4.5 From the biplanar X-rays, (**a**) longitudinal skeleton, (**b**) 3D reconstruction of the external envelope and barycentremetry allowing estimation of the gravity line, passing through the global center of mass of the subject. Center of mass of various body segments, such as the head, thorax, or abdomen, can be computed

biomechanical models requires taking into account mechanical properties of spine components, particularly vertebrae and intervertebral discs.

4.2 Focus on Vertebrae and Intervertebral Discs

4.2.1 Vertebrae

Vertebrae are constituted of an outer shell of cortical bone and inner spongy component. AIS is characterized by local vertebral deformities that were first described qualitatively and then quantitatively.

Anterior overgrowth of the vertebral body with regard to the posterior spine could play a role in the rotational phenomena that characterize spinal curvatures [32, 33]). Vertebral wedging progressively appears with the development of the deformity [34, 35]. Intravertebral torsion is also described [36]. Pedicle asymmetry is observed particularly at the apical level, with smaller and shorter pedicles on the concave side [37]. The mechanisms of such deformation are not yet fully understood and are probably multifactorial: among the observations on AIS bone, bone mineral density (BMD) may be lower than that of healthy subjects [38, 39], which means greater bone deformability as BMD is directly correlated to material properties [40]. Bone undergoes physiological changes during growth; together with the Hueter-Volkmann law, which relates bone formation-resorption to the mechanical stress, these changes could explain the asymmetrical vertebral shape modifications that appear in AIS. However, such vertebral deformity is probably a secondary phenomenon, and disc alteration probably plays a major role in curve progression.

4.2.2 Intervertebral Discs

Intervertebral discs are highly specialized structures that sit between adjacent vertebrae and constitute six degrees of freedom links between vertebral bodies, allowing three displacements (axial, posteroanterior, and lateral) and three rotations (sagittal, lateral, axial), in relation with the six load components, forces (compression/traction, anteroposterior, and lateral shear) and moments (flexion/extension, lateral bending, and axial torsion). Because of the geometry of the vertebrae, their ligaments, and posterior joints, the disc usually undergoes complex coupling of loads in different planes. In everyday activities, the disc is subjected to high and repeated loads, while absorbing shocks and giving spine its flexibility. The loading curve of a functional unit in a given direction shows a nonlinear behavior that is characteristic of biological samples (Fig. 4.6). The curve also shows hysteresis, which is characteristic of the dissipative/viscoelastic behavior of the disc.

4.2.2.1 Normal Intervertebral Discs

Each disc consists of two regions: a strong fibrous ring of tissue, the *annulus fibrosus*, retaining a gel-like core, the *nucleus pulposus*. Although the two regions have a very different structure and composition, the transition between them is not well defined, but it is more of a gradual change. The disc is almost entirely avascular, apart from fine capillaries that radially penetrate the periphery of the disc [41], and it exchanges nutrition and metabolic by-products through the adjacent vertebral end plates. Its main components are collagen, proteoglycans, and water, making up 90–95% of the disc's extracellular matrix.

The mechanical role of the *nucleus* is to resist compressive loads while exerting a hydrostatic pressure against the *annulus* that is therefore loaded radially [42, 43].

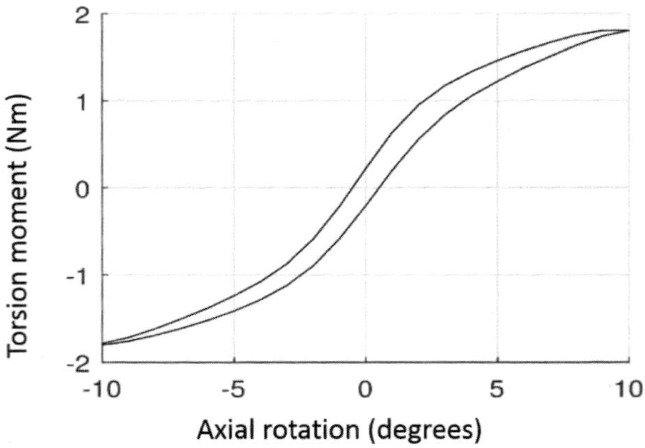

Fig. 4.6 Typical mechanical test of a L4/L5 human intervertebral disc loaded in axial rotation

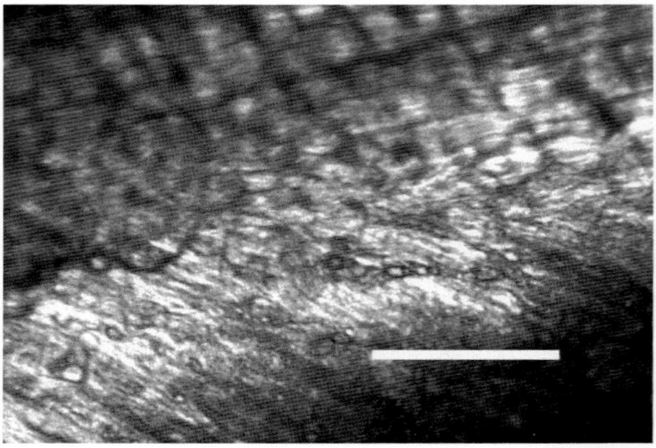

Fig. 4.7 Collagen arrangement of bovine tail intervertebral disc. Two lamellae with different collagen orientations are visible, as well as the crimping of the fibers. Image obtained by second harmonic generation microscopy (size bar represents 100 μm)

At higher loads, the *annulus* is actively engaged in bearing the load, being directly compressed between the two adjacent end plates.

The *annulus* is formed by a series of concentric lamellae which do not continuously encircle the disc: they are incomplete curved sheets [44, 45]. Collagen fibers have a repeating oblique arrangement within a lamella, with different angles in adjacent lamellae (Fig. 4.7). Collagen fibers are crimped in healthy disc [46], and they are organized in tightly packed bundles. These bundles are surrounded by a highly organized elastic fiber network that is spread throughout the annulus. Elastic fibers are aligned to the collagen bundles and encircle them, penetrating in the bundles themselves to integrate the two structures [47]. Translamellar radial bridges span multiple lamellae, passing between collagen bundles and thus maintaining interlamellar cohesion [48]. These bridges contain both elastin and type IV collagen [49]; the latter gives strength to the interlamellar bond [50], but it is also capable of interacting with hyaluronan, which could facilitate the lubrication of collagen bundles.

Micromechanical testing showed complex pattern of deformation within the annulus. When loaded, lamellae tend to skew, but no sliding occurs at the interlamellar junction [51]. The main mechanism of strain seems to lie in the sliding that occurs between bundles of fibers, which also limits the strain within the bundle itself [52, 53].

4.2.2.2 Disc Alterations in Scoliosis

Discs in the scoliotic curve undergo biochemical, metabolic, and morphological changes. Collagen and water content can be lower in the *annulus* of wedged discs, compared to healthy subjects, while glycosaminoglycan content can be higher. Collagen can also be asymmetrically distributed in the *annulus fibrosus*, with a decreased concentration in the concave aspect of the curve [54], although this asymmetry was not confirmed by more recent studies [55]. *Annulus* in scoliotic spine also presents a sparse network of elastic fibers, with a loss of lamellar structure and a different fiber arrangement [56, 57].

Nucleus in the scoliotic disc is characterized by a reduced content of glycosaminoglycans, which is accompanied by a dehydration of the tissue. A large number of apoptotic cells have also been reported in the nucleus, in particular of the apex disc [58].

Extended abnormal calcification of the vertebral end plate was observed in scoliotic specimens, which is likely to affect growth because of the altered nutrient supply to the disc [56, 59]. This could be a part of the "vicious cycle," which was described as the mechanism of deformity progression [60]: once a small lateral curvature is present, vertebral and disc growth can be affected by the asymmetrical loading on the vertebral end plates, leading to vertebral and disc wedging, which further increases the spinal curve and therefore the asymmetry of the load (Fig. 4.8).

The progression of AIS is strongly related to growth, as shown by the rapid progression of spinal deformity during peaks of skeletal growth velocity. The abovementioned geometric phenotype early associated to progressive scoliosis demonstrates specific characteristic concerning the intervertebral rotations in the transverse plane at the junctional area, suggesting that the disc is involved in the initial onset of the deformity. The cause of this early disc alteration, however, is still

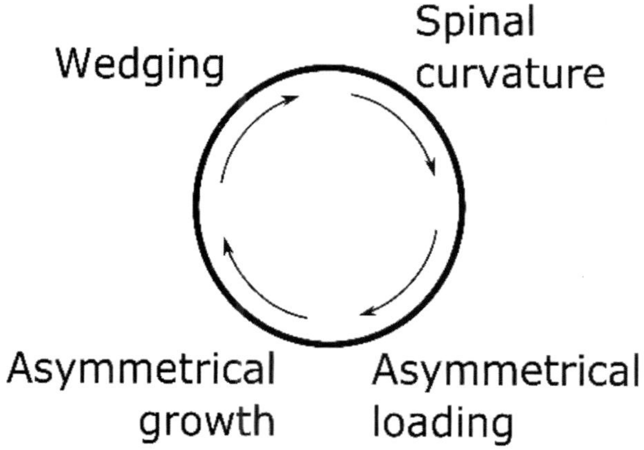

Fig. 4.8 Vicious cycle leading to spinal scoliotic deformity

unknown. In vivo characterization of the intervertebral discs is essential to progressively assess changes that may occur in intervertebral discs.

4.2.2.3 Intervertebral Disc Characterization In Vivo

The most diffused means of investigation of the disc in vivo is magnetic resonance imaging (MRI). Different imaging modalities allow quantifying disc morphology (its overall volume, the volume occupied by the *annulus* and *nucleus*, disc height, etc.) and its changes (for instance, physiological circadian changes or following corrective surgery), disc composition (water content and its diffusivity, proteoglycan concentration), and the presence of defects, such as tears or calcification [61–64].

In scoliosis, MRI was utilized to compare disc morphology before and after corrective surgery [64], which allowed quantifying the recovery of intervertebral space. MRI signal intensity of the disc is widely used to characterize disc degeneration, but more recently, it was suggested that MRI signal could also be a potential biomarker of early adolescent idiopathic scoliosis [65].

Radiography does not allow direct observation of the disc, although disc height can be inferred from the intervertebral space. Flexibility tests, fulcrum bending, and suspension have been used, in combination with radiographic imaging, to extrapolate spine stiffness and the distribution of disc mechanical properties along the spine [66–68]. This information can be used to plan corrective surgery, for instance, to appropriately select the vertebral levels to be fused in order to maximize postoperative mobility and restoration of trunk height.

Ultrasound is underexploited for the analysis of the intervertebral disc, although it would be a noninvasive simple method to characterize the disc in a standing position. Very preliminary work has been carried out to show the feasibility of ultrasound imaging for the characterization of disc structure [69, 70], while ultrasound elastography was used to noninvasively measure disc mechanical properties [71]. Measurements in the lumbar region of the scoliotic spine have been proven feasible and reliable, and work is in progress to evaluate clinical relevance of the technique to assess possible alterations in scoliotic spines.

Biomechanical models can help in understanding the impact of geometric and structural changes on the global mechanical behavior of the scoliotic construct.

4.3 Biomechanical Modeling and AIS

4.3.1 Spine Biomechanical Models

A biomechanical model is a simplified mathematical representation taking into account the geometry and the material properties of the structure of interest. It allows to virtually apply loads in order to investigate the mechanical response in terms of displacements, stress, and strains. The so-called finite element models allow taking into account the heterogeneity of the structure and its complex shape and are widely used in the general field of structural mechanics. Associated numerical simulation is more and more used in a wide range of applications and particularly in biomechanics. Spine models can be built at various scales, from very global models of the whole body to macroscopic or mesoscopic models for a more or less extended spine segment. Microscopic models aim to establish relationship between microarchitecture and macroscopic structural behavior [44, 72].

Figure 4.9 shows that the level of detail can vary a lot in the representation of the components, particularly vertebrae and intervertebral disc: in order to perform accurate disc stress analysis (e.g., to explore adjacent disc degeneration), intervertebral discs can be represented by a great number of elements including disc fibers with different material properties from the outer to inner annulus (Fig 4.9b). When modeling the whole spine to investigate realignment after bracing or surgical instrumentation, gross representation can be more cost-effective with vertebrae modeled as a series of stiff beams with contact surfaces at facet joints and discs as deformable beams with a torsional spring to represent the role of disc fibers (Fig 4.9d).

Since a model is a simplification of the real complex phenomena, it requires strong validation to determine its clinical relevance. Therefore, modeling is closely linked to experimental analysis, particularly checking through in vitro experiments that the virtual behavior consistently renders the experimentally observed one. Once the model is validated, it constitutes a powerful means of investigation: indeed, although building a validated finite element model represents a huge research effort, it opens a wide range of possibilities because changing the load conditions or numerical values of a given parameter is straightforward. Therefore, all other things remaining equal, the sensitivity of each parameter can be investigated. Such models can be built to provide the generic geometry of a spinal segment, allowing for conceptual analysis. Spine FEM has been developing for more than 30 years, and very detailed models of lumbar or cervical spine are used particularly for a better understanding of the intact and instrumented spines [73, 74].

4.3.2 Clinical Relevance of Spine Biomechanical Models

As for AIS, biomechanical models can be used in relation with various clinical issues. However, as each patient is unique, subject-specific modeling is essential. Getting subject-specific properties of tissues is still a challenge, although recent imaging techniques, such as ultrasound elastography or MRI, open new perspectives. However subject-specific geometry can now be routinely obtained using 3D reconstruction from low-dose biplanar X-rays, which allow a wide range of applications that will be illustrated hereafter.

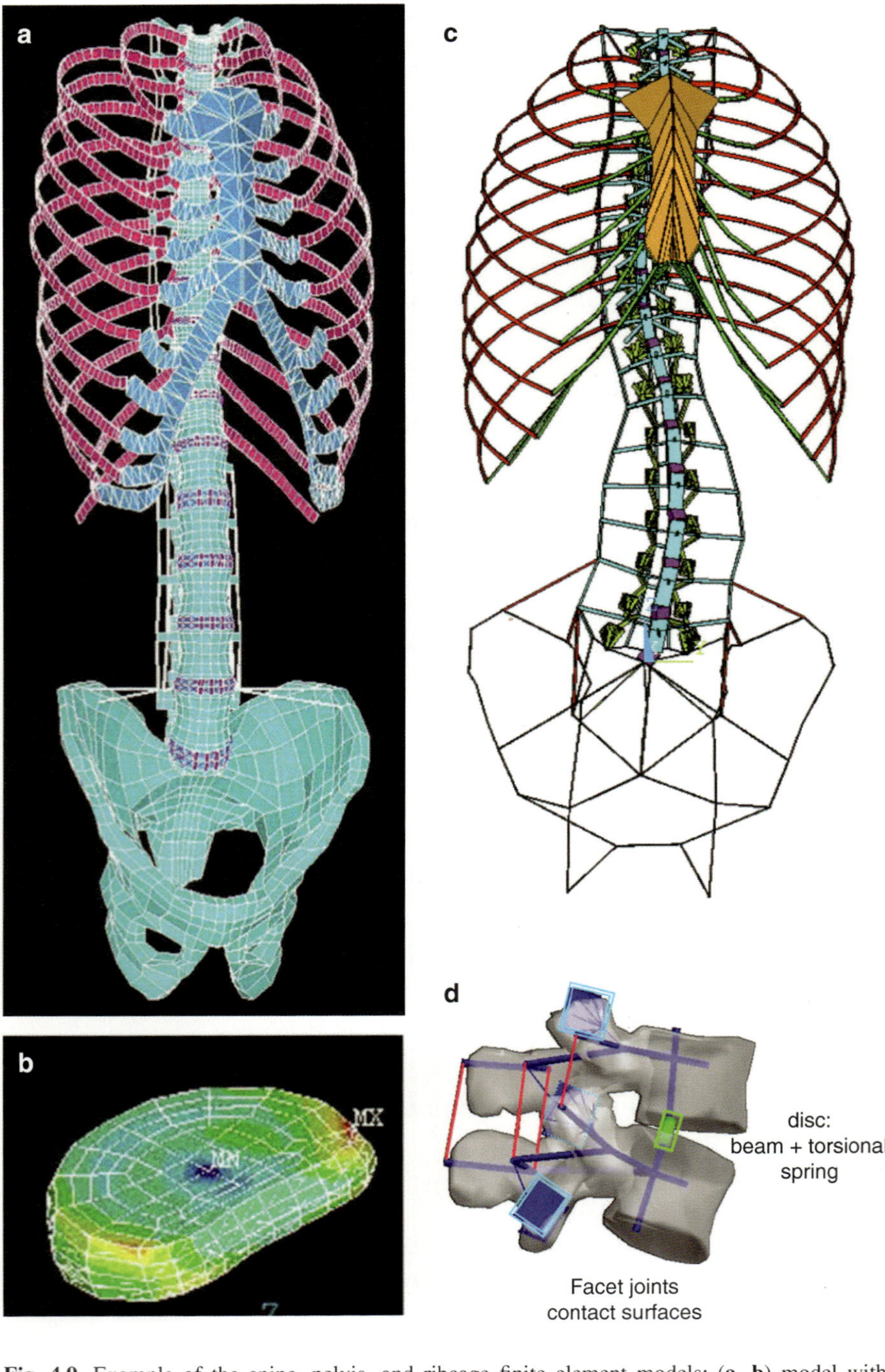

Fig. 4.9 Example of the spine, pelvis, and ribcage finite element models: (**a**, **b**) model with detailed representation of vertebrae and discs, including nucleus differentiation and disc fibers architecture and allowing for stress analysis; (**c**, **d**) model with gross representation of discs and vertebrae for numerical simulation of brace or surgery with reasonable numerical cost

4.3.2.1 Mechanism of Curve Progression

Because of the possibility to change a wide range of parameters, modeling can be used to explore mechanisms of progression of the curve [75–77]. The hypothesis is that 3D subject-specific biomechanical modeling should provide further understanding of the biomechanical cascade.

In Drevelle et al., a previously validated subject-specific spine model was used to simulate the spine of 18 adolescents, 12 with mild thoracolumbar scoliosis and 6 asymptomatic. Accurate 3D reconstructions were the basis of each model; then a large set of conditions were simulated in order to reproduce curve progression in relation with gravity loads, disc stiffness, and posteroanterior asymmetric vertebral growth. For some of the mild scoliosis curves, numerical simulation was able to mimic progression to severe scoliosis, with large rotations and torsion, thus providing possible explanations to the biomechanical cascade. Surprisingly, simulations never resulted in such scoliosis-like deformity for asymptomatic spines, clearly indicating that this biomechanical cascade is a secondary factor that can take place only once a specific deformation pattern is already there. Indeed, this conceptual analysis was an essential step in searching for such pattern at an early stage, thus yielding the definition of the severity index. This research also underlined the role of the intervertebral discs, which then was the driver for further basic research focused on in vivo assessment of intervertebral discs, particularly using ultrasound elastography. All these approaches are complementary and progressively converge to assess possible biomechanical pathomechanisms and key factors that could help for early detection of progression risk in mild scoliosis and for the assessment of treatment strategies.

4.3.2.2 Modeling of Brace Correction

Various models were proposed for brace simulation with first attempts to go toward clinical use of such models [21, 78–81]. Such models require the subject-specific modeling of trunk components including the spine, ribcage, costovertebral and costotransverse junction, pelvis, and associated soft tissues. However, since the model represents a simplification of the real complex mechanical properties of the bone and the soft tissues, model validation is an essential step for such models to assess their clinical relevance. The validation process has to consider the ability of the models to render not only the 2D Cobb angle change but also the full 3D behavior, particularly considering the effect of brace on the lordosis, kyphosis, transverse plane parameters, and rib hump. A framework for model validation from pre and post bracing has been recently proposed [82], and this framework has been used with promising results on 42 patients' data [71], Fig. 4.10. Biplanar X-rays and associated 3D reconstruction allowed getting subject-specific geometries in clinical routine. As ribs are essential components to transmit loads from the external trunk

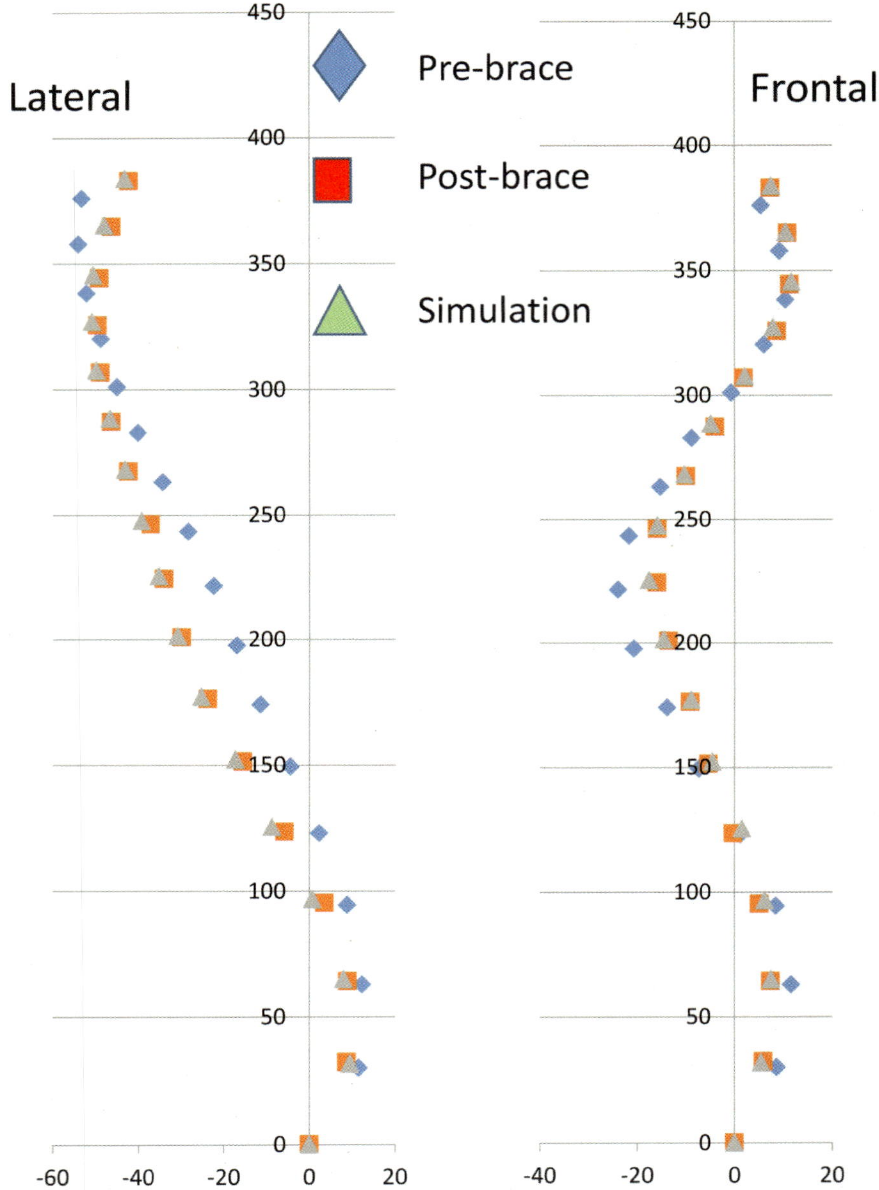

Fig. 4.10 Example of model evaluation for brace simulation: comparison of frontal body lines and clinical indices: real brace correction, computed from 3D reconstruction, vs simulated correction

	Real Pre-brace From 3D reconstruction	Real Post-brace From 3D reconstruction	Predicted Post-brace: From simulation
T1/T12 kyphosis	20	30	31
L1/L5 Lordosis	-55	-53	-54
Cobb angle	-33	-23	-25
Apical Axial rotation	-11	-8	-11
Torsion index	12	11	11
Max Rib hump	14	11	13

Fig. 4.10 (continued)

to the spine, their material properties were adapted taking into account age-based mechanical properties. Post brace data were used to control the relevance of the model's prediction for the abovementioned clinical indices, and 87% of them were within measurement uncertainty. Although still preliminary and requiring both improvements and extensive validation, such models progressively get mature enough to be used in a routine clinical environment.

4.3.2.3 Modeling of Surgical Correction

Like brace modeling, numerical simulation can also be of paramount importance for surgery planning. Indeed, defining the appropriate strategy for a given patient is still a challenge, and being able to provide a computer-assisted surgery planning using a subject-specific validated model would represent a definite progress to lower mechanical complications.

This topic represents a very active field of research, either for understanding basic phenomena [83], for conceptual thorough investigation of implant behavior [84], or for surgery planning. Subject-specific geometry can now be routinely obtained from preoperative biplanar X-rays, and model thorough validation can be performed by comparing the numerical prediction to the real effect of surgery, not only for the Cobb angle but on all the relevant clinical indices, inside and outside the fused area. As for brace simulation, extensive evaluation is essential before using such models in a routine environment. Because of local alterations of disc stiffness in severe preoperative scoliosis, getting subject-specific disc stiffness is necessary. Indirect techniques using bending tests quantitative analysis are used for preoperative estimation of disc stiffness: once the model is built, the bending test motion is simulated, and an optimization process is performed to change the disc stiffness at various levels until the model is able to properly render the material properties [85–86]. Simulating the correction gesture requires an in-depth dialogue between clinician and engineers, and first proofs of concept of providing reliable predictive models have been proposed, both for rotation techniques [87] and for in situ contouring technique [85]. Such models allow detailed analysis of each step of the surgical gesture, which can improve the understanding of the main mechanisms involved in the scoliosis surgical correction.

Such examples show the potential of subject-specific biomechanical models for scoliosis. All those approaches are still currently in clinical research, and routine clinical use still requires extensive validation and improvement of numerical procedures and software so that processing time is decreased and robust friendly used process is proposed. However drastic progress occurred in the last 10 years. All these approaches are complementary and progressively converge to assess possible pathomechanisms and key factors that could help for early detection of progression risk in mild scoliosis and for the assessment of strategies for improving treatment.

4.4 Conclusion

Adolescent idiopathic scoliosis is the result of complex multifactorial phenomena, and biomechanical analysis may help in better understanding mechanisms of progression and principles of correction. To that aim, quantitative measurements are essential, and head to feet accurate 3D reconstruction from low-dose biplanar X-rays now allows routine thorough exploration of the scoliotic spine. Such exploration already opens promising perspectives in early detection of progressive scoliosis which can be of paramount importance for diagnosis and early therapeutic management. It also allows objective assessment of the effects of orthopedic or surgical treatment, thus promising future improvement in the practice, together with better understanding of the key parameters in relation with clinical outcome. Head to feet investigation also should help our basic understanding of the compensation mechanisms that occur during progression of the curve. While such 3D analysis can already be already used in clinical routine, other fields of research are very active, both for noninvasive characterization of material properties of soft tissues, particularly intervertebral discs, and for building reliable predictive models for a computer-aided planning of correction strategy. Such research is conducted in very close collaboration between clinicians and engineers, and the quality of the pluridisciplinary dialogue is the key for future translation of such models for use in AIS management based on biomechanical principles.

Acknowledgments The authors gratefully thank all the spine team of the Institut de Biomécanique Humaine Georges Charpak and the clinical partners who participated to research on scoliosis.

Recent research was supported by the ParisTech Foundation within the BiomecAM chair program on subject-specific musculoskeletal modeling, with the participation of Cotrel Foundation, Proteor Company, Société Générale, and Covea.

References

1. Vital JM, Senegas J. Anatomical bases of the study of the constraints to which the cervical spine is subject in the sagittal plane A study of the center of gravity of the head. Surg Radiol Anat. 1986;8:169–73.
2. Dubousset J. Three-dimensional analysis of the scoliotic deformity, in: the pediatric spine: principles and practice. New York, NY: Raven Press; 1994.
3. Perdriolle R, Vidal J. Morphology of scoliosis: three-dimensional evolution. Orthopedics. 1987;10:909–15.
4. Meir AR, Fairbank JCT, Jones DA, McNally DS, Urban JPG. High pressures and asymmetrical stresses in the scoliotic disc in the absence of muscle loading. Scoliosis. 2007;2:4.
5. Brenner DJ, Hall EJ. Computed tomography. an increasing source of radiation exposure. N Engl J Med. 2007;357:2277–84.
6. Skalli W, Lavaste F, Descrimes JL. Quantification of three-dimensional vertebral rotations in scoliosis: what are the true values? Spine. 1995;20(5):546–53.
7. Aubert B, Vergari C, Ilharreborde B, Courvoisier A, Skalli W. 3D reconstruction of rib cage geometry from biplanar radiographs using a statistical parametric model approach. Comput Methods Biomech Biomed Eng Imag Vis. 2016;4:281–95.
8. Chaibi Y, Cresson T, Aubert B, Hausselle J, Neyret P, Hauger O, de Guise JA, Skalli W. Fast 3D reconstruction of the lower limb using a parametric model and statistical inferences and clinical measurements calculation from biplanar X-rays. Comput Methods Biomech Biomed Engin. 2012;15:457–66.
9. Dubousset J, Charpak G, Dorion I, Skalli W, Lavaste F, Deguise J, Kalifa G, Ferey S. A new 2D and 3D imaging approach to musculoskeletal physiology and pathology with low-dose radiation and the standing position: the EOS system. Bull Acad Natl Med. 2005;189:287–300.
10. Humbert L, De Guise JA, Aubert B, Godbout B, Skalli W. 3D reconstruction of the spine from biplanar X-rays using parametric models based on transversal and longitudinal inferences. Med Eng Phys. 2009;31:681–7.
11. Carreau JH, Bastrom T, Petcharaporn M, Schulte C, Marks M, Illés T, Somoskeöy S, Newton PO. Computer-generated, three-dimensional spine model from biplanar radiographs: a validity study in idiopathic scoliosis curves greater than 50 degrees. Spine Deform. 2014;2:81–8.
12. Ferrero E, Lafage R, Vira S, Rohan P-Y, Oren J, Delsole E, Guigui P, Schwab F, Lafage V, Skalli W. Three-dimensional reconstruction using stereoradiography for evaluating adult spinal deformity: a reproducibility study. Eur Spine J. 2016;26:2112–20.
13. Gille O, Champain N, Benchikh-El-Fegoun A, Vital J-M, Skalli W. Reliability of 3D reconstruction of the spine of mild scoliotic patients. Spine. 2007;32(5):568–73.
14. Glaser DA, Doan J, Newton PO. Comparison of 3-dimensional spinal reconstruction accuracy: biplanar radiographs with EOS versus computed tomography. Spine. 2012;37(16):1391–7.
15. Ilharreborde B, Steffen JS, Nectoux E, Vital JM, Mazda K, Skalli W, Obeid I. Angle measurement reproducibility using EOS three-dimensional reconstructions in adolescent idiopathic scoliosis treated by posterior instrumentation. Spine. 2011;36:E1306–13.
16. Illés T, Tunyogi-Csapó M, Somoskeöy S. Breakthrough in three-dimensional scoliosis diagnosis: significance of horizontal plane view and vertebra vectors. Eur Spine J. 2011;20:135–43. https://doi.org/10.1007/s00586-010-1566-8.

17. Steib JP, Dumas R, Mitton D, Skalli W. Surgical correction of scoliosis by in situ contouring: a detorsion analysis. Spine. 2004;29:193–9.
18. Courvoisier A, Drevelle X, Dubousset J, Skalli W. Transverse plane 3D analysis of mild scoliosis. Eur Spine J. 2013;22:2427–32.
19. Skalli W, Vergari C, Ebermeyer E, Courtois I, Drevelle X, Abelin-Genevois K, Kohler R, Dubousset J. Early detection of progressive adolescent idiopathic scoliosis: a severity index. Spine (Phila Pa 1976). 2017;42(11):823–30.
20. Courvoisier A, Drevelle X, Vialle R, Dubousset J, Skalli W. 3D analysis of brace treatment in idiopathic scoliosis. Eur Spine J. 2013;22:PMC3886497.
21. Vergari C, Mansfield J, Meakin JR, Winlove PC. Lamellar and fibre bundle mechanics of the annulus fibrosus in bovine intervertebral disc. Acta Biomater. 2016;37:14–20.
22. Donzelli S, Zaina F, Lusini M, Minnella S, Respizzi S, Balzarini L, Poma S, Negrini S. The three dimensional analysis of the Sforzesco brace correction. Scoliosis Spinal Disord. 2016;11:34. https://doi.org/10.1186/s13013-016-0092-9.
23. Ilharreborde B, Sebag G, Skalli W, Mazda K. Adolescent idiopathic scoliosis treated with posteromedial translation: radiologic evaluation with a 3D low-dose system. Eur Spine J. 2013;22:2382–91. https://doi.org/10.1007/s00586-013-2776-7.
24. Dubousset J, Wicart P, Pomero V, Barois A, Estournet B. Spinal penetration index: new three-dimensional quantified reference for lordoscoliosis and other spinal deformities. J Orthop Sci. 2003;8:41–9. https://doi.org/10.1007/s007760300007.
25. Pietton R, Bouloussa H, Vergari C, Skalli W, Vialle R. Rib cage measurement reproducibility using biplanar stereoradiographic 3D reconstructions in adolescent idiopathic scoliosis. J Pediatr Orthop. 2017. https://doi.org/10.1097/BPO.0000000000001095. Epub available.
26. Amabile C, Pillet H, Lafage V, Barrey C, Vital J-M, Skalli W. A new quasi-invariant parameter characterizing the postural alignment of young asymptomatic adults. Eur Spine J. 2016;25:3666–74. https://doi.org/10.1007/s00586-016-4552-y.
27. Steffen J-S, Obeid I, Aurouer N, Hauger O, Vital J-M, Dubousset J, Skalli W. 3D postural balance with regard to gravity line: an evaluation in the transversal plane on 93 patients and 23 asymptomatic volunteers. Eur Spine J. 2010;19:760–7. https://doi.org/10.1007/s00586-009-1249-5.
28. Sandoz B, Laporte S, Skalli W, Mitton D. Subject-specific body segment parameters' estimation using biplanar X-rays: a feasibility study. Comput Methods Biomech Biomed Engin. 2010;13:649–54. https://doi.org/10.1080/10255841003717608.
29. Nérot A, Choisne J, Amabile C, Travert C, Pillet H, Wang X, Skalli W. A 3D reconstruction method of the body envelope from biplanar X-rays: evaluation of its accuracy and reliability. J Biomech. 2015;48:4322–6. https://doi.org/10.1016/j.jbiomech.2015.10.044.
30. Amabile C, Choisne J, Nérot A, Pillet H, Skalli W. Determination of a new uniform thorax density representative of the living population from 3D external body shape modeling. J Biomech. 2016;49:1162–9.
31. Faro FD, Marks MC, Pawelek J, Newton PO. Evaluation of a functional position for lateral radiograph acquisition in adolescent idiopathic scoliosis. Spine (Phila Pa 1976). 2004;29:2284–9. http://www.ncbi.nlm.nih.gov/pubmed/15480143.
32. Guo X, Chau WW, Chan YL, Cheng JC, Burwell RG, Dangerfield PH. Relative anterior spinal overgrowth in adolescent idiopathic scoliosis—result of disproportionate endochondral-membranous bone growth? Eur Spine J. 2005;14(9):862–73.
33. Schlösser TPC, van Stralen M, Chu WCW, Lam T-P, Ng BKW, Vincken KL, Cheng JCY, Castelein RM. Anterior overgrowth in primary curves, compensatory curves and junctional segments in adolescent idiopathic scoliosis. PLoS One. 2016;11:1–11. https://doi.org/10.1371/journal.pone.0160267.
34. Perdriolle R, Becchetti S, Vidal J, Lopez P. Mechanical process and growth cartilages; Essential factors in the progression of scoliosis. Spine (Phila. Pa. 1976). 1993;18:343–9. http://journals.lww.com/spinejournal/Fulltext/1993/03000/Mechanical_Process_and_Growth_Cartilages_.7.aspx.
35. Parent S, Labelle H, Skalli W, de Guise J. Vertebral wedging characteristic changes in scoliotic spines. Spine. 2004;29(20):e455–62.

36. Schlösser TPC, van Stralen M, Brink RC, Chu WCW, Lam T-P, Vincken KL, Castelein RM, Cheng JCY. Three-dimensional characterization of torsion and asymmetry of the intervertebral discs versus vertebral bodies in adolescent idiopathic scoliosis. Spine (Phila. Pa. 1976). 2014;39:E1159–66. http://journals.lww.com/spinejournal/Fulltext/2014/09010/Three_Dimensional_Characterization_of_Torsion_and.16.aspx.
37. Parent S, Labelle H, Skalli W, Latimer B, de Guise J. Morphometric analysis of anatomic scoliotic specimens. Spine (Phila. Pa. 1976). 2002;27:2305–11. http://journals.lww.com/spinejournal/Fulltext/2002/11010/Morphometric_Analysis_of_Anatomic_Scoliotic.2.aspx.
38. Courtois I, Collet P, Mouilleseaux B, Alexandre C. Bone mineral density at the femur and lumbar spine in a population of young women treated for scoliosis in adolescence. Rev Rhum Engl Ed. 1999;66(12):705–10.
39. Cheng JC, Qin L, Cheung CS, Sher AH, Lee KM, Ng SW, Guo X. Generalized low areal and volumetric bone mineral density in adolescent idiopathic scoliosis. J Bone Miner Res. 2000;15(18):1587–95.
40. Kopperdahl DL, Morgan EF, Keaveny TM. Quantitative computed tomography estimates of the mechanical properties of human vertebral trabecular bone. J Orthop Res. 2002;20:801–5. https://doi.org/10.1016/S0736-0266(01)00185-1.
41. Crock HV. An atlas of vascular anatomy of the skeleton & spinal cord. London: Martin Dunitz Ltd; 1996.
42. Cannella M, Arthur A, Allen S, Keane M, Joshi A, Vresilovic E, Marcolongo M. The role of the nucleus pulposus in neutral zone human lumbar intervertebral disc mechanics. J Biomech. 2008;41:2104–11.
43. Shea M, Takeuchi TY, Wittenberg RH, White AA III, Hayes WC. A comparison of the effects of automated percutaneous diskectomy and conventional diskectomy on intradiscal pressure, disk geometry, and stiffness. J Spinal Disord. 1994;7:317–25.
44. Adam C, Rouch P, Skalli W. Inter-lamellar shear resistance confers compressive stiffness in the intervertebral disc: an image-based modelling study on the bovine caudal disc. J Biomech. 2015;48:4303–8.
45. Marchand F, Ahmed AM. Investigation of the laminate structure of lumbar disc anulus fibrosus. Spine. 1990;15:402–10.
46. Gruber HE, Hanley EN. Observations on morphologic changes in the aging and degenerating human disc: secondary collagen alterations. BMC Musculoskelet Disord. 2002;3:9.
47. Yu J, Schollum ML, Wade KR, Broom ND, Urban J. ISSLS Prize Winner: a detailed examination of the elastic network leads to a new understanding of annulus fibrosus organization. Spine. 2012;37:1490–6.
48. Pezowicz CA, Robertson PA, Broom ND. The structural basis of interlamellar cohesion in the intervertebral disc wall. J Anat. 2006;208:317–30.
49. Melrose J, Smith SM, Appleyard RC, Little CB. Aggrecan, versican and type VI collagen are components of annular translamellar crossbridges in the intervertebral disc. Eur Spine J. 2008;17:314–24.
50. Schollum ML, Robertson PA, Broom ND. ISSLS Prize Winner: microstructure and mechanical disruption of the lumbar disc annulus: part I: a microscopic investigation of the translamellar bridging network. Spine. 2008;33:2702–10.
51. Michalek AJ, Buckley MR, Bonassar LJ, Cohen I, Iatridis JC. Measurement of local strains in intervertebral disc anulus fibrosus tissue under dynamic shear: contributions of matrix fiber orientation and elastin content. J Biomech. 2009;42:2279–85.
52. Bruehlmann SB, Matyas JR, Duncan NA. ISSLS prize winner: collagen fibril sliding governs cell mechanics in the anulus fibrosus: an in situ confocal microscopy study of bovine discs. Spine. 2004;29:2612–20.
53. Vergari C, Dubois G, Vialle R, Gennisson J-L, Tanter M, Dubousset J, Rouch P, Skalli W. Lumbar annulus fibrosus biomechanical characterization in healthy children by ultrasound shear wave elastography. Eur Radiol. 2016;26:1213–7.
54. Bushell GR, Ghosh P, Taylor TKF, Sutherland JM. The collagen of the intervertebral disc in adolescent idiopathic scoliosis. J Bone Joint Surg. 1979;61-B:501–8.

55. Antoniou J, Arlet V, Goswami T, Aebi M, Alini M. Elevated synthetic activity in the convex side of scoliotic intervertebral discs and endplates compared with normal tissues. Spine. 2001;26(10):E198–206.
56. Roberts S, Menage J, Eisenstein SM. The cartilage end-plate and intervertebral disc in scoliosis: calcification and other sequelae. J Orthop Res. 1993;11:747–57.
57. Yu J, Fairbank JC, Roberts S, Urban JP. The elastic fiber network of the anulus fibrosus of the normal and scoliotic human intervertebral disc. Spine. 2005;30:1815–20.
58. Chen B, Fellenberg J, Wang H, Carstens C, Richter W. Occurrence and regional distribution of apoptosis in scoliotic discs. Spine. 2005;30(5):519–24.
59. Urban MR, Fairbank JCT, Etherington PJ, Loh Lawrence F, Winlove CP, Urban JPG. Electrochemical measurement of transport into scoliotic intervertebral discs invivo using nitrous oxide as a tracer. Spine. 2001;26:984–90.
60. Stokes IA, Spence H, Aronsson DD, Kilmer N. Mechanical modulation of vertebral body growth. Implications for scoliosis progression. Spine. 1996;21:1162–7.
61. Benneker L, Heini P, Anderson S, Alini M, Ito K. Correlation of radiographic and MRI parameters to morphological and biochemical assessment of intervertebral disc degeneration. Eur Spine J. 2005;14:27–35.
62. Ludescher B, Effelsberg J, Martirosian P, Steidle G, Markert B, Claussen C, Schick F. T2- and diffusion-maps reveal diurnal changes of intervertebral disc composition: An in vivo MRI study at 1.5 Tesla. J Magn Reson Imaging. 2008;28:252–7.
63. Osti OL, Fraser RD. MRI and discography of annular tears and intervertebral disc degeneration. A prospective clinical comparison. J Bone Joint Surg Br. 1992;74-B:431 LP–435.
64. Violas P, Estivalezes E, Briot J, Sales de Gauzy J, Swider P. Objective quantification of intervertebral disc volume properties using MRI in idiopathic scoliosis surgery. Magn Reson Imaging. 2007;25:386–91.
65. Gervais J, Périé D, Parent S, Labelle H, Aubin C-E. MRI signal distribution within the intervertebral disc as a biomarker of adolescent idiopathic scoliosis and spondylolisthesis. BMC Musculoskelet Disord. 2012;13:1–10.
66. Hirsch C, Ilharreborde B, Mazda K. EOS suspension test for the assessment of spinal flexibility in adolescent idiopathic scoliosis. Eur Spine J. 2015;24:1408–14.
67. Klepps SJ, Lenke LG, Bridwell KH, Bassett GS, Whorton J. Prospective comparison of flexibility radiographs in adolescent idiopathic scoliosis. Spine. 2001;26:E74–9.
68. Little JP, Adam CJ. The effect of soft tissue properties on spinal flexibility in scoliosis: biomechanical simulation of fulcrum bending. Spine. 2009;34:E76–82.
69. Kakitsubata Y, Theodorou SJ, Theodorou DJ, Nabeshima K, Kakitsubata S, Tamura S. Sonographic characterization of the lumbar intervertebral disk with anatomic correlation and histopathologic findings. J Ultrasound Med. 2005;24:489–99.
70. Naish C, Mitchell R, Innes J, Halliwell M, McNally D. Ultrasound imaging of the intervertebral disc. Spine. 2003;28:107–13.
71. Vergari C, Courtois I, Ebermeyer E, Bouloussa H, Vialle R, Skalli W. Experimental validation of a patient-specific model of orthotic action in adolescent idiopathic scoliosis. Eur Spine J. 2016;25:3049–55.
72. Prot M, Saletti D, Pattofatto S, Bousson V, Laporte S. Links between mechanical behavior of cancellous bone and its microstructural properties under dynamic loading. J Biomech. 2015;48:498–503. https://doi.org/10.1016/j.jbiomech.2014.12.002.
73. Charles YP, Lima LV, Persohn S, Rouch P, Steib JP, Skalli W. Influence of an auxiliary facet system on intervertebral discs and adjacent facet joints. Spine J. 2013;13(10):1293–300.
74. Le Huec JC, Lafage V, Bonnet X, Lavaste F, Josse L, Liu M, Skalli W. Validated finite element analysis of the maverick total disc prosthesis. J Spinal Disord Tech. 2010;23(4):249–57.
75. Villemure I, Aubin CE, Dansereau J, Labelle H. Biomechanical simulations of the spine deformation process in adolescent idiopathic scoliosis from different pathogenesis hypotheses. Eur Spine J. 2004;13:83–90. https://doi.org/10.1007/s00586-003-0565-4.
76. Drevelle X, Lafon Y, Ebermeyer E, Courtois I, Dubousset J, Skalli W. Analysis of idiopathic scoliosis progression by using numerical simulation. Spine (Phila Pa 1976). 2010;35:E407–12.

http://journals.lww.com/spinejournal/Fulltext/2010/05010/Analysis_of_Idiopathic_Scoliosis_Progression_by.21.aspx.
77. Shi L, Wang D, Driscoll M, Villemure I, Chu WC, Cheng JC, Aubin C-E. Biomechanical analysis and modeling of different vertebral growth patterns in adolescent idiopathic scoliosis and healthy subjects. Scoliosis. 2011;6:11. https://doi.org/10.1186/1748-7161-6-11.
78. Nie W-Z, Ye M, Liu Z-D, Wang C-T. The patient-specific brace design and biomechanical analysis of adolescent idiopathic scoliosis. J Biomech Eng. 2009;131:41007. https://doi.org/10.1115/1.3049843.
79. Desbiens-Blais F, Clin J, Parent S, Labelle H, Aubin C-E. New brace design combining CAD/CAM and biomechanical simulation for the treatment of adolescent idiopathic scoliosis. Clin Biomech. 2012;27:999–1005. https://doi.org/10.1016/j.clinbiomech.2012.08.006.
80. Rizza R, Liu X, Thometz J, Tassone C. Comparison of biomechanical behavior between a cast material torso jacket and a polyethylene based jacket. Scoliosis. 2015;10:S15. https://doi.org/10.1186/1748-7161-10-S2-S15.
81. Cobetto N, Aubin CE, Parent S, Clin J, Barchi S, Turgeon I, Labelle H. Effectiveness of braces designed using computer-aided design and manufacturing (CAD/CAM) and finite element simulation compared to CAD/CAM only for the conservative treatment of adolescent idiopathic scoliosis: a prospective randomized controlled trial. Eur Spine J. 2016;25(10):3056–64. https://doi.org/10.1007/s00586-016-4434-3.
82. Vergari C, Ribes G, Aubert B, Adam C, Miladi L, Ilharreborde B, Abelin-Genevois K, Rouch P, Skalli W. Evaluation of a patient-specific finite element model to simulate conservative treatment in adolescent idiopathic scoliosis. Spine Deform. 2015;3:4–11.
83. Little JP, Adam CJ. Geometric sensitivity of patient-specific finite element models of the spine to variability in user-selected anatomical landmarks. Comput Methods Biomech Biomed Engin. 2015;18(6):676–88.
84. Driscoll M, Aubin C-E, Moreau A, Parent S. Biomechanical comparison of fusionless growth modulation corrective techniques in pediatric scoliosis. Med Biol Eng Comput. 2011;49:1437–45. https://doi.org/10.1007/s11517-011-0801-8.
85. Lafon Y, Steib J-P, Skalli W. Intraoperative three dimensional correction during in situ contouring surgery by using a numerical model. Spine (Phila. Pa. 1976). 2010;35:453–9. https://doi.org/10.1097/BRS.0b013e3181b8eaca.
86. Berger S, Marcello O, Schuman S, Schneider J, Studer D, Hasler C, Zheng G, Büchler P. Patient-specific spinal stiffness in AIS: a preoperative and noninvasive method. Eur Spine J. 2015;24:249–55. https://doi.org/10.1007/s00586-014-3623-1.
87. Lafon Y, Lafage V, Dubousset J, Skalli W. Intraoperative three-dimensional correction during rod rotation technique. Spine (Phila Pa 1976). 2009;34:512–9. https://doi.org/10.1097/BRS.0b013e31819413ec.

Chapter 5
Biochemistry of Idiopathic Scoliosis: From Discovery to Diagnostic Biomarkers

Dina Nada and Alain Moreau

5.1 Introduction

Idiopathic scoliosis (IS) is a deformation of the spine, with an unknown cause or etiology [1]. Scoliosis has been predominantly observed in females during puberty and affects 1 to 4% of children. Nearly 80% of idiopathic scoliosis is in the form of adolescent idiopathic scoliosis (AIS) [1, 2]. Research into the causes of IS have unearthed evidence for potential biomarkers [1]. Until now, the diagnosis of IS relies solely on the measurement of the Cobb angle of the spinal curvature. A scoliosis diagnosis is given, when the value of the Cobb angle is ≥10°. However, physicians arrive at this diagnosis only after ruling out all other possible disorders [3]. Prior to the progression of the spinal curvature, it would be useful to identify markers in the body that could indicate the future onset or the progression of IS. In this chapter, we will cover the current research data on the biochemical factors

D. Nada, M.Sc
Viscogliosi Laboratory in Molecular Genetics of Musculoskeletal Diseases, Sainte-Justine University Hospital Research Center, Montreal, QC, Canada

Faculty of Medicine, Department of Biomedical Sciences, Université de Montréal, Montreal, QC, Canada

A. Moreau, Ph.D. (✉)
Faculty of Dentistry, Department of Stomatology, Université de Montréal, Montreal, QC, Canada

Faculty of Medicine, Department of Biochemistry and Molecular Medicine, Université de Montréal, Montreal, QC, Canada

Viscogliosi Laboratory in Molecular Genetics of Musculoskeletal Diseases, Sainte-Justine University Hospital Research Center, Montreal, QC, Canada

Faculty of Medicine, Department of Biomedical Sciences, Université de Montréal, Montreal, QC, Canada
e-mail: alain.moreau@recherche-ste-justine.qc.ca

M. Machida et al. (eds.), *Pathogenesis of Idiopathic Scoliosis*,
https://doi.org/10.1007/978-4-431-56541-3_5

associated with IS. We have classified the biomarkers into four main groups: hormones, systemic factors, hematological factors, and bone metabolism factors. Studies that cover all the key aspects of these factors have been included. Hence, gene association studies, protein function analyses, and protein interactions have been recorded. We will discuss the validity of the studies as well as the contradictory data for each factor. Through this process, we will understand the potential role of each factor in the pathogenesis of IS. We will also elaborate on the hypotheses associated with the biochemical factors and their potential relevance in the pathogenesis of IS.

5.2 Biochemical Factors

5.2.1 Hormonal Factors

5.2.1.1 Growth Hormone

The vast majority of IS cases occur during adolescence as the pubertal growth spurt occurs. The association of abnormal growth patterns with the development of scoliotic curves is well known [4]. A number of studies have confirmed that adolescent idiopathic scoliosis (AIS) patients are generally taller than age-matched controls [5, 6]. A study that involved 598 IS patients compared their growth patterns as well as other anthropometric parameters to those of normal controls at both the prepubertal and the postpubertal stages [7]. Prior to puberty, the length of the different body segments was significantly shorter in the IS patients compared with the normal controls. In contrast, following puberty, the length of the different body segments was significantly longer in the IS patients, and all the anthropometric parameters were greatly associated with the severity of the curve. This indicated that the abnormality in the growth rate of IS patients is specifically associated with the pubertal stage. The abnormal growth pattern in IS patients was further confirmed by another study that included 611 IS girls and 296 age-matched controls [8]. The study observed that the severe cases of spinal curve progression displayed late menarche and higher skeletal growth rates between the ages of 12 and 16 years.

Growth hormone (GH) is the hormone responsible for growth stimulation. The correlation of GH with IS has been studied since the 1970s, where Willner et al. observed significantly higher plasma levels of GH in IS girls compared with age-matched controls [9]. It has been shown that treatment with GHs could lead to scoliosis [10]. However, this observation was contradicted by other studies [11], and the results of other stimulating tests were inconclusive [9]. Later, Willner's group reported an increase in the morning fasting levels of the growth hormone in IS girls compared with the healthy controls [12]. Another study that compared the GH profile of scoliotic girls with matched controls over a 24-h period showed that only scoliotic girls exhibited higher levels of the hormone in the early stages of puberty, suggesting an early growth spurt in IS girls [13].

A genetic study that involved 30 IS patients and 30 matched controls identified a single nucleotide polymorphism (SNP) in the GH receptor gene as a predisposing factor to IS [14]. This was, however, contradicted by a large study of 510 IS patients and 363 controls, which investigated the GH receptor and found no association of GH receptor variants with IS [15].

Growth hormone itself is very variable and hard to assess, but its activity is correlated with insulin-like growth factor-1 (IGF-1), which in turn is associated with puberty [16, 17]. Insulin-like growth factor is known to play an important role in bone growth. One study suggested increased levels of IGF-1 and estrogen in IS patients after they achieved a growth spurt and recorded the maximum growth rate [18]. Another study demonstrated that IGF-1 and IGF binding protein-3 (IGFBP-3) were significantly associated with an accelerated rate of spinal curve progression in females with IS [19]. Yeung et al. studied two SNPs (rs5742612 and rs2288377) in the *IGF-1* promoter in a Chinese cohort of 506 IS girls and 227 healthy girls. They observed that the two SNPs affected the progression of the spinal curve but did not initiate or predispose individuals to IS [20]. Similarly, a Korean study reported an association between a SNP upstream of *IGF-1*, rs5742612, and the onset and progression of IS [21]. However, other studies failed to find any association between IGF-1 and IS. One study observed that SNPs found in the GH receptor and *IGF-1* were not associated with IS in a Han Chinese population [22]. This was confirmed by another report that failed to find an association between *IGF-1* and IS in a Japanese population [23]. Liu et al. reported in a study of 200 patients and 200 controls that SNPs in *IGF-1R* were not associated with either IS susceptibility or the severity of curve progression [24]. This conflict between different reports may warrant additional large-scale genetic studies that have sufficient statistical power, in different populations to validate the involvement of *IGF-1* and its receptor genes in IS.

5.2.1.2 Estrogens

The occurrence of scoliosis in females is almost double that of males, and this ratio reaches 10:1 for Cobb angles ≥30° [25]. Considering the high prevalence of this disorder in females and the concurrent onset of scoliosis with sexual maturation, it is plausible to hypothesize the involvement of estrogen and/or its receptors in the pathophysiology of the disease. Indeed, some studies report that estrogens and estrogen antagonists have a direct effect on the onset of scoliosis [26, 27]. Estrogen is critical for puberty [28]. Some researchers have studied blood estrogen levels in IS, but their results are inconclusive. Kulis et al. reported a reduction of plasma estrogen levels in females with scoliosis [29]. This was supported by another study that demonstrated lower average estrogen and progesterone levels in IS females compared with healthy controls of the same age [30]. It was also reported that low levels of estrogen increase the susceptibility of ballet dancers to scoliosis [31]. It was suggested that the effect of estrogen on IS was not due to its concentration but due to its interaction with target cells [32], specifically bone cells [33]. Interestingly, one study reported that there were elevated levels of testosterone in IS girls relative to age-matched controls [34].

As mentioned earlier, most IS cases occur at puberty. This stage involves significant bone remodeling [35]. The involvement of estrogen in bone remodeling is well known [36]. Estrogen plays a role in the formation of bones; it enhances the activity of alkaline phosphatase, the synthesis of collagen, and the deposition of calcium in the extracellular matrix [37]. It also affects bone growth, maturation, and turnover. Reduced estrogen levels lead to a reduced differentiation of osteoblasts, which affects both bone mineralization and its mechanical properties [32]. Estrogen plays a role in bone metabolism by affecting both bone cell types: osteoblasts and osteoclasts [38]. Additionally, estrogen affects the secretion of cytokines needed for the formation of osteoclasts [39] and inhibits IL-6 cytokine, which enhances bone resorption and activates osteoclasts [32].

The association between osteopenia and IS is widely recognized [40], but it has been mainly demonstrated in different Asian pediatric populations. It has been reported by many researchers that osteopenia occurs at a high frequency in IS [41, 42]. Moreover, osteopenia or osteoporosis has been shown to be involved in the progression of the spinal curvature [42]. A persistent lower bone mineral density was reported in IS patients compared with healthy controls [43]. The severity of scoliosis has been inversely correlated with bone mineral density and bone mineral content [44]. Defects in estrogen function or reduced estrogen levels should be taken into account as driving factors for osteopenia and reduced bone mineralization in IS girls [32].

Letellier et al. demonstrated the important role of estrogen in the functioning of osteoblasts. The interaction between estrogen and melatonin hormones and their subsequent effect on osteoblasts were established [33]. The involvement of melatonin in the pathogenesis of IS has been thoroughly investigated and will be discussed in detail later. Briefly, melatonin exerts its functions through Gi protein-coupled receptors with the subsequent inhibition of cAMP. The occurrence of a differential melatonin signaling dysfunction in the osteoblasts isolated from IS patients resulted in an intracellular elevation of cAMP levels [45]. In a certain subset of IS patients, this effect was due to a switch in the coupling of melatonin receptors from Gi to Gs [33]. Interestingly, osteoblasts obtained from this IS subgroup and treated with 17β-estradiol together with melatonin resulted in a significant reduction of cAMP levels compared with melatonin treatment alone. These results can be explained by the fact that Gi proteins are also known to be regulated by estrogen activity [46]. Indeed, exposure to 17β-estradiol is known to decrease Gi, Gs and Gq alpha subunit expression.

The interaction of estrogen with the melatonin signaling pathway was supported by the works from Acaroglu's group [47]. In this study, they treated melatonin-deficient mice models that were rendered bipedal, with both tamoxifen and raloxifene, which are selective estrogen receptor modulators (SERM) and have estrogen agonistic effects. Treatment of mice with tamoxifen or raloxifene did not prevent the occurrence of scoliosis but interfered with the aggravation of the scoliotic curves. Previous studies have shown the effectiveness of tamoxifen in reducing the severity of scoliotic curves in experimental mice models [48]. However, it is unclear whether tamoxifen's effects were solely due to its role as estrogen agonist or through off-target effects, since tamoxifen also acts as a nonspecific calmodulin inhibitor [49], where calmodulin was previously implicated in scoliosis severity [50, 51].

Estrogen stimulates the maturation of the physis, which leads to a linear growth spurt [28, 52, 53]. This action is mediated through its receptors, estrogen receptor α (ERα) and estrogen receptor β (ERβ), which are expressed in the growth plate [54]. At low levels, estrogen stimulates growth by enhancing the secretion of GH, while at high levels, estrogen interferes with GH secretion and subsequently terminates longitudinal growth [32]. This interplay with GH could affect patients with IS, who are known to be taller than healthy subjects of the same age.

Polymorphisms in the gene encoding ERα (*ESR1*) were shown to be associated with bone mineral density, a factor which is known to be abnormal in many IS cases [55]. Skeletal abnormalities have been shown to be associated with mutations in both *ESR1* and *CYP19* [56, 57]. The *CYP19* encodes the aromatase enzyme involved in estrogen synthesis. During the last decade, there has been extensive research on the polymorphisms of genes encoding estrogen receptors, in an effort to detect a genetic correlation between these receptors and IS. However, there is a high discrepancy among published studies, and this genetic correlation remains debated. A summary of these studies is presented in Table 5.1.

Table 5.1 Summary of the genetic studies performed on ERs and their correlation to IS

Reference	Study	Conclusions
Inoue et al. [59]	SNPs PvuII and XbaI in *ERα* were studied in 304 IS girls	An association between the SNP XbaI and curve progression was observed
Wu et al. [60]	The polymorphism XbaI in *ERα* was studied in 202 IS patients and 174 controls	This SNP was shown to be correlated with IS susceptibility
Tang et al. [61]	SNPs PvuII and XbaI in *ERα* were studied in a Chinese cohort of 540 IS patients and 260 controls	The two SNPs did not show any correlation with IS or its severity
Zhang et al. [62]	Polymorphism in the exon ØK of *ERβ* was studied in 218 IS patients and 140 controls	The studied polymorphism appeared to be correlated with IS predisposition and severity of the curves
Esposito et al. [30]	Detected four SNPs in the exons that encode the steroid-binding domain and two SNPs in the exons that encode the transactivation domain of *ERα*	Association with clinical manifestations of IS patients
Zhao et al. [63]	rs2234693 (PvuII) and rs9340799 (XbaI) in *ERα* were studied in 67 Chinese IS patients and 100 controls	rs2234693 (PvuII) was found to be associated with the double curve pattern, the thoracic curve, and the severity of IS
Takahashi et al. [64]	rs9340799 and rs1256120 in the estrogen receptor genes were studied in a Japanese cohort of 798 IS patients and 637 controls	Neither of the two SNPs was found to be associated with either susceptibility or progression of IS

(continued)

Table 5.1 (continued)

Reference	Study	Conclusions
Xu et al. [65]	SNPs in the *ERα* and *ERβ* together with other genes were tested as to whether they can be used as markers for predicting the outcome of brace treatment. This study included 312 IS patients	rs9340799 in *ERα* appeared to play a role in predicting the efficiency of brace treatment
Peng et al. [66]	16 SNPs in the G protein-coupled estrogen receptor 1 (*GPER1*) were studied in a total of 389 IS patients and 338 controls	Three SNPs (rs3808351, rs10269151, and rs426655s3) were found to be associated with curve progression in IS patients
Ogura et al. [67]	rs3808351, rs10269151, and rs4266553 in the G protein-coupled estrogen receptor (*GPER)* were studied in a Japanese cohort of 2117 IS patients	No association was observed between the studied SNPs and curve progression severity
Janusz et al. [68]	rs9340799 (XbaI) and rs2234693 (PvuII) in the *ERα* were studied in 287 Caucasian IS females and 182 controls	No association was found between either of the studied SNPs and severity of IS
Yang et al. [69]	This meta-analysis includes the results of six previous articles that studied the polymorphisms XbaI and PvuII in *ERα*	No association between the studied SNPs and IS
Chen et al. [70]	This meta-analysis included the results of four previous studies that studied the SNP rs9340799 of *ERα*	No association between the studied SNP and predisposition to IS
Kotwicki et al. [71]	rs1256120, rs4986938, and rs1256049 in *ERβ* were studied in 248 Caucasian IS females and 243 controls	None of the studied SNPs showed association with IS susceptibility
Janusz et al. [72]	rs9340799 (XbaI) and rs2234693 (PvuII) in *ERα* and rs4986938 (AluI) and rs1256049 (RasI) in *ERβ* were studied in 208 IS Caucasian females to test their association with age at menarche	None of the studied SNPs showed any association with age at menarche

There has been an extended effort by Fendri et al. to uncover the role of estrogen in IS. Osteoblasts from IS patients were treated with estrogen, and studied by microarray analysis. Fendri et al. identified a list of genes that were differentially expressed in IS cells compared to healthy control cells. Some of the genes are regulated by estrogen [58]. In general, it has been suggested that estrogens may not be involved in the etiology of IS but may play an important role in the progression or even the repression of the disease [32]. This is due to the interaction of estrogen with many factors that are involved in the etiopathogenesis of IS, bone modeling and remodeling, osteopenia, growth factors, the melatonin signaling pathway, and platelet regulatory factors (e.g., calmodulin that is discussed below) [32].

5.2.1.3 Leptin

Leptin is a hormone produced by adipose cells and plays a role in regulating the energy balance. Leptin also plays an important function in bone metabolism. Due to its role in the cross talk between energy and bone metabolism, it was hypothesized that it is most likely involved in the pathogenesis of scoliosis. Reduced leptin serum levels in IS patients are reported in many studies and are associated with a reduced bone mass [73–75], reduced bone strength [76], and abnormal growth parameters [75]. Moreover, the levels of sOB-R (soluble leptin receptor) are shown to be elevated in IS patients compared with controls [73, 74], which reflects an abnormal bioavailability of leptin and leptin signaling malfunction. This abnormal signaling was also described in a report where the osteoblasts of IS patients were significantly less responsive to leptin when compared with those of controls [77]. It was suggested that reduced serum leptin levels may be a result of the reduced ability of adipogenesis in IS [78].

A double neuro-osseous theory was proposed to explain the role of leptin in the pathogenesis of scoliosis [79]. This theory states that there is a distinct contribution of the autonomic as well as the somatic nervous systems to the development of IS. In the autonomic nervous system, due to the enhanced sensitivity of the hypothalamus to circulating leptin levels, the sympathetic nervous system causes a dissymmetry of the axial skeleton during growth, affecting the width of the trunk. That effect is enforced by the somatotropic (IGF/growth hormone) axis. In the somatic nervous system, spinal deformities may also be induced by a dysfunction in the postural mechanism. The postural mechanisms of the trunk and the spine are affected by the somatic nervous system [79].

On the other hand, other researchers suggest that the reduced levels of circulating leptin may result from a larger metabolic defect. It has been shown that melatonin signaling can lead to a reduction in the levels of leptin [80], where another study showed that the levels of leptin are reduced in pinealectomized rats and are elevated with melatonin administration [81]. It has also been shown that cytosolic cAMP inhibits leptin synthesis [82]. This finding is further strengthened by the fact that there is a generalized Gi signaling dysfunction in IS patients, which leads to the accumulation of cAMP [45, 83, 84]. Together these findings can help explain the reduced circulating levels of leptin that are observed in IS patients.

5.2.1.4 Ghrelin

Ghrelin is another hormone that plays a role in regulating energy as well as hunger. The ghrelin hormone is secreted by the ghrelin cells in the gastrointestinal tract [85]. Ghrelin also plays a role in bone metabolism [86]. The involvement of ghrelin in the pathogenesis of IS has recently been suggested. A study reported high circulating levels of ghrelin in IS patients compared with healthy subjects. The data of the study hypothesized the involvement of ghrelin in the pathophysiology of IS [87].

5.2.1.5 Melatonin

Melatonin is a hormone produced mostly by the pineal gland. It mainly functions in the regulation of the circadian rhythm and in the treatment of some sleep disorders. It plays a role in reproduction, aging, some cancers, and bone metabolism. It is also a potent antioxidant that helps in the protection of DNA. Melatonin is produced as a response to darkness and is inhibited by light. Upon the onset of darkness, the receptors of the retina secrete norepinephrine that increases the number of adrenergic receptors of the pineal gland. This stimulates the activity of the enzyme arylalkylamine *N*-acetyltransferase (AANAT), the key regulator of melatonin synthesis from tryptophan [88, 89]. Melatonin is mainly metabolized in the liver producing 6-sulfatoxymelatonin that is excreted in the urine. The level of 6-sulfatoxymelatonin in the urine correlates with serum melatonin levels [89]. Melatonin has two groups of receptors: melatonin receptor 1 (ML1) (high affinity) and melatonin receptor 2 (ML2) (low affinity) [90]. There are two subtypes of ML1 receptors known as melatonin receptor 1A (MTNR1A) and melatonin receptor 1B (MTNR1B) [91, 92]. Both receptors are Gi protein-coupled receptors that inhibit adenylate cyclase activity [89].

Pinealectomized animal models have been proposed as good models to study IS. In the late 1950s and early 1960s, Thillard et al. were the first to provide evidence on the development of deformities in the vertebral column in chickens by pinealectomy [93]. This was followed by the work of Dubousset et al. in the early 1980s, where scoliosis was induced in young chickens by provoking pineal and diencephalic damage [94]. This field of research was strongly supported thereafter by the work of Machida et al. The group of Machida et al. showed that if pinealectomy is performed shortly after hatching, chickens will consistently develop scoliosis similar to that in human IS. Moreover, these researchers showed that scoliosis could be prevented by intramuscular implantation of the pineal body in pinealectomized chickens [95]. They suggested that melatonin deficiency plays a role in the abnormal development of the asymmetry of the proprioceptive system, including the spine and the paraspinal muscles [96]. They then demonstrated that treating pinealectomized chickens with serotonin, the precursor of melatonin, leads to the development of scoliosis in 73.3% of the chickens, while treatment with melatonin leads to the development of scoliosis in only 20% of the chickens [96]. The ineffectiveness of serotonin to prevent scoliosis could be explained by the fact that serotonin is unable to cross the blood-brain barrier [97]. Thus, a precursor of serotonin, 5-hydroxytryptophan, which has the ability to cross the blood-brain barrier, was found to be more effective in scoliosis prevention in the chickens [98]. Machida et al. were also able to reinforce their findings by demonstrating that not only chickens, but bipedal pinealectomized rats developed scoliosis as well [99]. Moreover, the same group was able to demonstrate scoliosis in C57BL/6 mice (a strain of mice genetically deficient in melatonin), that were rendered bipedal [100]. Machida et al. also suggested that a melatonin deficiency has an effect on the prognosis of IS [101]. Bagnall et al. reinforced the observations of Machida et al. by demonstrating that the development of scoliosis in pinealectomized chickens is not a consequence of the surgical procedure [102].

However, the work of Machida et al. was later contradicted by data of other research groups [103–107]. The development of scoliosis in all pinealectomized chickens could not be reproduced in subsequent studies. Instead, the frequency of scoliosis was found to range from 50% to 60% [103, 104, 107]. Consistently, similar results were obtained in C57BL/6 mice and rat studies [48, 108]. The results then failed to be reproduced in primates, in a 2-year study using 18 pinealectomized monkeys, where none of the primated developed scoliosis, in the absence of circulating melatonin [109]. This raised the question of the appropriateness of using avian species and rodents as models for human idiopathic scoliosis. Furthermore, experiments that attempted to administer melatonin or transplant the pineal gland to inhibit the occurrence of scoliosis in chickens were unsuccessful [105, 106]. This conflict of data extended to human studies, where researchers disagreed with Machida's group [110, 111]. One of the studies observed elevated serum melatonin levels in IS patients in the early stage of the disease when compared with matched controls [111]. Additionally, the only way to mimic pinealectomized animal studies in humans was to examine patients who have pineal gland dysfunction, such as tumors or lesions [112]. In a study that included children with pineal lesions, only 2 out of 48 had scoliosis [113].

As a result, the hypothesis that melatonin deficiency produces scoliosis is not convincing. Yet, it is still accepted that melatonin does have a significant role in the pathogenesis of IS.

Qiu et al. studied the mRNA expression of melatonin receptors MTNR1A and MTNR1B in the paravertebral muscles of patients with IS, congenital scoliosis, and controls. They observed higher expression of MTNR1B mRNA on the concave side of the paravertebral muscle than on the convex side in IS patients, wheras no difference in expression of MTNR1A between both sides was observed [114]. They explained this asymmetry as a secondary effect. The expression of melatonin receptors in the osteoblasts of IS patients was also studied [115]. There was a reduced expression of MTNR1B receptors at the mRNA level and the protein level in those patients when compared with controls. This abnormal expression was associated with an abnormally long arm span.

The genetic regulation of melatonin synthesis and receptors in IS was also studied. Genetic association studies have been conducted on *TPH1* (tryptophan hydroxylase-1) and *AANAT* (arylalkylamine N-acetyltransferase), the two main enzymes involved in the biosynthesis of melatonin. Only polymorphisms in *TPH1* were found to be associated with the incidence of IS [116]. Qiu et al. studied the genetic association of the two melatonin receptors: *MTNR1A* and *MTNR1B*. They observed that a polymorphism in the promoter of *MTNR1B* is associated with IS [117], while no association was detected for *MTNR1A* [118]. However, these results were contradicted thereafter, by another meta-analysis study that reanalyzed *MTNR1B* polymorphisms and their correlation to IS in the collective data of 5 studies, consisting of 2395 IS cases and 3645 controls. They found no association in both the Asian and Caucasian populations [119].

Moreau et al. suggested the possibility of the involvement of a defect in the melatonin signaling pathway in the pathogenesis of scoliosis [45]. This will be discussed in detail in the following section on Gi proteins. The hypothesis of the presence of an abnormal melatonin signaling pathway was confirmed by the work of Wang et al. This group demonstrated that there was no effect of melatonin on the proliferation and differentiation of growth plate chondrocytes of IS patients as opposed to normal cells, indicating a melatonin signaling impairment [120]. This effect was suggested to be correlated with a defect in endochondral ossification in IS patients.

5.2.2 *Systemic Factors*

5.2.2.1 G Inhibitory Proteins

G proteins are a family of guanine nucleotide-binding proteins that play a role in signal transduction of another big family of membrane receptors known as GPCRs (G protein-coupled receptors). They act as molecular switches that help transmit signals from external stimuli to cells. G proteins are classified as monomeric small GTPases and heterotrimeric G proteins. The latter consist of three subunits: alpha (α), beta (β), and gamma (γ) [121]. The heterotrimeric G proteins are classified according to their subunits, Gαi/o (Gi), Gαs, Gαq, and Gα12/13. The G inhibitory (Gi) proteins have three different isoforms Gi1, Gi2, and Gi3. When an external stimulus interacts with one of the GPCRs, G proteins are activated and initiate a series of signaling events that ends with an altered cellular function. Cyclic adenosine monophosphate (cAMP) is a second messenger involved in these signaling events. When Gi proteins are activated, the formation of cAMP is normally inhibited. Gi proteins inhibit adenylate cyclases (AC) that catalyze the conversion of ATP (adenosine triphosphate) to cAMP and thus inhibit the intracellular accumulation of cAMP [122].

We previously mentioned that Moreau et al. suggested the role of a defect in the melatonin signaling pathway in the pathogenesis of IS. This group studied the effect of melatonin on osteoblasts isolated from IS patients. Owing to the fact that melatonin receptors are GPCRs that are preferentially conjugated to Gi proteins, they should be able to naturally prevent the accumulation of cAMP. In this study, it was demonstrated that melatonin failed to inhibit the accumulation of cAMP in all the osteoblasts isolated from IS patients compared with controls [45]. It is hypothesized that there is a defect in the downstream melatonin signaling pathway that may involve posttranslational modifications of Gi proteins. In another study that focused on Gi proteins, Azeddine et al. suggested an increased phosphorylation of serine residues in the Gi proteins in IS cells. This pointed to distinct protein-protein interactions that include those between MTNR1B melatonin receptors and PKC delta (protein kinase C delta) or the receptor for activated protein C kinase 1 and PKC delta [83]. In addition, this group was able to classify IS patients into three distinct groups based on their cellular response to melatonin [45, 83]. The same authors confirmed their findings by performing a cell-based screening test using the cellular dielectric spectroscopy technique which allows to measure the cellular response to Gi protein stimulation directly [123]. In their study, they confirmed their previous findings by obtaining the same patterns of reduced responses of IS cells to both melatonin and its derivative iodomelatonin. This indicates that Gi protein hypofunctionality is the key factor causing the observed defect in the melatonin signal transduction pathway [84]. The evidence to classify IS patients into three functional groups according to their differential responses to melatonin was also verified [84].

The same group further reported similar responses in different cell types isolated from IS patients, as observed with melatonin. They used osteoblasts, skeletal myoblasts, and PBMCs (peripheral blood mononuclear cells) from the same set of IS patients and controls. They concluded that the Gi protein hypofunctionality was not restricted to downstream melatonin receptors, but was in fact a generalized and systemic impairment of Gi protein-mediated receptor signaling. All IS cells showed a reduction in Gi-coupled receptor signaling, but to three different extents, which confirmed their previous classification into three functional groups or biological endophenotypes (FG1, FG2, and FG3) [84, 124]. They further studied the cause of this differential hypofunctionality and found distinctive phosphorylation patterns occurring at the serine residues of the Gi protein isoforms. Unlike the phenotypic variations that are observed in the measurement and site of the spinal curve in scoliotic patients, endophenotypes represent a conserved heritable trait. These endophenotypes can be used to stratify patients and serve as clinical prognostic indicators, which can be associated with the molecular signatures of a condition [125]. It has been observed that severe cases of IS individuals account for 60% of the FG2 endophenotype in the French-Canadian population, indicating an association with high risk of severe scoliosis in such individuals. In contrast, only 13% and 27% of IS individuals with the FG1 and FG3 endophenotypes respectively, have severe scoliosis [125].

Owing to the fact that Gi proteins are spread throughout the body in many different types of tissues, and act as an adaptor for different stimuli, molecules, hormones, and peptides to perform their function, Gi protein hypofunctionality thus represents a systemic defect, that would explain the larger picture of metabolic abnormalities in IS, rather than restricting them to a few molecules. For example, Alonso-Vale et al. showed that cAMP was able to inhibit leptin synthesis [82]. Therefore, the diminution of leptin, which has been documented in IS, may be correlated with the previously reported Gi signaling abnormality [45, 83, 84].

Additionally, the biggest challenge in studying IS is the complex nature of the disease and the high level of genotypic and phenotypic heterogeneity. The use of endophenotypes improves the stratification of IS patients at a molecular level since molecular signatures may be utilized to predict the risk of development of the condition or any associated symptoms.

5.2.2.2 Osteopontin

Osteopontin (OPN) is a multifunctional glycoprotein expressed by many different cell types and occurs throughout most of the biological systems in the body. OPN can exist either as a cytokine, which is expressed in all body fluids or as an extracellular matrix protein in mineralized tissues [126]. It has a wide variety of biological functions in both normal and pathological conditions [127–130].

Moreau's group previously reported high circulating plasma levels of OPN in patients with IS, which was associated with curve severity [131]. They further analyzed the role of OPN in scoliosis. They used C57BL/6 mice, a well-established model for studying scoliosis, which normally develop spinal deformities at a rate of approximately 60% following 40 weeks of bipedal ambulation, as previously mentioned [132]. They observed that the genetic depletion of OPN prevented spinal deformation in these mice [131] and enhanced the response to GiPCR stimulation in their osteoblasts [124].

The involvement of OPN in the pathogenesis of scoliosis was further supported by Yadav et al. who showed that OPN plasma levels were increased and the expression was enhanced in the vertebrae of Phospho1 KO (knockout) mice. Increased levels of OPN were associated with scoliosis and other skeletal abnormalities [133]. Furthermore, when OPN was genetically depleted from these mice, an improvement in their skeletal phenotype was observed. More evidence was provided by a recent study that investigated the involvement of OPN in the susceptibility and progression of scoliosis [134]. They used a new mouse model C3H/HeJ with elevated levels of OPN. The mice were divided into three groups: the first group was rendered bipedal and was treated with OPN; the second group was also rendered bipedal but treated with saline; and the third group was kept quadrupedal and treated with saline to serve as a control. 92.5% of the first group developed scoliosis with an average Cobb angle of 29.8°, 52.5% of the second group developed scoliosis with an average Cobb angle of 20.9°, while in the third group, 12% developed scoliosis with an average Cobb angle of 17.5°. Hence, we can conclude that there is consistent evidence for the potential involvement of OPN in the onset and progression of scoliosis.

5.2.3 Hematological factors (Platelet Regulatory Factors)

5.2.3.1 Calmodulin

Calmodulin (CaM—calcium modulated) is a protein that binds to calcium and acts as a messenger that transmits calcium signals and hence regulates the function of different enzymes [135, 136]. It plays a role in the contraction of muscles and platelets through calcium that regulates the interaction of actin and myosin. Since the early 1980s, a number of anomalies in platelets, calmodulin, and Ca transport in IS have been documented in the literature.

Elevated levels of intracellular phosphorus and calcium in platelets together with a defective structure of myosin chains [137, 138], reduction in the ATPase activity in the cytosol suggesting a dysfunctional calcium transport system [137], reduction in the functionality of the contractile system inside the cell [139], as well as a reduction in the aggregation of platelets [140] in IS patients have been reported. Another report demonstrated aberrant platelet maturation in IS patients and found differential expression of various Ca^{2+} ATPases in different groups of patients with different curve patterns [141]. These findings were challenged by two reports that demonstrated normal platelet behavior with respect to the different parameters that were previously studied [142, 143].

Platelet calmodulin levels were elevated in association to curve progression, while calmodulin levels in stabilized moderate curves and controls were similar [50]. These results were confirmed by another longitudinal study that followed calmodulin levels over time and demonstrated that there were elevated calmodulin levels in cases of curve progression, while levels did not change in stable cases [51]. Moreover, double-curved and severe cases showed higher levels of calmodulin than moderate cases. These levels were reduced in most cases following brace treatment or surgical intervention, which suggested calmodulin to be a potential biomarker for curve progression [51]. A Chinese group measured the protein expression levels of calmodulin in the paravertebral muscles of the curve apex of IS patients and observed significantly lower expression on the convex side compared with the concave side or normal muscles [144]. The asymmetric distribution of calmodulin in paravertebral muscles was also shown. However, in contrast, when the protein levels on the convex side were higher than the concave side of the scoliotic curve, there was no difference in the concentration of calmodulin in the platelets compared with the controls [145].

During the past few years, many genetic studies were performed to detect a genetic association between *CALM1* (the gene encoding for calmodulin) and IS. A study that involved 30 IS Chinese patients and 30 matched controls suggested a genetic correlation of a SNP in the promoter of *CALM1* and a predisposition to IS [14]. Another study that included 100 Chinese IS patients and 100 matched controls showed that different SNPs in *CALM1* may be correlated with different curve patterns. For example, *CALM1* rs12885713 was associated with double curves and lumbar curves, while rs5871 was associated with thoracic curves [146]. These findings were supported by another Chinese study involving 67 IS patients and 100 matched controls, where they confirmed the association of rs12885713 with double-curved cases and the association of rs5871with thoracic curve cases [63]. Recently, a Chinese study on 146 IS patients and 146 controls reported an association between three SNPs in *CALM1* (rs2300496, rs2300500, and rs3231718) and IS susceptibility [147]. None of the 12 studied SNPs were correlated with the severity of curve progression.

Akel et al. analyzed the effect of calmodulin antagonists, tamoxifen and trifluoperazine, on the onset and progression of scoliosis in experimental animal models. In the first study performed on pinealectomized chickens, both compounds were effective in preventing the deformity; tamoxifen was also effective in reducing the progression of the curve [49]. In the second study, C57BL/6 mice were used to confirm the efficiency of calmodulin antagonists in preventing scoliotic deformities [48]. It should be mentioned here that tamoxifen has an estrogen agonistic effect as well, and its action may be due to that effect.

As we previously mentioned, melatonin's involvement in IS is widely accepted since most of the pinealectomized and bipedal animal models develop scoliosis due to fluctuations in melatonin levels or a dysfunction in its signaling pathway. The interplay between melatonin and calmodulin is quite complex. It has been suggested that calmodulin is involved in regulating melatonin synthesis through adenylyl cyclases [148]. Melatonin also affects the activity of calmodulin by inhibiting calmodulin kinase II [149]. Moreover, downstream melatonin PKCα (protein kinase Cα) is activated, which induces calmodulin phosphorylation and subsequent inhibition [149]. Melatonin and calmodulin directly interact with each other, and melatonin exerts most of its effects through this interaction [149, 150]. As previously mentioned, calmodulin plays a role in regulating the contractile system in muscles and platelets. It was suggested that calmodulin may be involved in regulating the contractile proteins of the spinal cord as well, thus affecting the growth of neural cells [151]. This may correlate with the hypothesis that there is an imbalance in the growth of the spinal cord and the vertebrae, which may lead to the deformity observed in scoliosis [151]. The role of melatonin as a free radical scavenger is important in this hypothesis. If melatonin fails to combat the free radicals produced during stretching, damage to neural cells is probable, and consequently growth of the spinal cord will be affected [37, 151].

In summary, calmodulin is a potential modifying factor in IS. Calmodulin is not only involved in a cross talk with melatonin, but also plays a regulatory role in the contractile system of muscles and consequently the paraspinal muscle tone and spinal cord contractile system. This is in addition to the regulation of Ca^{2+} transport. It has been hypothesized that there may be a generalized defect in the calcium pump of scoliotic patients [151].

5.2.4 Bone Metabolism Factors

5.2.4.1 Receptor Activator of Nuclear Factor Kappa-B Ligand (RANKL)

Receptor activator of nuclear factor kappa-B ligand (RANKL) is also known as osteoprotegerin ligand (OPGL) or osteoclast differentiation factor (ODF). The protein RANKL is a member of the tumor necrosis factor (TNF) superfamily. It is well known that RANKL plays an important role in controlling bone resorption and remodeling [152]. The RANKL/RANK interaction induces the formation of osteoclasts from their precursor cells, maintains their survival, and helps in the activation of osteoclasts. Osteoprotegerin (OPG) hinders bone resorption by binding to RANKL and thus inhibiting its binding to RANK. Hence, the RANKL/OPG ratio is an important parameter which reflects bone quality [152].

The presence of osteopenia and reduced bone mass in the axial and peripheral skeleton of IS patients have been consistently reported. A number of researchers have thus studied the interrelationship between low bone mineral density (BMD) and its determinants in IS [153–155]. Suh et al. [153] reported an elevation of serum RANKL and the RANKL/OPG ratio, along with reduced BMD in 72 IS patients compared with 64 matched controls. This was later confirmed by a study which demonstrated higher levels of RANKL in both pre- and post-menarcheal girls with IS, when compared with corresponding control groups [156]. Another study involving 15 IS patients and 8 matched controls reported a significant elevation in the levels of RANKL and an imbalance in the RANKL/OPG ratio, suggesting that this imbalance plays a role in bone remodeling [157]. In agreement with these findings, Zhou et al. showed an elevation of both mRNA and protein levels of RANKL and an increased RANKL/OPG ratio in osteoblasts from 20 IS patients with low BMD, compared with 8 age-matched controls [155]. An association between a polymorphism in the OPG gene and LSBMD (lumbar spine BMD) in IS girls was also reported [154]. Lu et al. suggested that anti-osteoporotic treatments could effectively restore bone strength as well as the balance of the OPG/RANK/RANKL system [158].

5.2.4.2 Osteocalcin (OC)

Osteocalcin (OC, or bone gamma-carboxyglutamic acid protein, BGLAP) is a non-collagenous protein present in mineralized tissues. It is a hormone that is secreted by osteoblasts, odontoblasts and hypertrophic chondrocytes [159]. Osteocalcin is an important biochemical marker for bone formation in the case of uncoupled bone formation and resorption. In addition, osteocalcin is a marker for bone turnover in cases of high rates of bone resorption and formation [159]. It was observed that there was a significant elevation of osteocalcin levels in patients with IS compared with matched controls [156, 157]. This elevation reflects the high rate of bone remodeling and abnormal bone metabolism.

5.2.4.3 Matrilin-1 (MATN1)

Matrilin-1 or MATN1 is a protein known as cartilage matrix protein, which is encoded by *MATN1*. The MATN1 protein is a member of a family of matrix proteins that forms filamentous structures in the matrices of cartilage and many other types of tissues [160]. MATN1 helps in the organization of the extracellular matrix (ECM). The ECM is an important structure that supports the spinal column, and it has been hypothesized that a defect in the ECM could be involved in the pathogenesis of scoliosis [161]. A number of reports have studied the genetic association between IS and *MATN1*. However, the results of the reports are inconsistent. Montanaro et al. studied 81 IS trios (parents and their child with IS) and reported that microsatellite polymorphisms in *MATN1* were associated with familial IS [162]. Chen et al. studied a Chinese cohort involving a total of 419 IS cases and 750 controls and reported a significant association between a polymorphism in the promoter region of *MATN1* and the incidence and progression of scoliosis [163]. In another study that included a Korean cohort comprising 166 IS cases and 126 controls, a polymorphism in *MATN1* was found to be associated with a double major curve pattern [164].

Conversely, other studies have failed to reproduce the association of *MATN1* gene polymorphisms with IS susceptibility and/or curve progression [23, 165]. As a result of this discrepancy between different studies, a meta-analysis was recently conducted to assess the association of the rs1149048 SNP in *MATN1* with IS among different ethnic backgrounds [166]. This analysis included many studies consisting of a total of 1436 AIS patients and 1879 controls. It was shown that the association of this SNP in *MATN1* was restricted to the Asian cohort, as it was not observed in the Caucasian cohort.

Furthermore, Wang et al. reported a significant reduction in the plasma levels of MATN1 in IS patients compared to controls. This study involved 25 IS patients and 25 controls. The plasma MATN1 levels were significantly lower in cases of severe curve progression compared with non-severe cases, suggesting MATN1 as a potential biomarker for IS [167].

Single nucleotide polymorphisms as well as reduced expression levels of MATN1 have thus been found to be associated with the progression of IS. Besides being a potential biomarker, MATN1 also appears to be a selective marker for IS based on ethnic background.

5.2.4.4 Cartilage Oligomeric Matrix Protein (COMP)

Cartilage oligomeric matrix protein (COMP) is an extracellular matrix protein whose exact function is yet to be determined. It is present in the cartilage, ligament, tendon [168], bone, synovium [169], intervertebral discs [170] and in the growth plate [171]. At the cellular level, COMP is found in chondrocytes and osteoblasts [171]. It has been suggested that COMP interacts with ECM1 (extracellular matrix protein 1), another protein in the extracellular matrix of the growth plate. This interaction may affect endochondral ossification [172]. The expression of *COMP* is elevated during the development of the skeleton and the growth of long bones [173]. It has been reported that mutations in *COMP* are associated with two skeletal disorders: pseudoachondroplasia (PSACH) and multiple epiphyseal dysplasia (MED) [174, 175].

One of the clinical features of PSACH is the development of scoliosis [175]. Defective COMP protein was found to accumulate inside chondrocytes and failed to be transported outside the cells, leading to the early cell death and interference with the normal bone growth [176]. Serum COMP levels were observed to be correlated with the growth rate in juvenile idiopathic arthritic patients [177]. In a microarray analysis that was performed on osteoblasts from IS patients, it was reported that *COMP* is one of the most downregulated genes in IS osteoblasts, where the expression of *COMP* is fourfold lower than that in the controls [58].

These findings were further supported by a recent study that involved 105 IS patients and 103 age-matched healthy controls [178]. The COMP serum levels were found to be significantly lower in IS cases. They also reported that COMP levels were associated with the speed of growth in IS patients. Hence, COMP is a potential biomarker that needs to be further investigated for its usefulness in the diagnostic screening of scoliosis.

5.3 Conclusion

Identifying potential biomarkers is an essential exercise in improving the diagnostic efficiency of a condition. It has been a challenge to identify significant biomarkers for idiopathic scoliosis. Considerable research has been conducted in different aspects of cell physiology to detect and confirm these biomarkers. In this book chapter, we consolidated the relevant studies for each molecule and provided a perspective on the potential role of these factors in diagnosing IS.

What is interesting is the cross talk between some of the candidate biomarkers. For example, the previously discussed cross talk between calmodulin and melatonin, and between Gi proteins and osteopontin, which provide multiple clues to detect IS. Given the scarcity of confirmed biomarkers for IS, identifying a connection between some of the candidate factors is an affirmation of the direction in which IS research is headed.

Although IS is observed in first-degree relatives, the genetic aspect of the condition has not been clearly understood. In such a scenario, it has been useful to identify single nucleotide polymorphisms (SNPs) in calmodulin and MATN1, which influence the incidence of the spinal curve. Microsatellite polymorphisms in the MATN1 gene have been shown to be associated with familial IS, while the SNP rs1149048 is associated with IS in the Asian population. Similarly, different SNPs in the calmodulin gene appear to regulate the development of curves in different sections of the spine (thoracic, lumbar).

The influence of hormones on the spinal curve progression has provided interesting candidates, one of which is melatonin. Pinealectomized animals develop scoliosis due to either a defect in the signaling pathway or variation in the concentration of melatonin. The role of melatonin is diverse as it interacts and inhibits the action of calmodulin on platelets and muscle cells. Melatonin also acts on reactive oxygen species preventing their damaging action on neural cells. Downregulation of this hormone may cause neural cell damage and subsequently the potential development of IS.

Several diagnostic candidates are involved in bone metabolism. Osteocalcin, RANKL, COMP, and MATN1 have been identified as potential diagnostic biomarkers of IS. While increased levels of osteopontin were associated with IS, reduced concentrations of MATN1 and COMP were implicated in IS.

It is clear that some studies are in their preliminary stages and additional research is required to confirm the status of these candidates as diagnostic biomarkers. The data on growth hormones and estrogen have been inconclusive. While these hormones appear to be relevant due to their effects on growth at puberty, growth hormones and estrogen have to be validated and confirmed as potential diagnostic biomarkers with a number of large-scale clinical studies.

Identifying these factors is only half the job. There are multiple facets to each factor that have to be considered. For example, calmodulin is a potential diagnostic marker for many reasons. It is upregulated in IS patients, and thus appears to be an indicator of spinal curve progression. There are single nucleotide polymorphisms within the calmodulin gene that appear to be correlated with different patterns of spinal curvature. And in addition, calmodulin regulates the synthesis of melatonin. In separate studies, melatonin has been identified as a potential diagnostic candidate of IS. Melatonin, in turn, interacts with the hormone leptin that is a diagnostic candidate for IS. It is interesting to observe that the data of independent research studies have provided candidates that are interconnected with each other, much like the pieces of a puzzle.

Acknowledgment The authors would like to thank Dr. Smitha S. Dutt and Ms. Anita Franco for their critical review, writing assistance, and technical editing of this book chapter. This work was supported in part by a research grant from the Yves Cotrel Foundation (Institut de France, Paris). Mrs. Dina Nada was the recipient of CHU Sainte-Justine Foundation Scholarship.

References

1. Cheng JC, Castelein RM, Chu WC, Danielsson AJ, Dobbs MB, Grivas TB, et al. Primer. Nature. 2015;
2. Noshchenko A, Hoffecker L, Lindley EM, Burger EL, Cain CM, Patel VV, et al. Predictors of spine deformity progression in adolescent idiopathic scoliosis: a systematic review with meta-analysis. World J Orthoped. 2015;6(7):537.
3. Weinstein SL, Dolan LA, Cheng JC, Danielsson A, Morcuende JA. Adolescent idiopathic scoliosis. Lancet. 2008;371(9623):1527–37.
4. Loncar-Dusek M, Pecina M, Prebeg Z. A longitudinal study of growth velocity and development of secondary gender characteristics versus onset of idiopathic scoliosis. Clin Orthop Relat Res. 1991;270:278–82.
5. Archer IA, Dickson RA. Stature and idiopathic scoliosis. A prospective study. J Bone Joint Surg Br. 1985;67(2):185–8.
6. Skogland LB, Steen H, Trygstad O. Spinal deformities in tall girls. Acta Orthop Scand. 1985;56(2):155–7.
7. Siu King Cheung C, Tak Keung Lee W, Kit Tse Y, Ping Tang S, Man Lee K, Guo X, et al. Abnormal peri-pubertal anthropometric measurements and growth pattern in adolescent idiopathic scoliosis: a study of 598 patients. Spine (Phila Pa 1976). 2003;28(18):2152–7.
8. Yim AP, Yeung HY, Hung VW, Lee KM, Lam TP, Ng BK, et al. Abnormal skeletal growth patterns in adolescent idiopathic scoliosis—a longitudinal study until skeletal maturity. Spine (Phila Pa 1976). 2012;37(18):E1148–54.
9. Willner S, Nilsson KO, Kastrup K, Bergstrand CG. Growth hormone and somatomedin A in girls with adolescent idiopathic scoliosis. Acta Paediatr Scand. 1976;65(5):547–52.
10. Dymling JF, Willner S. Progression of a structural scoliosis during treatment with growth hormone. A case report. Acta Orthop Scand. 1978;49(3):264–8.
11. de Lind van Wijngaarden RF, de Klerk LW, Festen DA, Duivenvoorden HJ, Otten BJ, Hokken-Koelega AC. Randomized controlled trial to investigate the effects of growth hormone treatment on scoliosis in children with Prader-Willi syndrome. J Clin Endocrinol Metab. 2009;94(4):1274–80.
12. Willner S, Johnell O. Study of biochemical and hormonal data in idiopathic scoliosis in girls. Arch Orthop Trauma Surg. 1981;98(4):251–5.
13. Ahl T, Albertsson-Wikland K, Kalen R. Twenty-four-hour growth hormone profiles in pubertal girls with idiopathic scoliosis. Spine (Phila Pa 1976). 1988;13(2):139–42.
14. Zhuang Q, Wu Z, Qiu G. Is polymorphism of CALM1 gene or growth hormone receptor gene associated with susceptibility to adolescent idiopathic scoliosis? Zhonghua Yi Xue Za Zhi. 2007;87(31):2198–202.

15. Qiu XS, Tang NL, Yeung HY, Qiu Y, Cheng JC. Genetic association study of growth hormone receptor and idiopathic scoliosis. Clin Orthop Relat Res. 2007;462:53–8.
16. Hesse V, Jahreis G, Schambach H, Vogel H, Vilser C, Seewald H, et al. Insulin-like growth factor I correlations to changes of the hormonal status in puberty and age. Exp Clin Endocrinol. 1993;102(4):289–98.
17. Juul A, Dalgaard P, Blum WF, Bang P, Hall K, Michaelsen KF, et al. Serum levels of insulin-like growth factor (IGF)-binding protein-3 (IGFBP-3) in healthy infants, children, and adolescents: the relation to IGF-I, IGF-II, IGFBP-1, IGFBP-2, age, sex, body mass index, and pubertal maturation. J Clin Endocrinol Metab. 1995;80(8):2534–42.
18. Sanders JO, Browne RH, Cooney TE, Finegold DN, McConnell SJ, Margraf SA. Correlates of the peak height velocity in girls with idiopathic scoliosis. Spine. 2006;31(20):2289–95.
19. Sanders JO, Browne RH, McConnell SJ, Margraf SA, Cooney TE, Finegold DN. Maturity assessment and curve progression in girls with idiopathic scoliosis. J Bone Joint Surg Am. 2007;89(1):64–73.
20. Yeung HY, Tang NL, Lee KM, Ng BK, Hung VW, Kwok R, et al. Genetic association study of insulin-like growth factor-I (IGF-I) gene with curve severity and osteopenia in adolescent idiopathic scoliosis. Stud Health Technol Inform. 2006;123:18–24.
21. Moon ES, Kim HS, Sharma V, Park JO, Lee HM, Moon SH, et al. Analysis of single nucleotide polymorphism in adolescent idiopathic scoliosis in Korea: for personalized treatment. Yonsei Med J. 2013;54(2):500–9.
22. Yang Y, Wu Z, Zhao T, Wang H, Zhao D, Zhang J, et al. Adolescent idiopathic scoliosis and the single-nucleotide polymorphism of the growth hormone receptor and IGF-1 genes. Orthopedics. 2009;32(6):411.
23. Takahashi Y, Matsumoto M, Karasugi T, Watanabe K, Chiba K, Kawakami N, et al. Lack of association between adolescent idiopathic scoliosis and previously reported single nucleotide polymorphisms in MATN1, MTNR1B, TPH1, and IGF1 in a Japanese population. J Orthop Res. 2011;29(7):1055–8.
24. Liu W, Qiu Y, Chen Z, Liu Z, Shu H, Wang X, et al. Association between insulin-like growth factor-1 receptor gene polymorphisms and with susceptibility to adolescent idiopathic scoliosis. Chin J Surg. 2009;47(23):1813–6.
25. Moldovan F, Letellier K, Azeddine F, Lacroix G, Wang D, Turgeon I, et al. The role of estrogens and estrogen receptors in the pathogenesis of adolescent idiopathic scoliosis (AIS). J Bone Joint Surg. 2008;90(Suppl III):431.
26. Iwamuro S, Sakakibara M, Terao M, Ozawa A, Kurobe C, Shigeura T, et al. Teratogenic and anti-metamorphic effects of bisphenol A on embryonic and larval Xenopus laevis. Gen Comp Endocrinol. 2003;133(2):189–98.
27. Boudreau M, Courtenay SC, Maclatchy DL, Bérubé CH, Parrott JL, Van Der Kraak GJ. Utility of morphological abnormalities during early-life development of the estuarine mummichog, Fundulus heteroclitus, as an indicator of estrogenic and antiestrogenic endocrine disruption. Environ Toxicol Chem. 2004;23(2):415–25.
28. Grumbach MM. Estrogen, bone, growth and sex: a sea change in conventional wisdom. J Pediatr Endocrinol Metab. 2000;13(Suppl 6):1439–55.
29. Kulis A, Zarzycki D, Jaśkiewicz J. Concentration of estradiol in girls with idiopathic scoliosis. Ortop Traumatol Rehabil. 2006;8(4):455–9.
30. Esposito T, Uccello R, Caliendo R, Di Martino G, Carnevale UG, Cuomo S, et al. Estrogen receptor polymorphism, estrogen content and idiopathic scoliosis in human: a possible genetic linkage. J Steroid Biochem Mol Biol. 2009;116(1):56–60.
31. Warren MP, Brooks-Gunn J, Hamilton LH, Warren LF, Hamilton WG. Scoliosis and fractures in young ballet dancers. Relation to delayed menarche and secondary amenorrhea. N Engl J Med. 1986;314(21):1348–53.
32. Leboeuf D, Letellier K, Alos N, Edery P, Moldovan F. Do estrogens impact adolescent idiopathic scoliosis? Trends Endocrinol Metabol. 2009;20(4):147–52.
33. Letellier K, Azeddine B, Parent S, Labelle H, Rompre PH, Moreau A, et al. Estrogen cross-talk with the melatonin signaling pathway in human osteoblasts derived from adolescent idiopathic scoliosis patients. J Pineal Res. 2008;45(4):383–93.

34. Raczkowski JW. The concentrations of testosterone and estradiol in girls with adolescent idiopathic scoliosis. Neuro Endocrinol Lett. 2007;28(3):302–4.
35. Slemenda CW, Reister TK, Hui SL, Miller JZ, Christian JC, Johnston CC Jr. Influences on skeletal mineralization in children and adolescents: evidence for varying effects of sexual maturation and physical activity. J Pediatr. 1994;125(2):201–7.
36. Riggs BL, Khosla S, Melton LJ III. Sex steroids and the construction and conservation of the adult skeleton. Endocr Rev. 2002;23(3):279–302.
37. Lombardi G, Akoume MY, Colombini A, Moreau A, Banfi G. Biochemistry of adolescent idiopathic scoliosis. Adv Clin Chem. 2011;54:165–82.
38. Eastell R. Role of oestrogen in the regulation of bone turnover at the menarche. J Endocrinol. 2005;185(2):223–34.
39. Manolagas SC, Jilka RL. Cytokines, hematopoiesis, osteoclastogenesis, and estrogens. Calcif Tissue Int. 1992;50(3):199–202.
40. Burner WL III, Badger VM, Sherman FC. Osteoporosis and acquired back deformities. J Pediatr Orthop. 1982;2(4):383–5.
41. Thomas KA, Cook SD, Skalley TC, Renshaw SV, Makuch RS, Gross M, et al. Lumbar spine and femoral neck bone mineral density in idiopathic scoliosis: a follow-up study. J Pediatr Orthop. 1992;12(2):235–40.
42. Hung VW, Qin L, Cheung CS, Lam TP, Ng BK, Tse YK, et al. Osteopenia: a new prognostic factor of curve progression in adolescent idiopathic scoliosis. J Bone Joint Surg Am. 2005;87(12):2709–16.
43. Cheng JC, Guo X, Sher AH. Persistent osteopenia in adolescent idiopathic scoliosis. A longitudinal follow up study. Spine (Phila Pa 1976). 1999;24(12):1218–22.
44. Lee WT, Cheung CS, Tse YK, Guo X, Qin L, Lam TP, et al. Association of osteopenia with curve severity in adolescent idiopathic scoliosis: a study of 919 girls. Osteoporos Int. 2005;16(12):1924–32.
45. Moreau A, Wang DS, Forget S, Azeddine B, Angeloni D, Fraschini F, et al. Melatonin signaling dysfunction in adolescent idiopathic scoliosis. Spine (Phila Pa 1976). 2004;29(16):1772–81.
46. Papaioannou S, Tumber AM, Meikle MC, McDonald F. G-protein signalling pathways and oestrogen: a role of balanced maintenance in osteoblasts. Biochim Biophys Acta. 1999;1449(3):284–92.
47. Demirkiran G, Dede O, Yalcin N, Akel I, Marcucio R, Acaroglu E. Selective estrogen receptor modulation prevents scoliotic curve progression: radiologic and histomorphometric study on a bipedal C57Bl6 mice model. Eur Spine J. 2014;23(2):455–62.
48. Akel I, Demirkıran G, Alanay A, Karahan S, Marcucio R, Acaroglu E. The effect of calmodulin antagonists on scoliosis: bipedal C57BL/6 mice model. Eur Spine J. 2009;18(4):499–505.
49. Akel I, Kocak O, Bozkurt G, Alanay A, Marcucio R, Acaroglu E. The effect of calmodulin antagonists on experimental scoliosis: a pinealectomized chicken model. Spine (Phila Pa 1976). 2009;34(6):533–8.
50. Kindsfater K, Lowe T, Lawellin D, Weinstein D, Akmakjian J. Levels of platelet calmodulin for the prediction of progression and severity of adolescent idiopathic scoliosis. J Bone Joint Surg Am. 1994;76(8):1186–92.
51. Lowe T, Lawellin D, Smith D, Price C, Haher T, Merola A, et al. Platelet calmodulin levels in adolescent idiopathic scoliosis: do the levels correlate with curve progression and severity? Spine. 2002;27(7):768–75.
52. Cutler GB Jr. The role of estrogen in bone growth and maturation during childhood and adolescence. J Steroid Biochem Mol Biol. 1997;61(3-6):141–4.
53. Lee PA, Witchel SF. The influence of estrogen on growth. Curr Opin Pediatr. 1997;9(4):431–6.
54. Nilsson O, Chrysis D, Pajulo O, Boman A, Holst M, Rubinstein J, et al. Localization of estrogen receptors-alpha and-beta and androgen receptor in the human growth plate at different pubertal stages. J Endocrinol. 2003;177(2):319–26.
55. Wang K, Shi D, Sun L, Jiang X, Lü Y, Dai J, et al. Association of estrogen receptor alpha gene polymorphisms with bone mineral density: a meta-analysis. Chin Med J. 2012;125(14):2589–97.

56. Grumbach MM, Auchus RJ. Estrogen: consequences and implications of human mutations in synthesis and action. J Clin Endocrinol Metab. 1999;84(12):4677–94.
57. Bilezikian JP, Morishima A, Bell J, Grumbach MM. Increased bone mass as a result of estrogen therapy in a man with aromatase deficiency. N Engl J Med. 1998;339(9):599–603.
58. Fendri K, Patten S, Zaouter C, Parent S, Kaufman G, Labelle H, et al. Recent advances in the study of candidate genes for adolescent idiopathic scoliosis. Stud Health Technol Inform. 2010;158:3–7.
59. Inoue M, Minami S, Nakata Y, Kitahara H, Otsuka Y, Isobe K, et al. Association between estrogen receptor gene polymorphisms and curve severity of idiopathic scoliosis. Spine. 2002;27(21):2357–62.
60. Wu J, Qiu Y, Zhang L, Sun Q, Qiu X, He Y. Association of estrogen receptor gene polymorphisms with susceptibility to adolescent idiopathic scoliosis. Spine (Phila Pa 1976). 2006;31(10):1131–6.
61. Tang NL-S, Yeung H-Y, Lee K-M, Hung VW-Y, Cheung CS-K, Ng BK-W, et al. A relook into the association of the estrogen receptor α gene (PvuII, XbaI) and adolescent idiopathic scoliosis: a study of 540 Chinese cases. Spine. 2006;31(21):2463–8.
62. Zhang HQ, Lu SJ, Tang MX, Chen LQ, Liu SH, Guo CF, et al. Association of estrogen receptor beta gene polymorphisms with susceptibility to adolescent idiopathic scoliosis. Spine (Phila Pa 1976). 2009;34(8):760–4.
63. Zhao D, Qiu GX, Wang YP, Zhang JG, Shen JX, Wu ZH. Association between adolescent idiopathic scoliosis with double curve and polymorphisms of calmodulin1 gene/estrogen receptor-α gene. Orthop Surg. 2009;1(3):222–30.
64. Takahashi Y, Matsumoto M, Karasugi T, Watanabe K, Chiba K, Kawakami N, et al. Replication study of the association between adolescent idiopathic scoliosis and two estrogen receptor genes. J Orthop Res. 2011;29(6):834–7.
65. Xu L, Qiu X, Sun X, Mao S, Liu Z, Qiao J, et al. Potential genetic markers predicting the outcome of brace treatment in patients with adolescent idiopathic scoliosis. Eur Spine J. 2011;20(10):1757–64.
66. Peng Y, Liang G, Pei Y, Ye W, Liang A, Su P. Genomic polymorphisms of G-protein estrogen receptor 1 are associated with severity of adolescent idiopathic scoliosis. Int Orthop. 2012;36(3):671–7.
67. Ogura Y, Takahashi Y, Kou I, Nakajima M, Kono K, Kawakami N, et al. A replication study for association of 5 single nucleotide polymorphisms with curve progression of adolescent idiopathic scoliosis in Japanese patients. Spine (Phila Pa 1976). 2013;38(7):571–5.
68. Janusz P, Kotwicki T, Andrusiewicz M, Kotwicka M. XbaI and PvuII polymorphisms of estrogen receptor 1 gene in females with idiopathic scoliosis: no association with occurrence or clinical form. PLoS One. 2013;8(10):e76806.
69. Yang M, Li C, Li M. The estrogen receptor alpha gene (XbaI, PvuII) polymorphisms and susceptibility to idiopathic scoliosis: a meta-analysis. J Orthop Sci. 2014;19(5):713–21.
70. Chen S, Zhao L, Roffey DM, Phan P, Wai EK. Association between the ESR1-351A> G single nucleotide polymorphism (rs9340799) and adolescent idiopathic scoliosis: a systematic review and meta-analysis. Eur Spine J. 2014;23(12):2586–93.
71. Kotwicki T, Janusz P, Andrusiewicz M, Chmielewska M, Kotwicka M. Estrogen receptor 2 gene polymorphism in idiopathic scoliosis. Spine (Phila Pa 1976). 2014;39(26):E1599–607.
72. Janusz P, Kotwicka M, Andrusiewicz M, Czaprowski D, Czubak J, Kotwicki T. Estrogen receptors genes polymorphisms and age at menarche in idiopathic scoliosis. BMC Musculoskelet Disord. 2014;15(1):383.
73. Liu Z, Tam EM, Sun GQ, Lam TP, Zhu ZZ, Sun X, et al. Abnormal leptin bioavailability in adolescent idiopathic scoliosis: an important new finding. Spine (Phila Pa 1976). 2012;37(7):599–604.
74. Tam E, Yu F, Hung V, Liu Z, Liu KL, Ng BK, et al. Are volumetric bone mineral density and bone micro-architecture associated with leptin and soluble leptin receptor levels in adolescent idiopathic scoliosis?--A case-control study. PLoS One. 2014;9(2):e87939.

75. Qiu Y, Sun X, Qiu X, Li W, Zhu Z, Zhu F, et al. Decreased circulating leptin level and its association with body and bone mass in girls with adolescent idiopathic scoliosis. Spine (Phila Pa 1976). 2007;32(24):2703–10.
76. Elisa M, Lee W, Cheuk K-Y, Lam T-P, Ng BK, Lee SK, et al. Morphological and bone strength indices in girls with adolescent idiopathic scoliosis and their correlations with leptin and soluble leptin receptor. Scoliosis. 2015;10(Suppl 1):O13.
77. Tam EM, Yeung K-H, Tang S, Lam T-P, Ng BK, Lee SK, et al. Abnormal functional responses of osteoblasts to leptin in adolescent idiopathic scoliosis. Scoliosis. 2015;10(Suppl 1):O6.
78. Liang G, Gao W, Liang A, Ye W, Peng Y, Zhang L, et al. Normal leptin expression, lower adipogenic ability, decreased leptin receptor and hyposensitivity to leptin in adolescent idiopathic scoliosis. PLoS One. 2012;7(5):e36648.
79. Burwell RG, Aujla RK, Grevitt MP, Dangerfield PH, Moulton A, Randell TL, et al. Pathogenesis of adolescent idiopathic scoliosis in girls-a double neuro-osseous theory involving disharmony between two nervous systems, somatic and autonomic expressed in the spine and trunk: possible dependency on sympathetic nervous system and hormones with implications for medical therapy. Scoliosis. 2009;4(1):24.
80. Canpolat S, Sandal S, Yilmaz B, Yasar A, Kutlu S, Baydas G, et al. Effects of pinealectomy and exogenous melatonin on serum leptin levels in male rat. Eur J Pharmacol. 2001;428(1):145–8.
81. Baltaci A, Mogulkoc R. Pinealectomy and melatonin administration in rats: their effects on plasma leptin levels and relationship with zinc. Acta Biol Hung. 2007;58(4):335–43.
82. Alonso-Vale MI, Andreotti S, Peres SB, Anhe GF, das Neves Borges-Silva C, Neto JC, et al. Melatonin enhances leptin expression by rat adipocytes in the presence of insulin. Am J Physiol Endocrinol Metab. 2005;288(4):E805–12.
83. Azeddine B, Letellier K, Wang da S, Moldovan F, Moreau A. Molecular determinants of melatonin signaling dysfunction in adolescent idiopathic scoliosis. Clin Orthop Relat Res. 2007;462:45–52.
84. Akoume M-Y, Azeddine B, Turgeon I, Franco A, Labelle H, Poitras B, et al. Cell-based screening test for idiopathic scoliosis using cellular dielectric spectroscopy. Spine. 2010;35(13):E601–E8.
85. Sakata I, Sakai T. Ghrelin cells in the gastrointestinal tract. Int J Pept. 2010;2010:945056.
86. Maccarinelli G, Sibilia V, Torsello A, Raimondo F, Pitto M, Giustina A, et al. Ghrelin regulates proliferation and differentiation of osteoblastic cells. J Endocrinol. 2005;184(1):249–56.
87. Gennero I, Conte-Auriol F, Mus M, Molinas-Cazals C, Accadbled F, Tauber M, et al. Fasting total ghrelin levels are increased in patients with adolescent idiopathic scoliosis. Bone. 2013;2:122.
88. Brzezinski A. Melatonin in humans. N Engl J Med. 1997;336(3):186–95.
89. Grivas TB, Savvidou OD. Melatonin the "light of night" in human biology and adolescent idiopathic scoliosis. Scoliosis. 2007;2(6):1–14.
90. Morgan PJ, Barrett P, Howell HE, Helliwell R. Melatonin receptors: localization, molecular pharmacology and physiological significance. Neurochem Int. 1994;24(2):101–46.
91. Arendt J. Melatonin and the pineal gland: influence on mammalian seasonal and circadian physiology. Rev Reprod. 1998;3(1):13–22.
92. Reppert SM, Godson C, Mahle CD, Weaver DR, Slaugenhaupt SA, Gusella JF. Molecular characterization of a second melatonin receptor expressed in human retina and brain: the Mel1b melatonin receptor. Proc Natl Acad Sci. 1995;92(19):8734–8.
93. Thillard MJ. Vertebral column deformities following epiphysectomy in the chick. C R Hebd Seances Acad Sci. 1959;248(8):1238–40.
94. Dubousset J, Queneau P, Thillard M. Experimental scoliosis induced by pineal and diencephalic lesions in young chickens: its relation with clinical findings. Orthop Trans. 1983;7(7):4.
95. Machida M, Dubousset J, Imamura Y, Iwaya T, Yamada T, Kimura J. An experimental study in chickens for the pathogenesis of idiopathic scoliosis. Spine. 1993;18(12):1609–15.
96. Machida M, Dubousset J, Imamura Y, Iwaya T, Yamada T, Kimura J. Role of melatonin deficiency in the development of scoliosis in pinealectomised chickens. J Bone Joint Surg Br. 1995;77(1):134–8.

97. Acaroglu E, Bobe R, Enouf J, Marcucio R, Moldovan F, Moreau A. The metabolic basis of adolescent idiopathic scoliosis: 2011 report of the "metabolic" workgroup of the Fondation Yves Cotrel. Eur Spine J. 2012;21(6):1033–42.
98. Machida M, Miyashita Y, Murai I, Dubousset J, Yamada T, Kimura J. Role of serotonin for scoliotic deformity in pinealectomized chicken. Spine. 1997;22(12):1297–301.
99. Machida M, Murai I, Miyashita Y, Dubousset J, Yamada T, Kimura J. Pathogenesis of idiopathic scoliosis. Experimental study in rats. Spine (Phila Pa 1976). 1999;24(19):1985–9.
100. Machida M, Dubousset J, Yamada T, Kimura J, Saito M, Shiraishi T, et al. Experimental scoliosis in melatonin-deficient C57BL/6J mice without pinealectomy. J Pineal Res. 2006;41(1):1–7.
101. Machida M, Dubousset J, Yamada T, Kimura J. Serum melatonin levels in adolescent idiopathic scoliosis prediction and prevention for curve progression—a prospective study. J Pineal Res. 2009;46(3):344–8.
102. Bagnall K, Raso J, Moreau M, Mahood J, Wang X, Beuerlein M. The development of scoliosis following pinealectomy in young chickens is not the result of an artifact of the surgical. Res Spinal Deform. 2002;3:3.
103. Turgut M, Yenisey C, Uysal A, Bozkurt M, Yurtseven ME. The effects of pineal gland transplantation on the production of spinal deformity and serum melatonin level following pinealectomy in the chicken. Eur Spine J. 2003;12(5):487–94.
104. Turhan E, Acaroglu E, Bozkurt G, Alanay A, Yazici M, Surat A. Unilateral enucleation affects the laterality but not the incidence of scoliosis in pinealectomized chicken. Spine. 2006;31(2):133–8.
105. Bagnall K, Raso VJ, Moreau M, Mahood J, Wang X, Zhao J. The effects of melatonin therapy on the development of scoliosis after pinealectomy in the chicken. J Bone Joint Surg Am. 1999;81(2):191–9.
106. Bagnall KM, Beuerlein M, Johnson P, Wilson J, Raso VJ, Moreau M. Pineal transplantation after pinealectomy in young chickens has no effect on the development of scoliosis. Spine. 2001;26(9):1022–7.
107. Wang X, Moreau M, Raso VJ, Zhao J, Jiang H, Mahood J, et al. Changes in serum melatonin levels in response to pinealectomy in the chicken and its correlation with development of scoliosis. Spine (Phila Pa 1976). 1998;23(22):2377–81. discussion 82
108. Dede O, Akel I, Demirkiran G, Yalcin N, Marcucio R, Acaroglu E. Is decreased bone mineral density associated with development of scoliosis? A bipedal osteopenic rat model. Scoliosis. 2011;6(1):24.
109. Cheung KM, Wang T, Poon AM, Carl A, Tranmer B, Hu Y, et al. The effect of pinealectomy on scoliosis development in young nonhuman primates. Spine (Phila Pa 1976). 2005;30(18):2009–13.
110. Bagnall KM, Raso VJ, Hill DL, Moreau M, Mahood JK, Jiang H, et al. Melatonin levels in idiopathic scoliosis: diurnal and nocturnal serum melatonin levels in girls with adolescent idiopathic scoliosis. Spine. 1996;21(17):1974–8.
111. Goultidis TT, Papavasiliou KA, Petropoulos AS, Philippopoulos A, Kapetanos GA. Higher levels of melatonin in early stages of adolescent idiopathic scoliosis: toward a new scenario. J Pediatr Orthop. 2014;34(8):768–73.
112. Girardo M, Bettini N, Dema E, Cervellati S. The role of melatonin in the pathogenesis of adolescent idiopathic scoliosis (AIS). Eur Spine J. 2011;20(Suppl 1):S68–74.
113. Day GA, McPhee IB, Tuffley J, Tomlinson F, Chaseling R, Kellie S, et al. Idiopathic scoliosis and pineal lesions in Australian children. J Orthop Surg (Hong Kong). 2007;15(3):327–33.
114. Qiu Y, Wu L, Wang B, Yu Y, Zhu Z. Asymmetric expression of melatonin receptor mRNA in bilateral paravertebral muscles in adolescent idiopathic scoliosis. Spine. 2007;32(6):667–72.
115. Yim AP-Y, Yeung H-Y, Sun G, Lee K-M, Ng T-B, Lam T-P, et al. Abnormal skeletal growth in adolescent idiopathic scoliosis is associated with abnormal quantitative expression of melatonin receptor, mt2. Int J Mol Sci. 2013;14(3):6345–58.
116. Wang H, Wu Z, Zhuang Q, Fei Q, Zhang J, Liu Y, et al. Association study of tryptophan hydroxylase 1 and arylalkylamine N-acetyltransferase polymorphisms with adolescent idiopathic scoliosis in Han Chinese. Spine. 2008;33(20):2199–203.

117. Qiu XS, Tang NL, Yeung HY, Lee K-M, Hung VW, Ng BK, et al. Melatonin receptor 1B (MTNR1B) gene polymorphism is associated with the occurrence of adolescent idiopathic scoliosis. Spine. 2007;32(16):1748–53.
118. Qiu X-S, Tang NL, Yeung H-Y, Cheng JC, Qiu Y. Lack of association between the promoter polymorphism of the MTNR1A gene and adolescent idiopathic scoliosis. Spine. 2008;33(20):2204–7.
119. Yang M, Wei X, Yang W, Li Y, Ni H, Zhao Y, et al. The polymorphisms of melatonin receptor 1B gene (MTNR1B) (rs4753426 and rs10830963) and susceptibility to adolescent idiopathic scoliosis: a meta-analysis. J Orthop Sci. 2015;20(4):593–600.
120. Wang WW, Man GC, Wong JH, Ng TB, Lee KM, Ng BK, et al. Abnormal response of the proliferation and differentiation of growth plate chondrocytes to melatonin in adolescent idiopathic scoliosis. Int J Mol Sci. 2014;15(9):17100–14.
121. Hamm HE, Gilchrist A. Heterotrimeric G proteins. Curr Opin Cell Biol. 1996;8(2):189–96.
122. Gilman AG. G Proteins and dual control of adenylate cyclase. Cell. 1984;36(3):577–9.
123. Verdonk E, Johnson K, McGuinness R, Leung G, Chen YW, Tang HR, et al. Cellular dielectric spectroscopy: a label-free comprehensive platform for functional evaluation of endogenous receptors. Assay Drug Dev Technol. 2006;4(5):609–19.
124. Akoume M-Y, Franco A, Moreau A. Cell-based assay protocol for the prognostic prediction of idiopathic scoliosis using cellular dielectric spectroscopy. J Vis Exp. 2013;80:50768.
125. Julien C, Gorman KF, Akoume M-Y, Moreau A. Towards a comprehensive diagnostic assay for scoliosis. Pers Med. 2013;10(1):97–103.
126. Denhardt DT, Noda M, O'Regan AW, Pavlin D, Berman JS. Osteopontin as a means to cope with environmental insults: regulation of inflammation, tissue remodeling, and cell survival. J Clin Investig. 2001;107(9):1055.
127. Weintraub AS, Schnapp LM, Lin X, Taubman MB. Osteopontin deficiency in rat vascular smooth muscle cells is associated with an inability to adhere to collagen and increased apoptosis. Lab Investig. 2000;80(11):1603–15.
128. Mazzali M, Kipari T, Ophascharoensuk V, Wesson J, Johnson R, Hughes J. Osteopontin—a molecule for all seasons. Int J Med. 2002;95(1):3–13.
129. Standal T, Borset M, Sundan A. Role of osteopontin in adhesion, migration, cell survival and bone remodeling. Exp Oncol. 2004;26(3):179–84.
130. Terai K, Takano-Yamamoto T, Ohba Y, Hiura K, Sugimoto M, Sato M, et al. Role of osteopontin in bone remodeling caused by mechanical stress. J Bone Miner Res. 1999;14(6):839–49.
131. Moreau A, Franco A, Azeddine B, Rompré PH, Gagnon M-HR, Bagnall KM, et al. High circulating levels of osteopontin are associated with idiopathic scoliosis onset and spinal deformity progression 7. In: Aubin C-E, Stokes IAF, Labelle H, Moreau A, editors. Research into spinal deformities. Amsterdam: IOS Press BV; 2010.
132. Oyama J, Murai I, Kanazawa K, Machida M. Bipedal ambulation induces experimental scoliosis in C57BL/6J mice with reduced plasma and pineal melatonin levels. J Pineal Res. 2006;40(3):219–24.
133. Yadav MC, Huesa C, Narisawa S, Hoylaerts MF, Moreau A, Farquharson C, et al. Ablation of osteopontin improves the skeletal phenotype of phospho1−/− mice. J Bone Miner Res. 2014;29(11):2369–81.
134. Xie N, Li M, Wu T, Liu J, Wang B, Tang F. Does elevated osteopontin level play an important role in the development of scoliosis in bipedal mice? Spine J. 2015;15(7):1660–4.
135. Stevens FC. Calmodulin: an introduction. Can J Biochem Cell Biol. 1983;61(8):906–10.
136. Chin D, Means AR. Calmodulin: a prototypical calcium sensor. Trends Cell Biol. 2000;10(8):322–8.
137. Yarom R, Muhlrad A, Hodges S, Robin G. Platelet pathology in patients with idiopathic scoliosis: ultrastructural morphometry, aggregations, x-ray spectrometry, and biochemical analysis. Lab Investig. 1980;43(3):208–16.
138. Peleg I, Eldor A, Kahane I, Muhlrad A, Liebergall M, Floman Y. Altered structural and functional properties of myosins, from platelets of idiopathic scoliosis patients. J Orthop Res. 1989;7(2):260–5.

139. Muhlrad A, Yarom R. Contractile protein studies on platelets from patients with idiopathic scoliosis. Pathophysiol Haemost Thromb. 1982;11(3):154–60.
140. Sabato S, Rotman A, Robin GC, Floman Y. Platelet aggregation abnormalities in idiopathic scoliosis. J Pediatr Orthop. 1985;5(5):558–63.
141. Bredoux R, Corvazier E, Dally S, Chaabane C, Bobe R, Raies A, et al. Human platelet Ca2+–ATPases: new markers of cell differentiation as illustrated in idiopathic scoliosis. Platelets. 2006;17(6):421–33.
142. Kahmann RD, Donohue JM, Bradford DS, White JG, Rao GH. Platelet function in adolescent idiopathic scoliosis. Spine. 1992;17(2):145–8.
143. Suk S, Kim I, Lee C, Koh Y, Yeom J. A study on platelet function in idiopathic scoliosis. Orthopedics. 1991;14(10):1079–83.
144. Zhao Y, Qiu GX. Expression of calmodulin and nNOS in the paraspinal muscles in idiopathic scoliosis. Zhonghua Yi Xue Za Zhi. 2004;84(16):1358–61.
145. Acaroglu E, Akel I, Alanay A, Yazici M, Marcucio R. Comparison of the melatonin and calmodulin in paravertebral muscle and platelets of patients with or without adolescent idiopathic scoliosis. Spine. 2009;34(18):E659–E63.
146. Zhao D, Qiu GX, Wang YP, Zhang JG, Shen JX, Wu ZH, et al. Association of calmodulin1 gene polymorphisms with susceptibility to adolescent idiopathic scoliosis. Orthop Surg. 2009;1(1):58–65.
147. Zhang Y, Gu Z, Qiu G. The association study of calmodulin 1 gene polymorphisms with susceptibility to adolescent idiopathic scoliosis. Biomed Res Int. 2014;2014:168106.
148. Xia Z, Storm DR. Calmodulin-regulated adenylyl cyclases and neuromodulation. Curr Opin Neurobiol. 1997;7(3):391–6.
149. Hardeland R. Melatonin, hormone of darkness and more–occurrence, control mechanisms, actions and bioactive metabolites. Cell Mol Life Sci. 2008;65(13):2001–18.
150. Benítez-King G. Melatonin as a cytoskeletal modulator: implications for cell physiology and disease. J Pineal Res. 2006;40(1):1–9.
151. Porter RW. The pathogenesis of idiopathic scoliosis: uncoupled neuro-osseous growth? Eur Spine J. 2001;10(6):473–81.
152. Boyce BF, Xing L. Biology of RANK, RANKL, and osteoprotegerin. Arthritis Res Ther. 2007;9(1):S1.
153. Suh KT, Lee S-S, Hwang SH, Kim S-J, Lee JS. Elevated soluble receptor activator of nuclear factor-κB ligand and reduced bone mineral density in patients with adolescent idiopathic scoliosis. Eur Spine J. 2007;16(10):1563–9.
154. Eun I-S, Park WW, Suh KT, Kim JI, Lee JS. Association between osteoprotegerin gene polymorphism and bone mineral density in patients with adolescent idiopathic scoliosis. Eur Spine J. 2009;18(12):1936–40.
155. Zhou S, Wang W, Zhu Z, Sun X, Zhu F, Yu Y, et al. Increased expression of receptor activator of nuclear factor-κB ligand in osteoblasts from adolescent idiopathic scoliosis patients with low bone mineral density. J Huazhong Univ Sci Technol. 2012;32:686–90.
156. Kulis A, Gozdzialska A, Drag J, Jaskiewicz J, Knapik-Czajka M, Lipik E, et al. Participation of sex hormones in multifactorial pathogenesis of adolescent idiopathic scoliosis. Int Orthop. 2015;39(6):1227–36.
157. Chiru M. Adolescent idiopathic scoliosis and osteopenia. Maedica (Buchar). 2011;6(1):17–22.
158. Lu L, Dai Z, Lv G, Kang Y, Jiang Y. A novel therapeutic strategy for adolescent idiopathic scoliosis based on osteoporotic concept. Med Hypotheses. 2013;80(6):773–5.
159. Ram VS, Parthiban SU, Mithradas N, Prabhakar R. Bone biomarkers in periodontal disease: a review article. J Clin Diagn Res. 2015;9(1):ZE07–10.
160. Wagener R, Ehlen HW, Ko YP, Kobbe B, Mann HH, Sengle G, et al. The matrilins—adaptor proteins in the extracellular matrix. FEBS Lett. 2005;579(15):3323–9.
161. Lowe TG, Edgar M, Margulies JY, Miller NH, Raso VJ, Reinker KA, et al. Etiology of idiopathic scoliosis: current trends in research. J Bone Joint Surg. 2000;82(8):1157.
162. Montanaro L, Parisini P, Greggi T, Di Silvestre M, Campoccia D, Rizzi S, et al. Evidence of a linkage between matrilin-1 gene (MATN1) and idiopathic scoliosis. Scoliosis. 2006;1(1):21.

163. Chen Z, Tang NL, Cao X, Qiao D, Yi L, Cheng JC, et al. Promoter polymorphism of matrilin-1 gene predisposes to adolescent idiopathic scoliosis in a Chinese population. Eur J Hum Genet. 2009;17(4):525–32.
164. Bae JW, Cho C-H, Min W-K, Kim U-K. Associations between matrilin-1 gene polymorphisms and adolescent idiopathic scoliosis curve patterns in a Korean population. Mol Biol Rep. 2012;39(5):5561–7.
165. Yilmaz H, Zateri C, Uludag A, Bakar C, Kosar S, Ozdemir O. Single-nucleotide polymorphism in Turkish patients with adolescent idiopathic scoliosis: curve progression is not related with MATN-1, LCT C/T-13910, and VDR BsmI. J Orthop Res. 2012;30(9):1459–63.
166. Zhang H, Zhao S, Zhao Z, Tang L, Guo Q, Liu S, et al. The association of rs1149048 polymorphism in matrilin-1(MATN1) gene with adolescent idiopathic scoliosis susceptibility: a meta-analysis. Mol Biol Rep. 2014;41(4):2543–9.
167. Wang B, Chen ZJ, Qiu Y, Liu WJ. Decreased circulating matrilin-1 levels in adolescent idiopathic scoliosis. Zhonghua Wai Ke Za Zhi. 2009;47(21):1638–41.
168. Posey KL, Hecht JT. The role of cartilage oligomeric matrix protein (COMP) in skeletal disease. Curr Drug Targets. 2008;9(10):869–77.
169. Xu K, Zhang Y, Ilalov K, Carlson CS, Feng JQ, Di Cesare PE, et al. Cartilage oligomeric matrix protein associates with granulin-epithelin precursor (GEP) and potentiates GEP-stimulated chondrocyte proliferation. J Biol Chem. 2007;282(15):11347–55.
170. Ishii Y, Thomas AO, Guo XE, Hung CT, Chen FH. Localization and distribution of cartilage oligomeric matrix protein in the rat intervertebral disc. Spine (Phila Pa 1976). 2006;31(14):1539–46.
171. Di Cesare PE, Fang C, Leslie MP, Tulli H, Perris R, Carlson CS. Expression of cartilage oligomeric matrix protein (COMP) by embryonic and adult osteoblasts. J Orthop Res. 2000;18(5):713–20.
172. Kong L, Tian Q, Guo F, Mucignat MT, Perris R, Sercu S, et al. Interaction between cartilage oligomeric matrix protein and extracellular matrix protein 1 mediates endochondral bone growth. Matrix Biol. 2010;29(4):276–86.
173. Fendri K, Moldovan F. Potential role of COMP as a biomarker for adolescent idiopathic scoliosis. Med Hypotheses. 2011;76(5):762–3.
174. Hecht JT, Nelson LD, Crowder E, Wang Y, Elder FF, Harrison WR, et al. Mutations in exon 17B of cartilage oligomeric matrix protein (COMP) cause pseudoachondroplasia. Nat Genet. 1995;10(3):325–9.
175. Briggs M, Hoffman S, King L, Olsen A, Mohrenweiser H, Leroy J, et al. Pseudoachondroplasia and multiple epiphyseal dysplasia due to mutations in the cartilage oligomeric matrix protein gene. Nat Genet. 1995;10(3):330–6.
176. Hecht JT, Makitie O, Hayes E, Haynes R, Susic M, Montufar-Solis D, et al. Chondrocyte cell death and intracellular distribution of COMP and type IX collagen in the pseudoachondroplasia growth plate. J Orthop Res. 2004;22(4):759–67.
177. Bjornhart B, Juul A, Nielsen S, Zak M, Svenningsen P, Muller K. Cartilage oligomeric matrix protein in patients with juvenile idiopathic arthritis: relation to growth and disease activity. J Rheumatol. 2009;36(8):1749–54.
178. Gerdhem P, Topalis C, Grauers A, Stubendorff J, Ohlin A, Karlsson K. Serum level of cartilage oligomeric matrix protein is lower in children with idiopathic scoliosis than in non-scoliotic controls. Eur Spine J. 2015;24(2):256–61.

Chapter 6
Bone Metabolism in AIS

Jack C. Y. Cheng, Wayne Y. W. Lee, Elisa M. S. Tam, and T. P. Lam

6.1 Skeletal Growth and Bone Metabolism

6.1.1 Overview of Adolescent Skeletal Growth

Adolescence is a period of rapid skeletal growth; the skeletal mass nearly doubles at the end of adolescence [1]. During puberty the process of bone formation predominates, resulting in a steady increase of bone mass. This life stage represents an important opportunity for influencing peak bone mass and thus reducing the risk of osteoporotic fractures occurring later in life. Peak bone mass occurs from ages as early as 16–18 years at the lumbar spine, femoral neck, and midshaft, to as late as 35 years at the radius, skull, and whole body [2]. During puberty, a transient period of bone fragility at metaphysis was reported [3]. Previous studies on growth pattern showed asynchrony in bone mass accretion and growth, resulting in a transient decline in bone mineral density (BMD) and cortical weakness [4, 5].

J. C. Y. Cheng (✉) • W. Y. W. Lee • E. M. S. Tam • T. P. Lam
Department of Orthopaedics and Traumatology, SH Ho Scoliosis Research Laboratory, Prince of Wales Hospital, The Chinese University of Hong Kong, Shatin, NT, Hong Kong, China

Joint Scoliosis Research Center of the Chinese University of Hong Kong and Nanjing University, Hong Kong, China
e-mail: jackcheng@cuhk.edu.hk

M. Machida et al. (eds.), *Pathogenesis of Idiopathic Scoliosis*,
https://doi.org/10.1007/978-4-431-56541-3_6

Bone mass is the net result of the bone modeling and remodeling processes which are affected by complex hormonal changes that are programmed by genetics and also interact with nutritional and environmental factors. Endocrine factors that may influence bone mass during adolescence include insulin-like growth factor-1 (IGF-1), which stimulates systemic body growth; growth hormone, which promotes growth and cell reproduction and regeneration; gonadotropic hormones, which promote epiphyseal maturation; and sex hormones, which mediate calcium accretion, decrease bone resorption with estrogen, and increase bone thickness and periosteal bone formation with testosterone [6]. The gender differences in bone mass and geometry are noted during puberty. In general, boys have larger cortical cross-sectional areas and higher trabecular bone volume ratios, while girls have higher cortical density and less cortical porosity [7].

6.1.2 Bone Modeling and Remodeling

Bone is a metabolically active tissue undergoing modeling and remodeling which are highly coordinated by osteoblasts, osteoclasts, and osteocytes. Bone modeling is bone gain without previous bone resorption resulting in changes in size and shape of the bone. Bone remodeling is a structural replacement or repair to maintain bone integrity and strength in response to mechanical stimulation and damage. Bone remodeling takes place in basic multicellular unit (BMU) encased with a canopy of cells within an anatomical structure known as bone remodeling compartment (BRC) [8]. In normal bone remodeling, the amount of resorbed bone is often completely replaced by newly formed bone. Osteopenia and osteoporosis are the result of net bone loss, while in osteopetrosis, bone formation dominates.

Osteoblasts arise from the differentiation of mesenchymal stem cells. Runt-related transcription factor 2 (Runx2) is a critical transcription factor regulating osteogenic differentiation and encoding genes for the synthesis of bone matrix and mineralization [9]. Mature osteoblasts commit its function by laying down organic osteoid followed by mineralization and extracellular matrix formation. Along this process, some osteoblasts further differentiate into osteocytes or become lining cells or undergo apoptotic cell death. Osteoclasts are terminally differentiated myeloid cells from either adjacent bone marrow in trabecular bone or vasculature in cortical bone. The RANKL/RANK/NF-κB pathway is the main signaling pathway regulating osteoclasts differentiation. RANKL (*r*eceptor *a*ctivator of *N*F-κB *l*igand) from osteoblasts binds to RANK expressing osteoclast precursor cells. Osteoprotegerin (OPG), released by osteoblasts, is a soluble decoy receptor for RANKL which plays as a physiological negative feedback regulation of bone resorption [10]. The RANKL/OPG ratio has been suggested to indicate the extent of osteoclasts differentiation and activation [11]. Osteocytes are the most abundant cell type (over 90%) in bone, and its death is suggested to initiate the formation of BRC wherein resorption and formation are activated [12]. Recent evidence suggests the modulatory roles of osteocytes in bone remodeling through the release of sclerostin, RANKL, and OPG. Sclerostin is a potent inhibitor of bone formation through the binding to low-density lipoprotein receptor-related protein 5/6 (LRP5/LRP6) and thus abolishing canonical Wnt/β-catenin signaling [13]. The Wnt signaling is the prime target for many bone anabolic drugs through the inhibition of Wnt antagonists such as sclerostin and dickkopf WNT signaling pathway inhibitor 1 (Dkk1).

6.1.3 Bone Mineralization

Bone is a bioceramic composite consisting of intimate organization of organic substances (collagenous proteins and non-collagenous proteins), minerals (mainly calcium phosphate of apatite structure), and water. The complex bone structure can be divided into seven hierarchical levels of organization [14] which is speculated to provide optimal strength and toughness [15]. Bone formation is composed of two main stages known as primary and secondary osteogenesis resulting in the formation of woven and lamellar bone, respectively [16]. The mineralization in woven bone is relatively rapid and unorganized and serves as a transient stage during endochondral ossification. The woven bone is remodeled into lamellar bone which in human is organized into osteons for the construction of cortical bone or cancellous bone. During lamellar bone formation, osteoblasts secrete collagen fibrils assembled in a highly organized, close-packed lamellar structure. The organization of crystals is directed along the collagen fibrils leading to intrafibrillar crystallization. Osteoblasts also secrete non-collagenous proteins, such as osteonectin, osteopontin, osteocalcin, and bone sialoprotein, which are enriched with acidic amino acids and promote mineral nucleation in collagen fibrils [17].

6.2 Abnormal Skeletal Growth and Maturation in AIS

AIS occurs in children during their pubertal growth spurt. Rapid growth is associated with the development and progression of scoliotic curves, with the curves stabilized at skeletal maturity [18]. These observations have led researchers to investigate growth and growth-related endocrine factors and their possible contribution to the etiopathogenesis of AIS.

6.2.1 Body Height and Proportion

Patients with AIS were found to be taller and leaner [19, 20]. Some studies reported that the tall stature returns to normal by skeletal maturity [21], while others have shown it to persist into adulthood [22]. Cheung et al. reported that girls with AIS were shorter before menarche but caught up and became taller, with higher sitting height and longer arm span and leg length during growth spurt when compared with control subjects [20]. To calculate the height loss due to the spinal deformity, different equations have been suggested, and it appeared that no formula can fit every curve of different severities [23]. In another study, linear correlation between arm span and standing height in healthy children and adolescents was found to be very high ($r^2 = 0.99$) [24]. Therefore, the use of arm span as a surrogate for body height might be a better solution in the estimation of height loss due to the scoliosis.

In addition to abnormal lengths, asymmetries in the limb length and segmental length were also reported [25, 26]. While the asymmetry in arm length was not found in patients with lumbar curves, asymmetry in iliac height and leg length inequality were reported instead [27, 28]. Researchers have interpreted these findings to be (a) secondary to the scoliosis curve, (b) nonspecific manifestations of developmental instability due to natural left-right asymmetry in humans [29], and (c) sentinels in paired bones of vertebral growth plate asymmetries implying putative pathogenic significance [30].

6.2.2 Growth Pattern and Skeletal Maturity

In a large cross-sectional study with 598 AIS girls and 307 healthy control girls stratified by chronological age and pubertal stage, abnormal growth was observed in scoliotic girls from ages 12 to 15 years or older and in all pubertal stages [20]. At prepubertal spurt, AIS girls were significantly shorter and leaner when compared with maturity-matched normal controls. After the onset of puberty, corrected height and sitting height were significantly greater in scoliotic girls than in controls. Segmental lengths, namely, arm span and leg length, were also significantly longer in AIS girls. These observations indicated that the abnormal development in the pattern of growth and anthropometric parameters coincided with the onset and progress of pubertal development during adolescence.

The age at onset of menarche is a widely used maturity indicator reflecting the growth potential in girls and is closely related to curve progression. Previous studies reported that risk of curve progression was markedly higher before the onset of menarche than after menarche has already started [31]. In addition, the age at onset of menarche was also reported to be associated with the incidence of AIS [32]. The age at the onset of menarche has been reported to be earlier, normal, and delayed in AIS girls [21, 33–35]. A large cross-sectional study conducted by Mao et al. reported delayed onset of menarche occurred more frequently in AIS girls with Chinese ethnicity [34], while Grivas et al. and Goldberg et al. reported no difference and earlier age at onset of menarche in Mediterranean and Irish girls with AIS, respectively [21, 35].

6.2.3 Body Composition

Apart from abnormal skeletal growth, many- studies have also reported lower body weight and lower body mass index (BMI) in patients with AIS [20–22]. The differences in height, weight, and BMI were found to be correlated with the curve severity [19]. The earlier studies on the body composition of AIS patients reported conflicting findings and were limited by their small sample sizes [36, 37]. Studies from different centers have all shown that the lower body weight and BMI in AIS girls were attributed to decrease in both body fat and fat-free mass [36–38]. The association of altered body composition with the occurrence of AIS was substantiated by a large population-based prospective cohort study which utilized the subjects recruited in the Avon Longitudinal Study of Parents and Children (ALSPAC) [39]. This important study have investigated the association between fat and lean mass at age 10 years as assessed by DXA, with the presence of scoliosis at age 15 years. 5299 children were included, of which 184 had developed scoliosis (Cobb angle ≥10°) at age 15. The study demonstrated that after adjustment for confounders, per SD decrease in lean mass at age 10 was associated with a 20% higher risk of scoliosis and per SD decrease in fat mass with a 13% higher risk.

Muscle mass was found to be closely and linearly correlated with bone mass particularly during growth and development [40]. In addition, muscle strength as assessed by grip strength was found to be strongly correlated with vBMD, cortical area, cortical thickness, and bone strength index assessed using pQCT [41–43]. Mechanical stimuli linked to body weight have been thought to underlie differences in bone mass [44]. The hypothesis that the bone adapts to mechanical forces was first postulated by Wolff [45]. Experiments have demonstrated that dynamic loads resulting from the use of the muscle could promote bone formation and that the response of the bone is governed by the amplitude and frequency of these stimuli which can greatly exceed the static gravitational loads resulting from body weight [44, 46]. In AIS, the reduced lean and fat mass might affect the mechanical stimuli and result in reduced bone formation and lower bone mass.

6.3 Abnormal Bone Mineral Density in AIS

The general goals of bone densitometry in adults are to identify patients at greatest risk of skeletal fragility fractures, to guide decisions regarding treatment, and to monitor responses to therapy. The bone health of an individual could be assessed quantitatively by the following approaches.

6.3.1 Bone Densitometry in Pediatric Patients

6.3.1.1 Dual-Energy X-Ray Absorptiometry (DXA)

DXA uses low-dose X-ray source with two different energy peaks. One energy peak is absorbed more by the soft tissue, while the other is absorbed more by the bone, and then the soft tissue component is subtracted to determine the BMD. DXA can be used to scan both central and peripheral skeletal sites. Due to its low radiation, high precision, and accessibility, DXA is widely used for BMD assessment

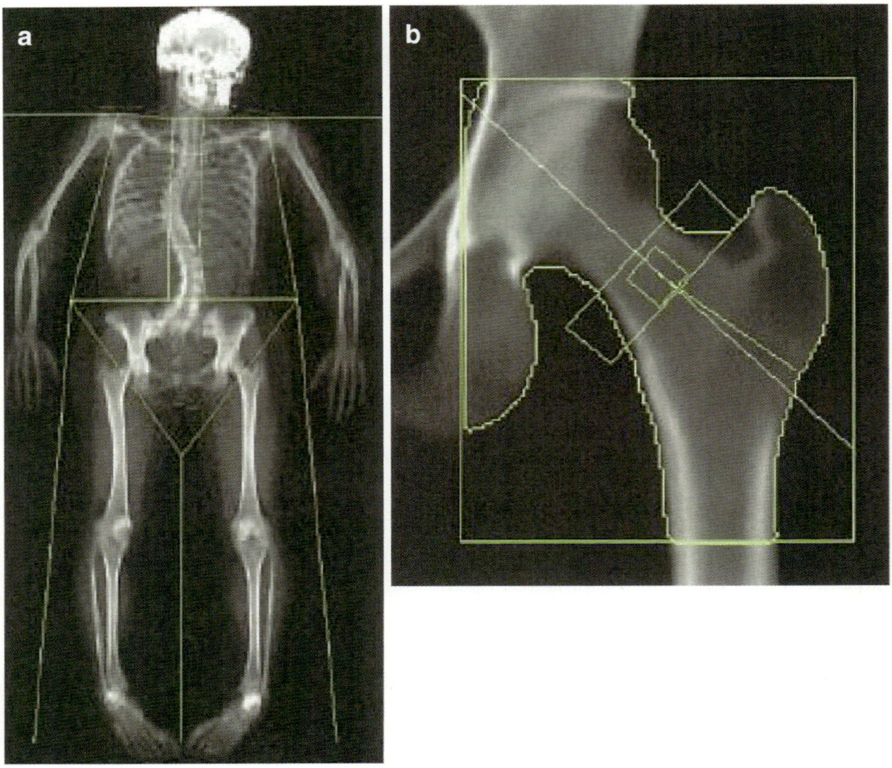

Fig. 6.1 Whole-body less head (**a**) and hip (**b**) DXA scans of an AIS patient

nowadays and is regarded as the gold standard for clinical assessment of osteoporosis by World Health Organization, and for the evaluation and management of adult bone diseases [47]. Bone densitometry assessments have been recommended for children with recurrent fractures, bone pain, bone deformities, osteopenia on standard radiographs, or to monitor therapy [48]. Examples of whole-body less head and hip DXA scans of an AIS patient are shown in Fig. 6.1. The projectional nature of the areal BMD (aBMD) measurement by DXA was confounded by bone sizes and bone geometry [49]; when DXA is being used for the study of pediatric bone health, adjustments for the smaller size of children must be made, and caution must be taken as the bones of the children change markedly in size and shape as they grow, especially during puberty. Researchers have attempted to account for the effect of bone size on the DXA result and minimize the effect of growing skeleton on the BMD value using various methods of size adjustment [50]. On the other hand, because of its reproducibility and lack of areal density-related errors, the total body bone mineral content (BMC) is sometimes preferred for the assessment of bone mineral status by some researchers [51].

6.3.1.2 Quantitative Computed Tomography (QCT)

Although not as widely utilized as DXA, QCT allows separate measurements of cortical and trabecular bone compartments; provides volumetric, as opposed to areal BMD measurement, thus avoiding the problems associated with changes in bone size; and allows measurement of geometric and structural parameters which contribute to bone strength [52]. The term central QCT is used when the technique is being applied to the spine and proximal femur, while pQCT is the application of QCT to peripheral skeletal sites. High-resolution peripheral quantitative computed tomography (HR-pQCT) is also a pQCT method but has resolution high enough to allow the quantification of trabecular micro-architecture and cortical porosity [53, 54]. Central QCT can be used in children, however, it is largely limited to research use because of limited reference databases being available for the spine and femur and higher dose of ionizing radiation involved [52].

6.3.1.3 Peripheral Quantitative Computed Tomography (pQCT)

pQCT evaluates the bone geometry and true volumetric BMD (vBMD) for the cortical and trabecular bone compartments separately in peripheral sites such as radius and tibia. It is used more widely than central QCT in growing children and adolescents, largely because of the significantly lower dose of ionizing radiation, and availability and easy access of pQCT scanners in centers dedicated to research and clinical care of children with bone disorders [52, 53]. However, pQCT is not as widely available compared with DXA and is used primarily for research purposes only. It was noted that meaningful and effective use of pQCT for assessing BMD and overall bone health in all age groups will require better defined normative data derived with common measuring techniques, equipment, and analytical approaches.

6.3.1.4 High-Resolution Peripheral Quantitative Computed Tomography (HR-pQCT)

The resolution of HR-pQCT is high enough that when computer-based finite element analysis (FEA) is being used to assess bone strength, the structure can be represented directly by the elements in the model. FE models based on HR-pQCT images have been validated against micro-CT models [55] and mechanical testing [56]. It is important to recognize that HR-pQCT only assesses the distal radius and distal tibia typically, and there is a concern whether measurements at these sites could reflect the bone mineral status and bone strength at the hip and spine. The few studies that have examined the relationship between HR-pQCT measurements of the peripheral skeleton have shown a moderate correlation ($r = 0.56–0.70$) to the axial skeleton [57, 58].

6.3.2 Low Bone Mass (Osteopenia) in AIS

Special attention is required when performing DXA scan on patients with scoliosis, because the measured aBMD in the spine is likely to be affected by any deformity or axial rotation of the vertebrae, which commonly occurs in scoliosis subjects [59]. In addition, patients with scoliosis cannot be positioned with the spine straight on the DXA table, and in those with severe scoliosis, degenerative changes can lead to invalid spine measurement [60].

Many previous studies had reported the association between AIS and low BMD. Burner et al. was the first to report the relationship between osteoporosis and acquired back deformity in 1982 [61]. Healey and Lane reported a higher prevalence of scoliosis in biopsy-proven osteoporotic women (48%) [62]. Cook et al. noted that AIS subjects had significantly lower lumbar spine and proximal femur BMD when compared with age-matched control subjects [63]. Cheng et al. investigated a large cohort of AIS and reported 36–38% of cases had generalized osteopenia (Z-score < -1) [59]. In a cross-sectional study on 919 girls with AIS, Lee et al. reported an inverse relationship between curve severity and BMD [64]. Lower vBMD has also been reported in AIS patients with pQCT study [65]. In general, the average BMD value of AIS girls was 4.5% lower than the age- and sex-matched controls [59, 66]. Previous studies have reported that osteopenia in AIS girls is systemic in nature and could affect the whole body including the spine, hip, distal radius, distal tibia, and calcaneus [22, 59, 63, 67]. This systemic low bone mass is also likely to associate with lower bone strength and peak bone mass [63], which might contribute to osteoporosis, osteoporotic fracture, progression of scoliosis, and other associated complications in late adulthood.

6.3.3 Is Osteopenia a Transient or Persistent Problem?

A few researchers have continued further and questioned whether this osteopenic status could persist into skeletal maturity, thus affecting the acquisition of peak bone mass. Thomas et al. have conducted a follow-up study of the BMD of 22 AIS girls with an average age of 11.5 years for an average follow-up period of 30.8 months [68]. Compared to the initial scans, at the follow-up evaluation, the prevalence of BMD below two SDs in the AIS group increased from 38% to 60% for the BMD measured from different standard sites. Cheng et al. have conducted a longitudinal follow-up study on the aBMD of bilateral proximal femurs in 14 AIS girls with significant osteopenia with more than two SDs below the mean normal value and 70 healthy control subjects using DXA for an average follow-up period of 29 months [66]. The study has found that the follow-up aBMD decreased from the initial evaluation of -2.96 to -3.84 SD in the follow-up visit. The same group of researchers have subsequently conducted a larger longitudinal 2-year follow-up study on the

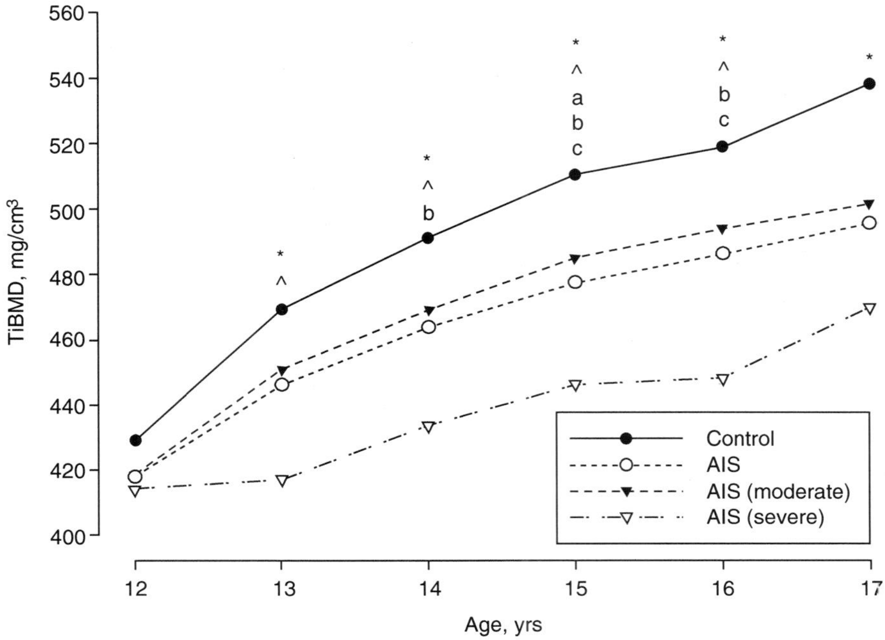

Fig. 6.2 Mean volumetric BMD of distal tibia of AIS (moderate and severe curve severity) and controls by age. $*p < 0.05$ comparison between AIS and control by *t*-test; $^\wedge p < 0.05$ comparison among AIS moderate, severe, and control by one-way ANOVA; post hoc Bonferroni multiple comparison: $^{a}p < 0.05$ (control vs. moderate), $^{b}p < 0.05$ (control vs. severe), $^{c}p < 0.05$ (moderate vs. severe) [33]

aBMD of proximal neck of femur and lumbar spinal BMC using DXA, and the vBMD of distal tibia using pQCT in 196 AIS girls and 122 healthy girls aged 12–15 years [33]. The vBMD of distal tibia in AIS group was persistently and significantly lower than the controls from 13 to 16 years (Fig. 6.2). Similarly, lumbar spinal BMC and femoral neck aBMD were persistently and significantly lower among AIS (moderate and severe severity) than the controls from age 13 to 17 years. This study indicated that both axial and peripheral BMD of AIS were persistently lower than the healthy girls throughout age 12–17 years.

Could the lower rate of increase of BMD in the AIS group a result of bracing during the follow-up period? Snyder et al. have conducted a follow-up study on 52 AIS girls with brace treatment and found the annual rate of bone density accumulation was similar to the reported normal values [69]. Summarizing the evidence, the osteopenic condition found in AIS girls appeared to be a persistent rather than a transient phenomenon. It is likely that the persistent osteopenia in AIS girls could lead to significantly lower peak bone mass and manifest with complications of osteoporosis in adult life.

6.3.4 *Clinical Relevance: BMD as a Prognostic Factor of Curve Progression in AIS*

One recurrent important clinical question in the management of AIS is whether one can predict and prognosticate which curves will deteriorate so that appropriate and timely treatment can be started [18]. The widely accepted prognostic factors include chronologic age, menarchal status, Risser sign, degree of curvatures at presentation, and the curve pattern [18, 70]. The widely reported association between osteopenia and AIS has led researchers to investigate the prognostic value of BMD and bone quality in the prediction of curve progression in girls with AIS.

Hung et al. followed a cohort of 324 AIS girls until skeletal maturity or until the curve had progressed ≥6°. Osteopenia with a *Z*-score ≤ -1 in the femoral neck of the hip on the side of the concavity was identified as a significant prognostic factor for curve progression with an adjusted odds ratio of 2.3 [71]. A predictive model was established in the study, and the area under the receiver operating characteristic (ROC) curve of the model was 0.80. Subsequently, Lam et al. have conducted a prospective cohort study with 294 AIS girls being followed beyond skeletal maturity in order to investigate the use of quantitative ultrasound in predicting curve progression. The study has reported stiffness index (SI) was a significant and independent prognostic factor for curve progression with an odds ratio of 2.0 after adjustment for age, puberty, and curve severity [72]. The area under the ROC curve was reported to be 0.831. Recently, the same group has conducted a longitudinal cohort study of 513 newly diagnosed AIS girls to validate the prognostic value of osteopenia on the risk of curve progression to surgical threshold defined as Cobb angle ≥45° and/or undergone surgery. The results showed that osteopenic patients had significantly higher risk of surgery with a hazard ratio of 2.25 after adjustment for confounders [73]. Despite the fact that osteopenia represents a promising new prognostic factor for curve progression in clinical management, its use has not been popularized, probably due to the lack of multicenters validation study, availability and cost of DXA, and other bone densitometry machines in scoliosis clinics.

6.3.5 *Factors Contributing to Low BMD in AIS*

6.3.5.1 Environmental Lifestyle: Physical Activities

The importance of physical activity and mechanical loading on bone mass accrual has been well documented, particularly in children and adolescents. Slemenda et al. found that the weight bearing activity level was positively correlated to BMD of the radius and hip in children and adolescents between 5 and 14 years old [74]. Besides, Rubin et al. found a positive correlation between physical activity and lumbar spine BMD [75]. Lee et al. in a large-scale cross-sectional study have found lower physical activity level in AIS during the pubertal period, which was also significantly correlated with both the aBMD and vBMD at various sites as measured by DXA and pQCT, respectively [76]. Yu et al. studied 214 AIS girls and 187 healthy girls aged 11–13 years old and have also found lower physical activity level in the AIS group [77]. Physical activity level was found to be positively and independently associated with greater cortical area and total vBMD with multivariate analysis.

6.3.5.2 Calcium and Vitamin D

Calcium is required for normal growth and development as well as maintenance of the skeleton. During adolescence, there is nearly a doubling of body mineral stores due to increase in the size of the skeleton, with minor changes in volumetric BMD [78]. This increase in demand must be met through dietary intake for the optimum bone mineral accretion. Vitamin D is essential for intestinal calcium absorption and plays a central role in maintaining calcium homeostasis and skeletal integrity. Vitamin D insufficiency and deficiency are highly prevalent among children and adolescents worldwide, and calcium intake often falls below recommended levels [48].

It was suggested that the osteopenia in AIS could be a result of suboptimal bone mineralization both qualitatively and quantitatively, and thus fails to catch up with abnormally escalated bone growth during the peri-pubertal period. Lee et al. studied 596 AIS girls and 302 healthy control girls aged 11–16 years old and found that the mean calcium intake of both AIS and control groups have reached only 36% and 32% of the Chinese calcium Dietary Reference Intake (DRI) of 1000 mg/day, respectively [79], and there was no difference between the AIS and controls [76]. Yu et al. have reported slightly higher calcium intake in a case-control study of 214 AIS and 187 healthy girls aged 11–13 years old [77]. The median calcium intake was found to be 571.9 mg/day in the AIS group and 587.9 mg/day in the control group, with no difference between the two groups.

Despite the importance of vitamin D in bone mineralization, there was only one study reporting the dietary vitamin D intake in AIS patients and with small sample size. Akseer et al. have studied the daily dietary vitamin D intake including supplement in 15 women with AIS who had no treatment, 15 women with AIS who had brace treatment, and 19 healthy controls [80], and reported no differences between the three groups. Our recent longitudinal study revealed a significant improvement of BMD in AIS with supplementary calcium and vitamin D. The result is discussed further in Sect. 6. With the rising interest in the involvement of vitamin D deficiency in various diseases, researchers have also looked into the serum levels of 25-hydroxyvitamin D (25(OH)Vit-D, the main circulating form of Vit-D) in patients with AIS [81, 82]. A study from Poland by Gozdzialska et al. have compared the serum 25(OH)Vit-D levels in four groups of 50 girls aged 11–14. The groups were premenarchal and postmenarchal girls with AIS vs. matched controls. The study reported significantly lower serum 25(OH)Vit-D levels in both groups of AIS patients when compared with controls of matched menarchal status, with levels reaching the status of deficiency [81].

Balioglu et al. have compared the serum 25(OH)Vit-D levels in 229 AIS patients aged 10–22 years old and 389 age-matched comparison group of athletes without scoliosis. The results indicated significantly lower serum 25(OH)Vit-D levels in AIS patients, and the vitamin D level was correlated negatively ($R = -0.147$) with Cobb angle, which suggested a possible role of vitamin D in the etiopathogenesis of AIS [82].

6.3.5.3 Genetics

Twin and family studies have consistently shown that peak bone mass, ultrasound properties of the bone, skeletal geometry, bone turnover, and fracture are heritable [83]. Candidate gene association studies have been widely used in investigating the genetic factors associated with variations in BMD and osteoporosis. About 150 candidate genes related to osteoporosis have currently been identified [84]. The most widely studied among these genes include type I collagen, vitamin D receptor, estrogen receptor, androgen receptor, aromatase, LRP5 and LRP6, sclerostin, transforming growth factor β1, interleukin-6, and insulin growth factor-1. These factors act by inhibiting osteoblast activation and/or increasing osteoclast function, leading to osteoporosis. However, findings from a large consortium of five population-based studies involving 19,195 participants suggested that most of the previously studied candidate genes were not replicated in a well-powered study with standardized phenotyping and genotyping [85, 86]. Subsequent genome-wide association studies (GWASs) have identified 62 loci that are genome-wide significant for BMD at either the lumbar spine or the femoral neck [86].

6.4 Abnormal Bone Quality and Bone Strength in AIS

The critical role of bone quality in determination of bone strength has been well recognized, and bone quality has been taken as one of the key elements in the clinical definition of osteoporosis. Since then a large number of evidence have been published, supporting the theory that bone quality is of paramount importance for bone strength. Previous investigations with detailed bone geometry and micro-architecture parameters had enhanced predictive power for osteoporotic fracture and could better explain the mechanism underlying fragility fractures [87]. Bone geometry such as cortical thickness has been established as crucial factors for determining bone strength [88]. Recent studies have also suggested the importance of trabecular bone micro-architecture in the determination of bone quality and bone strength [87, 89]. In 2001, the NIH reinforced the theory that bone strength reflects both bone quality and BMD by defining osteoporosis as "A skeletal disorder characterized by compromised bone strength predisposing to an increased rate of fracture. Bone strength reflects the integration of two main features: bone density and bone quality" [90].

6.4.1 *Studies on Bone Quality in AIS*

At the time of writing, there were only a few studies which have reported the bone quality of AIS patients. It was speculated that the low bone mass and deranged bone quality could lead to mechanically weakened spinal column in the osteopenic patients, who might be more susceptible to the development of scoliosis and curve progression during the rapid growth in peri-pubertal period.

6.4.1.1 Bone Geometry

Yu et al. performed HR-pQCT assessment in the non-dominant distal radius of 214 newly diagnosed AIS girls between the age of 11 and 13 and 187 healthy age- and gender-matched controls [77]. The trabecular area, cortical area, cortical perimeter, and mean cortical thickness were measured. AIS girls were found to have lower cortical area (% difference = −8.88%) and cortical thickness (% difference = −8.53%) (Table 6.1). Cortical area remained significantly lower after adjustment for age, but not after adjustment for age, calcium intake, and physical activity level (Table 6.2).

Table 6.1 Comparison of bone geometry, volumetric bone mineral density, and trabecular bone micro-architecture between AIS and control girls

		AIS, $N = 214$	Control, $N = 187$	% Difference	p Value
Bone geometry	Ct.Area (mm^2)	25.5 ± 11.6	27.9 ± 12.5	−8.88%	0.043
	Ct.Th (mm)	0.512 ± 0.226	0.690 ± 0.221	−8.53%	0.053
	Ct.Pm (mm)	55.0 ± 4.32	54.6 ± 4.40	0.64%	0.363
	Trab.Area (mm^2)	148.7 ± 28.5	146.3 ± 28.2	1.68%	0.342
vBMD	D_{tot} (mg HA/cm^3)	256.0 ± 54.2	266.6 ± 51.8	−3.97%	0.042
	D_{cort} (mg HA/cm^3)	689.3 ± 76.6	708.1 ± 73.7	−2.65%	0.014
	D_{trab} (mg HA/cm^3)	148.9 ± 27.6	152.2 ± 25.3	−2.14%	0.181
Trabecular bone micro-architecture	BV/TV	0.124 ± 0.023	0.127 ± 0.021	−2.14%	0.181
	Tb.N (mm^{-1})	1.71 ± 0.22	1.77 ± 0.22	−3.50%	0.004
	Tb.Sp (mm)	0.524 ± 0.090	0.502 ± 0.075	4.26%	0.008
	Tb.Th (mm)	0.072 ± 0.009	0.072 ± 0.008	1.25%	0.325

Two-tailed Student's t-test was performed. Data was expressed as mean ± SD
Ct.Area cortical area, *Ct.Th* cortical thickness, *Ct.Pm* cortical perimeter, *Trab.Area* trabecular area, D_{tot} total vBMD, D_{cort} cortical bone vBMD, D_{trab} trabecular bone vBMD, *BV/TV* trabecular bone-volume-to-tissue-volume ratio, *Tb.N* trabecular number, *Tb.Sp* trabecular separation, *Tb.Th* trabecular thickness

Table 6.2 Multivariate linear regression analysis for comparing bone geometry, volumetric bone mineral density, and trabecular bone micro-architecture between AIS and control girls

			Model 1			Model 2				
			Group (AIS/Ctrl)	Age	R^2	Group (AIS/Ctrl)	Age	Ca intake	Physical activity level	R^2
Bone geometry	Ct.Area (mm^2)	B	−2.251	7.465	0.127	−1.888	7.581	<0.001	1.200	0.14
		p	0.048	<0.001		0.098	<0.00*	0.924	0.042	
	Ct.Th (mm)	B	−0.040	0.135	0.12	−0.033	0.136	<0.001	0.021	0.13
		p	0.060	<0.001		0.119	<0.001	0.718	0.059	
	Ct.Pm (mm)	B	0.400	0.111	0.002	0.404	0.237	0.001	0.071	0.01
		p	0.361	0.779		0.361	0.553	0.077	0.757	
vBMD (mgHA/cm^3)	D_{tot}	B	−10.227	23.077	0.068	−8.573	23.370	<0.001	5.429	0.08
		p	0.048	<0.001		0.100	<0.001	0.962	0.044	
	D_{cort}	B	−17.310	50.808	0.153	−15.144	50.819	−0.006	6.938	0.16
		p	0.014	<0.001		0.032	<0.001	0.489	0.057	
Trabecular micro-architecture	Tb.N (mm^{-1})	B	−0.066	−0.062	0.043	−0.062	−0.055	<0.001	0.01	0.06
		p	0.003	0.002		0.005	0.007	0.012	0.401	
	Tb.Sp (mm)	B	0.023	0.02	0.034	0.022	0.017	<0.001	−0.004	0.05
		p	0.006	0.009		0.010	0.022	0.025	0.401	

Group: the status of the subject (control subject is assigned a value of "0" and AIS subject is assigned a value of "1"); Model 1: multivariate linear regression model adjusting for age; Model 2: multivariate linear regression model adjusting for age, Ca intake, and physical activity level; B: regression coefficient for the independent variable; p: *p* value for the regression coefficient B

Ct.Area cortical area, *Ct.Th* cortical thickness, *Ct.Pm* cortical perimeter, *Trab.Area* trabecular area, D_{tot} total vBMD, D_{cort} cortical bone vBMD, *Tb.N* trabecular number, *Tb.Sp* trabecular separation

Table 6.3 Bone mineral status measured with SEM/EDX in AIS and controls

Parameters	AIS, $N = 9$	Control, $N = 5$	Difference%	p Value
$R_{Ca/P}$	1.55 ± 0.0542	1.56 ± 0.041	−0.64%	0.947
$R_{Ca/C}$	0.77 ± 0.13	1.05 ± 0.1	−26.67%	0.006

Independent t-test was used in the comparisons; difference % = (AIS value − control value)/(control value) %

6.4.1.2 Abnormal Bone Mineralization

Yu et al. have also assessed the total vBMD, cortical bone vBMD, and trabecular bone vBMD in their HR-pQCT study of 214 AIS girls and 187 healthy age- and gender-matched controls [77]. Total vBMD and cortical bone vBMD were significantly lower in the AIS group with mean difference of −3.97% and −2.65%, respectively (Table 6.1). No significant difference was found in the trabecular vBMD between AIS and control groups. Multivariate regression analysis indicated that AIS was associated with lower total vBMD and cortical bone vBMD after adjustment for age; cortical bone vBMD remained significantly lower after adjustment for age, calcium intake, and physical activity level (Table 6.2).

Due to the lack of good animal model that could mimic the 3D pathoanatomy of the spinal deformity in AIS, the mechanisms underlying abnormal bone mineralization remain unclear. A recent study by Wang et al. reported for the first time a comprehensive comparative study using SEM/EDX on iliac crest bone tissues collected from AIS and non-AIS controls undergoing bony fusion surgery [91]. Scanning electron microscopy coupled with energy-dispersive X-ray spectroscopy (SEM/EDX) is a sensitive tool to detect small difference in calcium content which is not distinguishable with conventional DXA and micro-CT. Previous studies suggested that the amount of carbon could be regarded as organic components and the ratio of calcium to carbon ($R_{Ca/C}$) was proportional to the BMD [92], while the ratio of carbon to phosphorus ($R_{Ca/P}$) could reflect the status of bone mineralization [92, 93]. The lower $R_{Ca/C}$ in AIS suggested decreased mineralization in AIS which was in agreement with the increased osteoid volume and width in the same study (Table 6.3).

6.4.1.3 Bone Micro-architecture

Quantitative ultrasound (QUS) offers a radiation-free and portable modality of investigation and can provide indirect assessment on material properties and micro-architecture of bone. Using QUS, Lam et al. reported significantly lower broadband ultrasound attenuation (BUA) and stiffness index (SI) at the non-dominant calcaneus of 635 AIS girls when compared to 269 controls [67], suggesting possibility of altered bone micro-architecture in AIS. The latest HR-pQCT can offer noninvasive measurement of trabecular bone micro-architecture, without

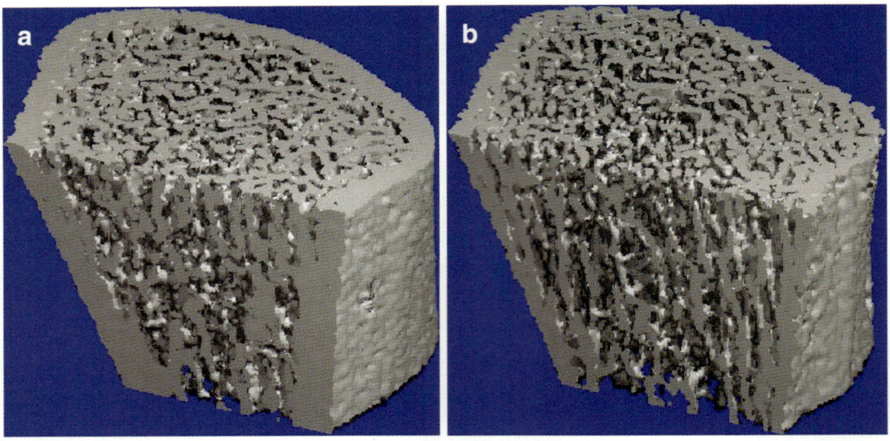

Fig. 6.3 Representative 3D reconstructions of trabecular and cortical bone of distal radius, as measured by HR-pQCT for (**a**) non-osteopenic AIS and (**b**) osteopenic AIS. Alterations of trabecular bone micro-architecture could be visualized in osteopenic AIS as shown in **b**

being confounded by bone size. Using this technique, Yu et al. assessed the trabecular bone micro-architecture in the non-dominant distal radius of 214 young AIS girls between the age of 11 and 13 and 187 healthy age- and gender-matched controls and have found lower trabecular number and higher trabecular separation in the AIS group after adjustment for age, calcium intake, and physical activity level (Table 6.2) [77]. In another study by Yu et al., where the bone qualities of osteopenic AIS girls, non-osteopenic AIS girls, osteopenic controls, and non-osteopenic controls were assessed with HR-pQCT, the osteopenic AIS girls had additional abnormal trabecular vBMD and micro-architecture that were not found in the osteopenic control girls [94]. This finding suggested the osteopenia is different between osteopenic AIS and osteopenic control girls, and that predominant changes of osteopenia in AIS girls occurred in the trabecular bone compartment (Fig. 6.3).

The measurements with HR-pQCT on distal radius dominated by cortical bone might underestimate particularly the changes in trabecular bone compartment. The micro-structure of plate and rod trabeculae is also critical in determining the bone strength and is associated with changes in BMD, which can be delineated with individual trabeculae segmentation (ITS) [95, 96]. Our current study on iliac crest bone biopsies with micro-CT40 and ITS analysis showed that AIS had significantly lower rod thickness (rTbTh) and number (rTbN) when compared with controls. Subsequent FEA also revealed significantly lower bone strength than controls (Table 6.4, [91]).

Table 6.4 Comparisons of trabeculae micro-architecture measured with ITS[a] in AIS and controls

Parameters	AIS, $N = 14$	Control, $N = 5$	Difference%	p Value
pBV/TV	0.16 ± 0.03	0.17 ± 0.03	−5.88	0.517
rBV/TV	0.021 ± 0.008	0.026 ± 0.014	−19.23	0.459
P-R ratio	7.93 ± 1.93	7.31 ± 2.31	8.48	0.781
pTb.N (mm^{-1})	4.10 ± 0.27	4.38 ± 0.39	−6.39	0.139
rTb.N (mm^{-1})	2.90 ± 0.32	3.26 ± 0.72	−11.04	0.229
pTb.Th (mm)	0.087 ± 0.003	0.082 ± 0.003	6.1	0.012
rTb.Th (mm)	0.065 ± 0.003	0.062 ± 0.004	4.84	0.052
pTb.S (mm^2)	0.026 ± 0.002	0.024 ± 0.003	8.33	0.165
rTb.L (mm)	0.215 ± 0.012	0.211 ± 0.004	1.9	0.926
R-R Junc.D (mm^{-3})	7.84 ± 2.57	18.19 ± 18.77	−56.9	0.033
R-P Junc.D (mm^{-3})	76.82 ± 24.62	103.82 ± 56.03	−26	0.267
P-P Junc.D (mm^{-3})	71.34 ± 18.53	94.57 ± 40.34	−24.56	0.229

Independent *t*-test was used; difference % = (AIS value − control value)/(control value) %

[a]Individual trabeculae segmentation (ITS) is a rigorous model-independent 3D morphological analysis that is capable of segmenting trabecular bone microstructure into individual trabecular plates and rods. Based on measurements of each individual trabecula, ITS-based morphological analyses enable separate assessments of trabecular plate and rod microstructure and have been used to elucidate the important but distinct roles of trabecular plates and rods in determining mechanical properties and failure mechanisms of trabecular bone

pBV/TV plate bone volume fraction, *rBV/TV* rod bone volume fraction, *P-R* ratio ratio of plate bone tissue to rod bone tissue, *pTb.N* plate trabeculae number density, *rTb.N* rod trabeculae number density, *pTb.Th* mean trabecular plate thickness, *rTb.Th* mean trabecular rod thickness, *pTb.S* mean trabecular plate surface area, *rTb.L* mean trabecular rod length, *R-R Junc.D* rod-rod junction density, *P-R Junc.D* plate-rod junction density, *P-P Junc.D* plate-plate junction density

6.5 Abnormal Bone Turnover and Hormonal Changes

6.5.1 Bone Turnover Markers

A previous study has shown serum bone-specific alkaline phosphatase (bALP) in AIS was 38.6% higher than that of controls [97]. Additionally, Suh et al. [98] reported higher serum-soluble RANKL levels and RANKL-to-OPG ratios in AIS. A recent study by Ishida et al. assessed the BMD and TRAP5b in 49 AIS girls aged 10–19. Sixty percent of AIS girls had osteopenia or osteoporosis at the femoral site, and 59% of AIS girls had high values of TRAP5b with >1.88 SDs. The AIS girls with high values of TRAP5b had lower *Z* scores, younger age, and lower BMI than those with normal values of TRAP5b. TRAP5b was also found to be positively correlated with Cobb angle. Apart from serological study, our recent study on iliac crest bone biopsies showed higher expression level of genes regulating bone formation markers, including collagen type I (*COL1*), osteocalcin (*BGLAP*) and osteopontin (*SPP1*), and bone resorption markers, including tartrate-resistant

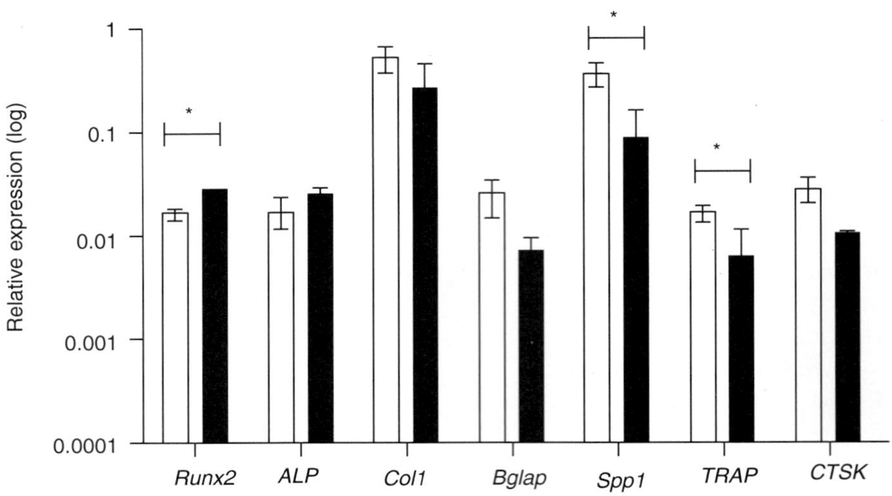

Fig. 6.4 Relative mRNA expression to GAPDH of bone formation and resorption genes in iliac crest bone biopsies collected from AIS (white bars; $N = 14$) and control (black bars; $N = 5$). Data is presented as mean ± SEM $*p < 0.05$

acid phosphatase (*TRAP*) and cathepsin K (*CTSK*), in AIS (Fig. 6.4). Taking these together, concurrent abnormal bone turnover in AIS might play a role in the etio-pathogenesis of AIS.

6.5.2 *Abnormal Hormonal Changes and Abnormal Responses in Primary Culture*

6.5.2.1 Melatonin

Melatonin is a secretory hormone mainly synthesized by pinealocytes in the pineal gland [99]. Melatonin plays an essential role in the physical health and skeletal development of the human body. Several animal studies shown that pinealectomy in chickens [100] and bipedal rats [101] lead to scoliosis, and this has led to the postulation that disturbance of melatonin production can be a potential cause of AIS [102]. In cellular models, Moreau et al. reported impaired melatonin signaling transduction in osteoblasts, myoblasts, and lymphocytes of progressive AIS and have linked the findings to the inactivation of Gi proteins [103, 104]. Man et al. reported a lack of response to the melatonin's stimulating effects on proliferation and differentiation in osteoblast cultures prepared from bone biopsies obtained intraoperatively during spine surgeries from girls with AIS [105], which could be partly explained by a low melatonin receptor 1B expression [106, 107]. Melatonin receptor 1B gene polymorphism was also reported to be associated with AIS [108]. Yim et al. have further linked the abnormal skeletal growth in AIS girls to abnormal quantitative expression of melatonin receptor 1B [107]. However, it remains unclear whether melatonin has a definite role in the etiopathogenesis of AIS.

6.5.2.2 Leptin

Leptin is a relatively new topic in AIS research, the first study related to leptin in AIS by Qiu et al. showed that the circulating leptin levels were significantly lower in AIS girls, even after adjustment for age and menstrual status [109]. Liu et al. in a study of 95 AIS girls and 46 healthy matched controls aged 11–16 years found abnormal leptin bioavailability with increased levels of soluble leptin receptor (sOB-R) and lower free leptin index (FLI) in AIS girls after adjusting for age and body weight [110]. Significant correlations were also found between sOB-R, FLI, and curve severity in AIS girls. Subsequently, Tam et al. showed that this abnormal leptin bioavailability was also associated with deranged bone quality and lower muscle and fat mass in AIS girls [38, 111]. Burwell et al. formulated an etiologic theory of autonomic nervous system and leptin-sympathetic nervous system (SNS) concept for AIS and hypothesized an altered sensitivity to leptin in the hypothalamus of AIS girls, resulted in increased SNS activity, which contributed to skeletal overgrowth, generalized osteopenia, lower BMI, asymmetric spinal growth, and other phenotypes of AIS [112].

6.5.2.3 Estrogen and Its Receptor

Several studies have suggested that estrogen and/or estrogen receptors could play an important role in the pathogenesis and progression of AIS [113]. This hypothesis is reasonable and appealing as it attempts to explain the increased occurrence of scoliosis in girls and also the manifestation of osteopenia in scoliotic individuals. Studies on the circulating estrogen levels in AIS girls have reported conflicting findings. In in vitro study involving human osteoblasts isolated from AIS and control patients, Letellier et al. have shown that the increased cAMP levels induced by melatonin can be corrected by the treatment of the cells with 17-β-estradiol, which suggested an interaction between 17-β-estradiol and the already defective melatonin signaling pathway in human AIS osteoblasts. It was also suggested that the melatonin receptor MT2, which is normally physiologically coupled with the Gi protein, could switch to the Gs protein in the osteoblasts of a specific group of AIS patients when their cells are exposed to 17-β-estradiol [104].

6.6 Potential Clinical Interventions

When managing patients with idiopathic scoliosis, apart from focusing on curve control, therapeutic measures for achieving good bone health should be considered. Despite the lack of high level evidence in favor of any particular regimen for treating low bone mass in AIS, the general principles of physical stimulation and nutritional measures for enhancing positive balance in bone metabolism should be followed. Physical stimulation refers to weight bearing exercise and, more recently, vibration treatment; and nutritional measures include vitamin D and calcium supplementation.

6.6.1 Whole-Body Vibration Therapy

While weight bearing exercise can be prescribed and recommended as an integral part of healthy lifestyles for good bone health, compliance with the advice and high variability in exercise characteristics can be an issue. On the other hand, a non-pharmacological and extracorporeal modality recently receiving attention is the low-magnitude high-frequency whole-body vibration therapy (WBV). Rubin et al. reported mechanical vibration at a magnitude of 0.3 g and a frequency of 30 Hz could lead to increased bone mineral content and improved bone quality when applied at the hind limb of sheep [114]. The effect of WBV in increasing aBMD of the femur [115, 116] and the spine [115, 116] without adverse outcomes [117] has been reported. Lee et al. reported low bone mass in AIS was related to inadequate weight bearing physical activity [76]. Given that mechanical loading is osteogenic especially for children [118], Lam et al. thus carried out a randomized controlled trial to evaluate whether WBV, as a form of mechanical loading simulating weight bearing physical activity [114], could improve low BMD and bone quality for osteopenia associated with AIS. AIS subjects between 15 and 25 years old and with BMD Z-score < -1 were recruited. The treatment group received low-magnitude (acceleration = 0.3 g) high-frequency (32–37 Hz) vibration therapy by standing on the WBV platform 20 min/day and 5 days/week for 12 months. The control group received observation alone. Bone parameters were measured at baseline and at the 12-month time-point using DXA at bilateral femoral necks and the lumbar spine (L2–L4), and HR-pQCT at bilateral distal tibiae and the non-dominant distal radius. Results showed that at the 12-month time-point, while there was no statistically significant difference on the changes in HR-pQCT parameters between the treatment and the control group, WBV was noted to have positive effects on increasing femoral neck aBMD at the convex leg but less obviously at the concave side [119]. To evaluate if there is other factor that modulates and enhances the therapeutic effect of WBV, a nested study was carried out to analyze the percentage changes in aBMD across the 1-year period for the treatment and control group through subgroup analysis according to 25-hydroxyvitamin D (25(OH)Vit-D) levels. Results indicated the presence of factor interaction between WBV and 25(OH)Vit-D on increment of aBMD with statistical significance noted at the concave side ($p = 0.027$). For the subgroup with 25(OH)Vit-D > 40 nmol/L, not only were the positive effects of WBV greater at both sides, the treatment effect was also more obviously seen at the concave side indicating interaction between mechanical loading and Vit-D on bone metabolism in alignment with results obtained from previous animal and in vitro studies.

6.6.2 Supplement Therapy

Apart from physical stimulation, vitamin D physiology in AIS deserves further attention. It has been reported that the prevalence of vitamin D insufficiency is higher in areas at high latitude [120]. This latitude dependence in prevalence is also found in AIS [121]. Lam et al. have reported a case-control study showing that both the AIS and control group had mean 25(OH)Vit-D levels at the insufficient range. The findings did not suggest AIS was associated with lower 25(OH)Vit-D level when compared with controls. On the other hand, the positive correlation between 25(OH)Vit-D and aBMD that was seen in normal controls was not present in AIS subjects, spelling out the possibility of certain degree of abnormal physiology with vitamin D being present in AIS [122].

Apart from having synergistic effects with WBV on bone anabolism mentioned earlier, vitamin D itself may play an important role in optimizing bone status in AIS. As reported at the 2016 Scoliosis Research Society Annual Meeting, Lam et al. carried out the first randomized controlled trial evaluating the therapeutic effects of vitamin D and calcium supplementation on improving bone health and controlling curve progression in AIS. Three hundred and thirty AIS girls (mean age: 12.9 ± 0.9 years) with femoral neck aBMD Z-score < 0 and radiological Cobb angle ≥15° were randomized to Group 1 ($N = 110$, placebo), Group 2 ($N = 110$, 600 mg Ca + 400 IU Vit-D3/day), and Group 3 ($N = 110$, 600 mg Ca + 800 IU Vit-D3/day). At baseline and at end of 2-year treatment, serum 25(OH)Vit-D, DXA of femoral necks, and HR-pQCT at distal radius were performed. Curve progression was defined as increase in Cobb angle ≥6°. Results showed that 270 (81.8%) subjects completed the 2-year treatment (91 in Group 1 and 2, 88 in Group 3). At baseline, mean serum 25(OH)Vit-D was 41.2 ± 14.7 nmol/L, and mean Cobb angle was $25.9 \pm 8.4°$. Mean increase in serum 25(OH)Vit-D at 2-year was 6.3 ± 15.3, 20.4 ± 19.6, and 28.0 ± 23.3 nmol/L for Group 1, 2, and 3, respectively ($p < 0.001$). Changes in aBMD, average and trabecular vBMD, and trabecular HR-pQCT parameters at the end of 2-year treatment showed improvement in bone health with Ca + Vit-D supplement ($p < 0.05$). At the latest follow-up for (1) those with initial Cobb angle ≤40° and (2) those who were not on brace treatment or never been braced ($N = 132$), 21.7% in Group 3 and 24.4% in Group 2 had curve progression as compared with 46.7% in Group 1 ($p < 0.05$). For those with baseline serum 25(OH) Vit-D ≤ 50 nmol/L ($N = 103$), 16.2% had curve progression in Group 3 as compared with 48.6% in Group 1 ($p = 0.003$). The study provided evidences that daily 600 mg Ca + 400/800 IU Vit-D3 can improve low bone mass and prevent curve progression in AIS. Vit-D status and bone density and quality should be assessed for AIS subjects and be followed with Ca + Vit-D supplementation as appropriate. This paper was well received during the conference and was granted the Russell A. Hibbs Clinical Research Award (http://www.srs.org/about-srs/news-and-announcements/winners-of-the-russell-a-hibbs-john-h-moe-louis-a-goldstein-awards).

In brief and as far as low bone mass in AIS is concerned, for those with low BMD, WBV and vitamin D and calcium supplementation can be recommended.

Further studies are warranted to confirm the roles of vitamin D and calcium supplementation and WBV, and their mutual synergistic effect in treating low bone mass in AIS; and to evaluate whether this anabolic bone effects can help to control curve progression through its positive effect on BMD [123].

6.7 Future Research Direction

We hypothesize that dysfunctional interaction of specific genetic and multiple environmental factors acting through different biochemical pathways could lead to abnormal regulation and modulation of systemic bone metabolism and growth, which are phenotypically manifested as abnormal mineralization and structure affecting bone strength and contributing to the initiation/progression of AIS (Fig. 6.5). More in-depth studies in collaboration with multidisciplinary experts will help to understand the underlying mechanisms better.

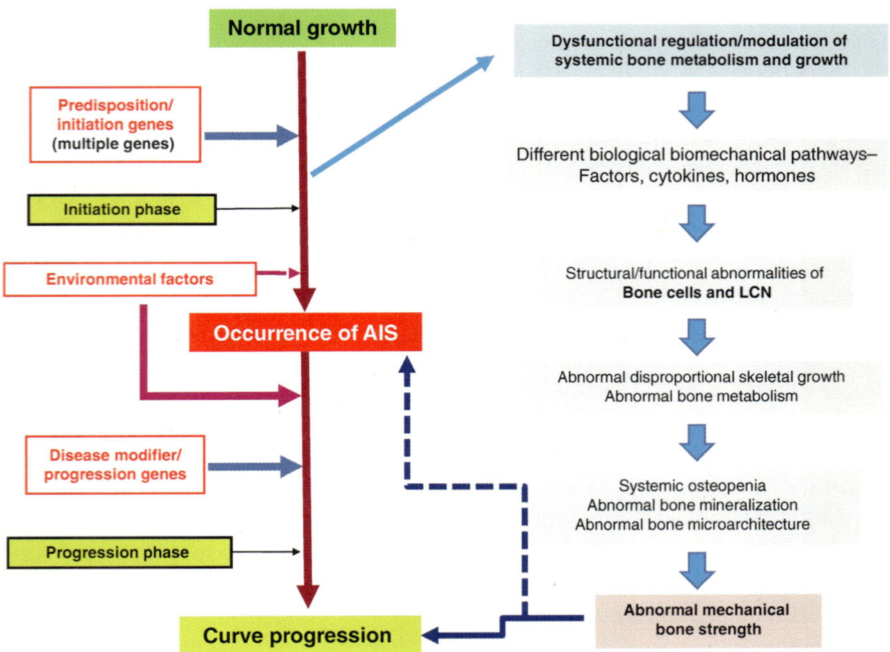

Fig. 6.5 Hypothesis on the link of abnormal bone metabolism to etiopathogenesis of AIS

6.7.1 Osteocytes: The Missing Link in AIS Bone Metabolism?

Osteocytes residing in mineralized matrix canals are interconnected with neighboring cells via multiple dendritic processes, resulting in a lacuno-canalicular network (LCN) [124]. Osteocytes regulate bone phosphate metabolism [125], and their viability is closely associated with bone quality [126]. Change in connectivity of the LCN is reported in diverse skeletal disorders such as osteoporosis, osteoarthritis, osteomalacia, and osteogenesis imperfecta [127, 128]. We have previously reported decreased osteocytes number in AIS trabecular bone [129] and have recently identified abnormal ultrastructure of osteocytes and LCN in severe AIS with SEM and FITC-Imaris technique [130]. Abnormal clusters of roundish irregular shape osteocytes with short and disorganized canaliculae were found in the AIS bone biopsies in contrast to the well-organized LCN and osteocytes with clearly spotted spindle-cell body and longer canaliculi protruded perpendicularly from the cell bodies in normal controls (Fig. 6.6). Abnormal morphology and function of the osteocyte and LCN could be a sign of impaired osteocyte functions. Recent evidence indicates that serum sclerostin level was correlated positively with BMD and micro-architecture [131]. It is of clinical interest to investigate if such change in serum sclerostin level is associated with curve severity and abnormal BMD in AIS, and could serve as a potential quantifiable prognostic factor for curve progression.

6.7.2 Time-Lapse Monitoring of Bone Remodeling in AIS Patients

The impact of bone remodeling in the etiopathogenesis in AIS remains a debatable issue because HR-pQCT scan and other measurements like serological biomarkers and primary osteoblast culture studies are not able to delineate bone formation and resorption at bone sites directly to unveil how the remodeling is affected in AIS. Conventional HR-pQCT parameters only depict the overview of bone quality from three different aspects, including geometry, vBMD, and micro-architecture, which are the consequences of many complicated cellular events. Recently, a new approach in image analysis emerges as a feasible solution for time-lapse monitoring of bone remodeling in human beings [132]. In vivo bone remodeling site quantification is done with a series of HR-pQCT images registered to corresponding baseline images using rigid 3D registration. Bone formation and resorption are determined using image processing language (IPL, Scanco) after density-based characterization and noise removal (Fig. 6.7). With this, we started a preliminary study using previous data on the effect of whole-body vibration on BMD in osteopenic AIS girls [119]. Although we did not find significant difference in global bone remodeling between the five treated and three nontreated subjects, it was noted that there were more endocortical and periosteal apposition and resorption in treatment group, which might increase mechanical integrity without affecting global bone density or

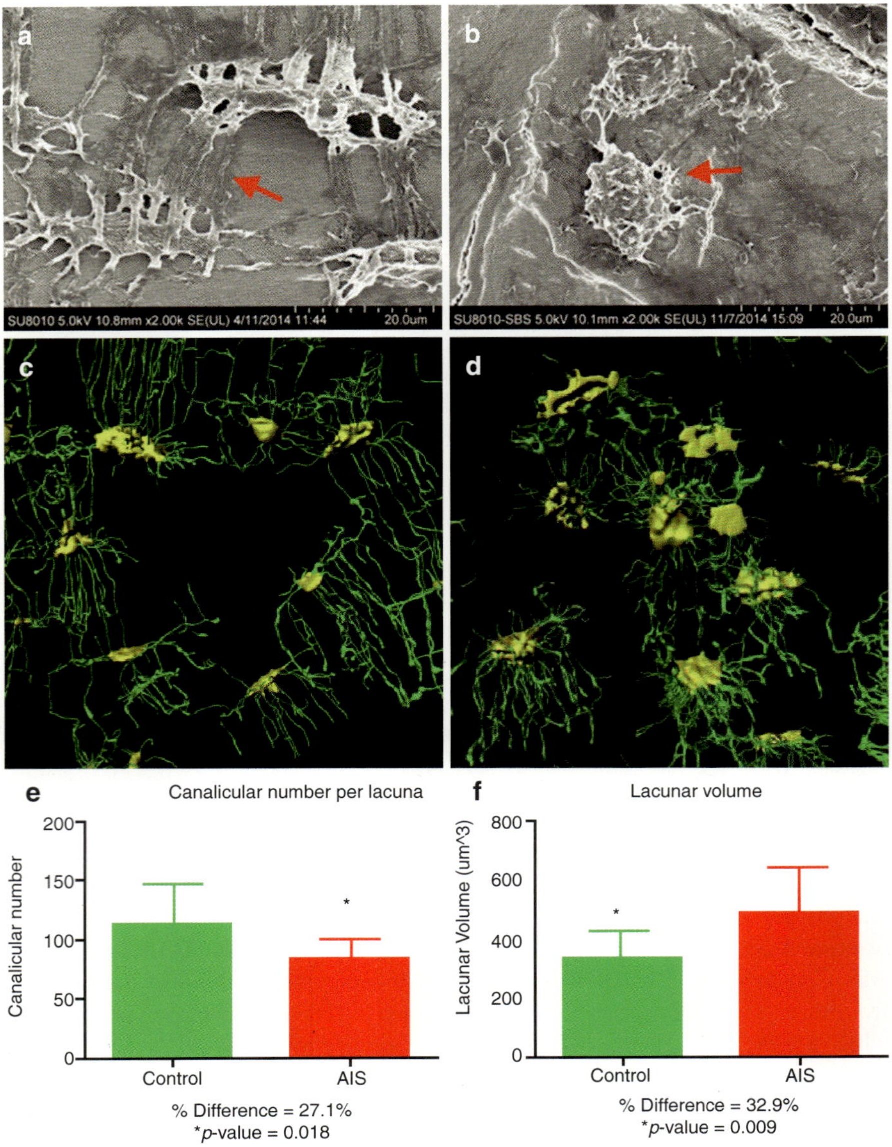

Fig. 6.6 Representative acid etched SEM images (2000×) of osteocytes in non-AIS control (**a**) and AIS (**b**) iliac crest bone biopsies. Canaliculi are indicated by red arrows. Confocal images (600×) of LCN (green) and osteocytes (presented as lacunar volume in yellow) in non-AIS control (**c**) and AIS (**d**) biopsies stained with FITC. Canalicular length and lacunar volume analyzed with Imaris are presented as mean ± SD $*p < 0.05$ compared with control (**e** and **f**, $N = 5$)

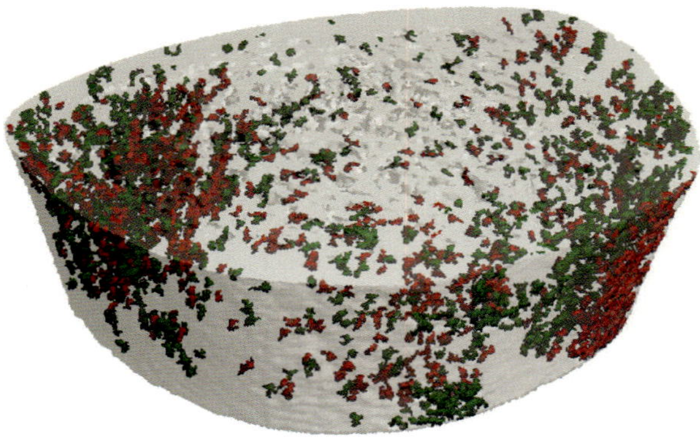

Fig. 6.7 Cross-sectional image of the non-dominant distal radius of an AIS subject with HR-pQCT showing bone geometry (gray transparent), bone formation (green), and bone resorption (red). Courtesy by Dr. Patrik Christen (ETH Zurich)

microstructural parameters. We admitted that this result should be interpreted with caution because of small sample size, but this advanced approach provides new research direction to elucidate how bone remodeling is affected in AIS.

References

1. Riggs BL, Khosla S, Melton LJ III. The assembly of the adult skeleton during growth and maturation: implications for senile osteoporosis. J Clin Invest. 1999;104(6):671–2.
2. Theintz G, Buchs B, Rizzoli R, Slosman D, Clavien H, Sizonenko PC, et al. Longitudinal monitoring of bone mass accumulation in healthy adolescents: evidence for a marked reduction after 16 years of age at the levels of lumbar spine and femoral neck in female subjects. J Clin Endocrinol Metab. 1992;75(4):1060–5.
3. Bailey DA, Wedge JH, McCulloch RG, Martin AD, Bernhardson SC. Epidemiology of fractures of the distal end of the radius in children as associated with growth. J Bone Joint Surg Am. 1989;71(8):1225–31.
4. Wang Q, Alen M, Nicholson P, Lyytikainen A, Suuriniemi M, Helkala E, et al. Growth patterns at distal radius and tibial shaft in pubertal girls: a 2-year longitudinal study. J Bone Miner Res. 2005;20(6):954–61.
5. Wang Q, Wang XF, Iuliano-Burns S, Ghasem-Zadeh A, Zebaze R, Seeman E. Rapid growth produces transient cortical weakness: a risk factor for metaphyseal fractures during puberty. J Bone Miner Res. 2010;25(7):1521–6.
6. Weaver CM. Adolescence: the period of dramatic bone growth. Endocrine. 2002;17(1):43–8.
7. Nishiyama KK, Macdonald HM, Moore SA, Fung T, Boyd SK, McKay HA. Cortical porosity is higher in boys compared with girls at the distal radius and distal tibia during pubertal growth: an HR-pQCT study. J Bone Miner Res. 2012;27(2):273–82.
8. Hauge EM, Qvesel D, Eriksen EF, Mosekilde L, Melsen F. Cancellous bone remodeling occurs in specialized compartments lined by cells expressing osteoblastic markers. J Bone Miner Res. 2001;16(9):1575–82.
9. Komori T. Regulation of osteoblast differentiation by Runx2. Adv Exp Med Biol. 2010;658:43–9.
10. Boyce BF, Xing L. Functions of RANKL/RANK/OPG in bone modeling and remodeling. Arch Biochem Biophys. 2008;473(2):139–46.

11. Hofbauer LC, Khosla S, Dunstan CR, Lacey DL, Boyle WJ, Riggs BL. The roles of osteoprotegerin and osteoprotegerin ligand in the paracrine regulation of bone resorption. J Bone Miner Res. 2000;15(1):2–12.
12. Bellido T. Osteocyte-driven bone remodeling. Calcif Tissue Int. 2014;94(1):25–34.
13. Li X, Zhang Y, Kang H, Liu W, Liu P, Zhang J, et al. Sclerostin binds to LRP5/6 and antagonizes canonical Wnt signaling. J Biol Chem. 2005;280(20):19883–7.
14. Weiner S, Wagner HD. The material bone: structure mechanical function relations. Annu Rev Mater Sci. 1998;28:271–98.
15. Zhang Z, Zhang YW, Gao H. On optimal hierarchy of load-bearing biological materials. Proc Biol Sci. 2011;278(1705):519–25.
16. Olszta MJ, Cheng XG, Jee SS, Kumar R, Kim YY, Kaufman MJ, et al. Bone structure and formation: a new perspective. Mat Sci Eng R. 2007;58(3–5):77–116.
17. Addadi L, Weiner S. Interactions between acidic proteins and crystals: stereochemical requirements in biomineralization. Proc Natl Acad Sci U S A. 1985;82(12):4110–4.
18. Lonstein JE, Carlson JM. The prediction of curve progression in untreated idiopathic scoliosis during growth. J Bone Joint Surg Ser A. 1984;66(7):1061–71.
19. Shohat M, Shohat T, Nitzan M, Mimouni M, Kedem R, Danon YL. Growth and ethnicity in scoliosis. Acta Orthop Scand. 1988;59(3):310–3.
20. Cheung CSK, Lee WTK, Tse YK, Tang SP, Lee KM, Guo X, et al. Abnormal peri-pubertal anthropometric measurements and growth pattern in adolescent idiopathic scoliosis: a study of 598 patients. Spine. 2003;28(18):2152–7.
21. Goldberg CJ, Dowling FE, Fogarty EE. Adolescent idiopathic scoliosis – early menarche, normal growth. Spine. 1993;18(5):529–35.
22. Cheung CSK, Lee WTK, Tse YK, Guo X, Qin L, Cheng JCY. Generalized osteopenia in adolescent idiopathic scoliosis – association with abnormal pubertal growth, bone turnover, and calcium intake? Spine. 2006;31(3):330–8.
23. Ylikoski M. Height of girls with adolescent idiopathic scoliosis. Eur Spine J. 2003;12(3): 288–91.
24. Cheng JCY, Leung SSF, Lau J. Anthropometric measurements and body proportions among Chinese children. Clin Orthop Relat Res. 1996;323:22–30.
25. Burwell RG, Freeman BJ, Dangerfield PH, Aujla RK, Cole AA, Kirby AS, et al. Left-right upper arm length asymmetry associated with apical vertebral rotation in subjects with thoracic scoliosis: anomaly of bilateral symmetry affecting vertebral, costal and upper arm physes? Stud Health Technol Inform. 2006;123:66–71.
26. Burwell RG, Aujla RK, Grevitt MP, Randell TL, Dangerfield PH, Cole AA, et al. Upper arm length model suggests transient bilateral asymmetry is associated with right thoracic adolescent idiopathic scoliosis (RT-AIS) with implications for pathogenesis and estimation of linear skeletal overgrowth. Stud Health Technol Inform. 2012;176:188–94.
27. Burwell RG, Aujla RK, Freeman BJ, Dangerfield PH, Cole AA, Kirby AS, et al. Patterns of extra-spinal left-right skeletal asymmetries in adolescent girls with lower spine scoliosis: relative lengthening of the ilium on the curve concavity & of right lower limb segments. Stud Health Technol Inform. 2006;123:57–65.
28. Schwender JD, Denis F. Coronal plane imbalance in adolescent idiopathic scoliosis with left lumbar curves exceeding 40°: the role of the lumbosacral hemicurve. Spine. 2000;25(18):2358–63.
29. Goldberg CJ, Fogarty EE, Moore DP, Dowling FE. Scoliosis and developmental theory: adolescent idiopathic scoliosis. Spine. 1997;22(19):2228–38.
30. Burwell RG, Aujla RK, Grevitt MP, Dangerfield PH, Moulton A, Randell TL, et al. Pathogenesis of adolescent idiopathic scoliosis in girls – a double neuro-osseous theory involving disharmony between two nervous systems, somatic and autonomic expressed in the spine and trunk: possible dependency on sympathetic nervous system and hormones with implications for medical therapy. Scoliosis. 2009;4:24.
31. Weinstein SL. Natural history. Spine (Phila Pa 1976). 1999;24(24):2592–600.

32. Grivas TB, Vasiliadis E, Mouzakis V, Mihas C, Koufopoulos G. Association between adolescent idiopathic scoliosis prevalence and age at menarche in different geographic latitudes. Scoliosis. 2006;1(1):9.
33. Lee WTK, Cheung CSK, Tse YK, Chau WW, Qin L, Cheng JCY. Persistent osteopenia in adolescent idiopathic scoliosis (AIS) – factors predisposing to generalized osteopenia, a cross-sectional and longitudinal investigation. Int Congr Ser. 2007;1297:25–31.
34. Mao SH, Jiang J, Sun X, Zhao Q, Qian BP, Liu Z, et al. Timing of menarche in Chinese girls with and without adolescent idiopathic scoliosis: current results and review of the literature. Eur Spine J. 2011;20(2):260–5.
35. Grivas TB, Samelis P, Pappa AS, Stavlas P, Polyzois D. Menarche in scoliotic and nonscoliotic Mediterranean girls. Is there any relation between menarche and laterality of scoliotic curves? Stud Health Technol Inform. 2002;88:30–6.
36. Ramirez M, Martinez-Llorens J, Sanchez JF, Bago J, Molina A, Gea J, et al. Body composition in adolescent idiopathic scoliosis. Eur Spine J. 2013;22(2):324–9.
37. Barrios C, Cortes S, Perez-Encinas C, Escriva MD, Benet I, Burgos J, et al. Anthropometry and body composition profile of girls with nonsurgically treated adolescent idiopathic scoliosis. Spine. 2011;36(18):1470–7.
38. Tam EM, Liu Z, Lam TP, Ting T, Cheung G, Ng BK, et al. Lower muscle mass and body fat in adolescent idiopathic scoliosis are associated with abnormal leptin bioavailability. Spine (Phila Pa 1976). 2016;41(11):940–6.
39. Clark EM, Taylor HJ, Harding I, Hutchinson J, Nelson I, Deanfield JE, et al. Association between components of body composition and scoliosis: a prospective cohort study reporting differences identifiable before the onset of scoliosis. J Bone Miner Res. 2014;29(8):1729–36.
40. Witzke KA, Snow CM. Lean body mass and leg power best predict bone mineral density in adolescent girls. Med Sci Sports Exerc. 1999;31(11):1558–63.
41. Schonau E. The development of the skeletal system in children and the influence of muscular strength. Horm Res. 1998;49(1):27–31.
42. Kaji H, Kosaka R, Yamauchi M, Kuno K, Chihara K, Sugimoto T. Effects of age, grip strength and smoking on forearm volumetric bone mineral density and bone geometry by peripheral quantitative computed tomography: comparisons between female and male. Endocr J. 2005;52(6):659–66.
43. Hasegawa Y, Schneider P, Reiners C. Age, sex, and grip strength determine architectural bone parameters assessed by peripheral quantitative computed tomography (pQCT) at the human radius. J Biomech. 2001;34(4):497–503.
44. Faje A, Klibanski A. Body composition and skeletal health: too heavy? Too thin? Curr Osteoporos Rep. 2012;10(3):208–16.
45. Wolff J. The law of bone remodeling. New York, NY: Springer; 1986.
46. Lanyon LE, Rubin CT. Static vs dynamic loads as an influence on bone remodelling. J Biomech. 1984;17(12):897–905.
47. World Health Organization W. Assessment of fracture risk and its application to screening for postmenopausal osteoporosis. Report of a WHO Study Group. World Health Organ Tech Rep Ser. 1994;843:1–129.
48. Endocrinology TSo. Bone densitometry in children and adolescents. Pediatrics. 2011;127(1):189–94.
49. Bacchetta J, Boutroy S, Vilayphiou N, Ranchin B, Fouque-Aubert A, Basmaison O, et al. Bone assessment in children with chronic kidney disease: data from two new bone imaging techniques in a single-center pilot study. Pediatr Nephrol. 2011;26(4):587–95.
50. Fewtrell MS, Gordon I, Biassoni L, Cole TJ. Dual X-ray absorptiometry (DXA) of the lumbar spine in a clinical paediatric setting: does the method of size-adjustment matter? Bone. 2005;37(3):413–9.
51. Binkovitz LA, Henwood MJ. Pediatric DXA: technique and interpretation. Pediatr Radiol. 2007;37(1):21–31.
52. Adams JE. Quantitative computed tomography. Eur J Radiol. 2009;71(3):415–24.

53. Adams JE, Engelke K, Zemel BS, Ward KA. Quantitative computer tomography in children and adolescents: the 2013 ISCD pediatric official positions. J Clin Densitom. 2014;17(2):258–74.
54. Nishiyama KK, Shane E. Clinical imaging of bone microarchitecture with HR-pQCT. Curr Osteoporos Rep. 2013;11(2):147–55.
55. Liu XS, Zhang XH, Sekhon KK, Adams MF, McMahon DJ, Bilezikian JP, et al. High-resolution peripheral quantitative computed tomography can assess microstructural and mechanical properties of human distal tibial bone. J Bone Miner Res. 2010;25(4):746–56.
56. Macneil JA, Boyd SK. Bone strength at the distal radius can be estimated from high-resolution peripheral quantitative computed tomography and the finite element method. Bone. 2008;42(6):1203–13.
57. Liu XS, Cohen A, Shane E, Yin PT, Stein EM, Rogers H, et al. Bone density, geometry, microstructure, and stiffness: relationships between peripheral and central skeletal sites assessed by DXA, HR-pQCT, and cQCT in premenopausal women. J Bone Miner Res. 2010;25(10):2229–38.
58. Cohen A, Dempster DW, Muller R, Guo XE, Nickolas TL, Liu XS, et al. Assessment of trabecular and cortical architecture and mechanical competence of bone by high-resolution peripheral computed tomography: comparison with transiliac bone biopsy. Osteoporos Int. 2010;21(2):263–73.
59. Cheng JCY, Qin L, Cheung CSK, Sher AHL, Lee KM, Ng SWE, et al. Generalized low areal and volumetric bone mineral density in adolescent idiopathic scoliosis. J Bone Miner Res. 2000;15(8):1587–95.
60. El Maghraoui A, Roux C. DXA scanning in clinical practice. QJM. 2008;101(8):605–17.
61. Burner WL III, Badger VM, Sherman FC. Osteoporosis and acquired back deformities. J Pediatr Orthop. 1982;2(4):383–5.
62. Healey JH, Lane JM. Structural scoliosis in osteoporotic women. Clin Orthop Relat Res. 1985;195:216–23.
63. Cook SD, Harding AF, Morgan EL, Nicholson RJ, Thomas KA, Whitecloud TS, et al. Trabecular bone mineral density in idiopathic scoliosis. J Pediatr Orthop. 1987;7(2):168–74.
64. Lee WTK, Cheung CSK, Tse YK, Guo X, Qin L, Lam TP, et al. Association of osteopenia with curve severity in adolescent idiopathic scoliosis: a study of 919 girls. Osteoporos Int. 2005;16:1924–32.
65. Yeung HY, Qin L, Hung VW, Lee KM, Guo X, Ng BW, et al. Lower degree of mineralization found in cortical bone of adolescent idiopathic scoliosis (AIS). Stud Health Technol Inform. 2006;123:599–604.
66. Cheng JCY, Guo X, Sher AHL. Persistent osteopenia in adolescent idiopathic scoliosis – a longitudinal follow-up study. Spine. 1999;24(12):1218–22.
67. Lam TP, Hung VW, Yeung HY, Tse YK, Chu WC, Ng BK, et al. Abnormal bone quality in adolescent idiopathic scoliosis: a case-control study on 635 subjects and 269 normal controls with bone densitometry and quantitative ultrasound. Spine (Phila Pa 1976). 2011;36(15):1211–7.
68. Thomas KA, Cook SD, Skalley TC, Renshaw SV, Makuch RS, Gross M, et al. Lumbar spine and femoral neck bone mineral density in idiopathic scoliosis: a follow-up study. J Pediatr Orthop. 1992;12(2):235–40.
69. Snyder BD, Katz DA, Myers ER, Breitenbach MA, Emans JB. Bone density accumulation is not affected by brace treatment of idiopathic scoliosis in adolescent girls. J Pediatr Orthop. 2005;25(4):423–8.
70. Soucacos PN, Zacharis K, Soultanis K, Gelalis J, Xenakis T, Beris AE. Risk factors for idiopathic scoliosis: review of a 6-year prospective study. Orthopedics. 2000;23(8):833–8.
71. Hung VWY, Qin L, Cheung CSK, Lam TP, Ng BKW, Tse YK, et al. Osteopenia: a new prognostic factor of curve progression in adolescent idiopathic scoliosis. J Bone Joint Surg. 2005;87(12):2709–16.
72. Lam TP, Hung VW, Yeung HY, Chu WC, Ng BK, Lee KM, et al. Quantitative ultrasound for predicting curve progression in adolescent idiopathic scoliosis: a prospective cohort study of 294 cases followed-up beyond skeletal maturity. Ultrasound Med Biol. 2013;39(3):381–7.

73. Yip BH, Yu FW, Wang Z, Hung VW, Lam TP, Ng BK, et al. Prognostic value of bone mineral density on curve progression: a longitudinal cohort study of 513 girls with adolescent idiopathic scoliosis. Sci Rep. 2016;6:39220.
74. Slemenda CW, Miller JZ, Hui SL, Reister TK, Johnston CC Jr. Role of physical activity in the development of skeletal mass in children. J Bone Miner Res. 1991;6(11):1227–33.
75. Rubin K, Schirduan V, Gendreau P, Sarfarazi M, Mendola R, Dalsky G. Predictors of axial and peripheral bone mineral density in healthy children and adolescents, with special attention to the role of puberty. J Pediatr. 1993;123(6):863–70.
76. Lee WTK, Cheung CSK, Tse YK, Guo X, Qin L, Ho SC, et al. Generalized low bone mass of girls with adolescent idiopathic scoliosis is related to inadequate calcium intake and weight bearing physical activity in peripubertal period. Osteoporos Int. 2005;16:1024–35.
77. Yu WS, Chan KY, Yu FW, Ng BK, Lee KM, Qin L, et al. Bone structural and mechanical indices in adolescent idiopathic scoliosis evaluated by high-resolution peripheral quantitative computed tomography (HR-pQCT). Bone. 2014;61C:109–15.
78. Rizzoli R, Bonjour JP. Physiology of calcium and phosphate homeostases. In: Seibel MJ, Robins SP, Bilezikian JP, editors. Dynamics of bone and cartilage metabolism. London: Academic; 2006. p. 345–60.
79. Society CN. Chinese dietary reference intakes. Beijing: Chinese Light Industry Press; 2000.
80. Akseer N, Kish K, Rigby WA, Greenway M, Klentrou P, Wilson PM, et al. Does bracing affect bone health in women with adolescent idiopathic scoliosis? Scoliosis. 2015;10:5.
81. Gozdzialska A, Jaskiewicz J, Knapik-Czajka M, Drag J, Gawlik M, Ciesla M, et al. Association of calcium and phosphate balance, vitamin D, PTH, and calcitonin in patients with adolescent idiopathic scoliosis. Spine (Phila Pa 1976). 2016;41(8):693–7.
82. Balioglu MB, Aydin C, Kargin D, Albayrak A, Atici Y, Tas SK, et al. Vitamin-D measurement in patients with adolescent idiopathic scoliosis. J Pediatr Orthop B. 2017;26(1):48–52.
83. Andrew T, Macgregor AJ. Genes and osteoporosis. Curr Osteoporos Rep. 2004;2(3):79–89.
84. Sobieszczanska M, Jonkisz J, Tabin M, Laszki-Szczachor K. Osteoporosis: genetic determinants and relationship with cardiovascular disease. Adv Clin Exp Med. 2013;22(1):119–24.
85. Richards JB, Kavvoura FK, Rivadeneira F, Styrkarsdottir U, Estrada K, Halldorsson BV, et al. Collaborative meta-analysis: associations of 150 candidate genes with osteoporosis and osteoporotic fracture. Ann Intern Med. 2009;151(8):528–37.
86. Richards JB, Zheng HF, Spector TD. Genetics of osteoporosis from genome-wide association studies: advances and challenges. Nat Rev Genet. 2012;13(8):576–88.
87. Pothuaud L, Van Rietbergen B, Mosekilde L, Beuf O, Levitz P, Benhamou CL, et al. Combination of topological parameters and bone volume fraction better predicts the mechanical properties of trabecular bone. J Biomech. 2002;35(8):1091–9.
88. Pistoia W, van Rietbergen B, Lochmuller EM, Lill CA, Eckstein F, Ruegsegger P. Estimation of distal radius failure load with micro-finite element analysis models based on three-dimensional peripheral quantitative computed tomography images. Bone. 2002;30(6):842–8.
89. Sornay-Rendu E, Boutroy S, Munoz F, Delmas PD. Alterations of cortical and trabecular architecture are associated with fractures in postmenopausal women, partially independent of decreased BMD measured by DXA: the OFELY study. J Bone Miner Res. 2007;22(3):425–33.
90. NIH Consensus Development Panel on Osteoporosis Prevention, Diagnosis, and Therapy. Osteoporosis prevention, diagnosis, and therapy. JAMA. 2001;285(6):785–95.
91. Wang Z, Chen H, Yu YE, Zhang J, Cheuk KY, Ng BK, et al. Unique local bone tissue characteristics in iliac crest bone biopsy from adolescent idiopathic scoliosis with severe spinal deformity. Sci Rep. 2017;7:40265.
92. Okata H, Nakamura M, Henmi A, Yamaguchi S, Mikami Y, Shimauchi H, et al. Calcification during bone healing in a standardised rat calvarial defect assessed by micro-CT and SEM-EDX. Oral Dis. 2015;21(1):74–82.
93. Tzaphlidou M, Speller R, Royle G, Griffiths J, Olivo A, Pani S, et al. High resolution Ca/P maps of bone architecture in 3D synchrotron radiation microtomographic images. Appl Rad Isotopes. 2005;62(4):569–75.

94. Yu W, Chan Ky YFWP, Hy Y, Ng BKW, Lee K, et al. Abnormal bone quality versus low bone mineral density in adolescent idiopathic scoliosis: a case-control study with in vivo high-resolution peripheral quantitative computed tomography. Spine J. 2013;13(11):1493–9.
95. Liu XS, Sajda P, Saha PK, Wehrli FW, Bevill G, Keaveny TM, et al. Complete volumetric decomposition of individual trabecular plates and rods and its morphological correlations with anisotropic elastic moduli in human trabecular bone. J Bone Miner Res. 2008;23(2):223–35.
96. Liu XS, Stein EM, Zhou B, Zhang CA, Nickolas TL, Cohen A, et al. Individual trabecula segmentation (ITS)-based morphological analyses and microfinite element analysis of HR-pQCT images discriminate postmenopausal fragility fractures independent of DXA measurements. J Bone Miner Res. 2012;27(2):263–72.
97. Cheung CS, Lee WT, Tse YK, Lee KM, Guo X, Qin L, et al. Generalized osteopenia in adolescent idiopathic scoliosis—association with abnormal pubertal growth, bone turnover, and calcium intake? Spine (Phila Pa 1976). 2006;31(3):330–8.
98. Suh KT, Lee SS, Hwang SH, Kim SJ, Lee JS. Elevated soluble receptor activator of nuclear factor-kappaB ligand and reduced bone mineral density in patients with adolescent idiopathic scoliosis. Eur Spine J. 2007;16(10):1563–9.
99. Brzezinski A. Melatonin in humans. N Engl J Med. 1997;336(3):186–95.
100. O'Kelly C, Wang X, Raso J, Moreau M, Mahood J, Zhao J, et al. The production of scoliosis after pinealectomy in young chickens, rats, and hamsters. Spine. 1999;24(1):35–43.
101. Machida M, Saito M, Dubousset J, Yamada T, Kimura J, Shibasaki K. Pathological mechanism of idiopathic scoliosis: Experimental scoliosis in pinealectomized rats. Eur Spine J. 2005;14(9):843–8.
102. Machida M, Dubousset J, Imamura Y, Iwaya T, Yamada T, Kimura J. An experimental study in chickens for the pathogenesis of idiopathic scoliosis. Spine. 1993;18(12):1609–15.
103. Moreau A, Wang DS, Forget S, Azeddine B, Angeloni D, Fraschini F, et al. Melatonin signaling dysfunction in adolescent idiopathic scoliosis. Spine. 2004;29(16):1772–81.
104. Moreau A, Akoumé Ndong MY, Azeddine B, Franco A, Rompré PH, Roy-Gagnon MH, et al. Molecular and genetic aspects of idiopathic scoliosis: Blood test for idiopathic scoliosis. Orthopade. 2009;38(2):114–21.
105. Man G, Wang W, Yeung B, Lee S, Ng B, Hung W-Y, et al. Abnormal proliferation and differentiation of osteoblasts from girls with adolescent idiopathic scoliosis to melatonin. J Pineal Res. 2010;49:69–77.
106. Man GCW, Wong JH, Wang WWJ, Sun GQ, Yeung BHY, Ng TB, et al. Abnormal melatonin receptor 1B expression in osteoblasts from girls with adolescent idiopathic scoliosis. J Pineal Res. 2011;50(4):395–402.
107. Yim AP, Yeung HY, Sun G, Lee KM, Ng TB, Lam TP, et al. Abnormal skeletal growth in adolescent idiopathic scoliosis is associated with abnormal quantitative expression of melatonin receptor, MT2. Int J Mol Sci. 2013;14(3):6345–58.
108. Qiu XS, Tang NLS, Yeung HY, Lee KM, Hung VWY, Ng BKW, et al. Melatonin receptor 1B (MTNR1B) gene polymorphism is associated with the occurrence of adolescent idiopathic scoliosis. Spine. 2007;32(16):1748–53.
109. Qiu Y, Sun X, Qiu X, Li W, Zhu Z, Zhu F, et al. Decreased circulating leptin level and its association with body and bone mass in girls with adolescent idiopathic scoliosis. Spine (Phila Pa 1976). 2007;32(24):2703–10.
110. Liu Z, Tam EM, Sun GQ, Lam TP, Zhu ZZ, Sun X, et al. Abnormal leptin bioavailability in adolescent idiopathic scoliosis: an important new finding. Spine (Phila Pa 1976). 2012;37(7):599–604.
111. Tam EM, Yu FW, Hung VW, Liu Z, Liu KL, Ng BK, et al. Are volumetric bone mineral density and bone micro-architecture associated with leptin and soluble leptin receptor levels in adolescent idiopathic scoliosis? A case-control study. PLoS One. 2014;9(2):e87939.
112. Burwell RG, Dangerfield PH, Moulton A, Anderson SI. Etiologic theories of idiopathic scoliosis: autonomic nervous system and the leptin-sympathetic nervous system con-

cept for the pathogenesis of adolescent idiopathic scoliosis. Stud Health Technol Inform. 2008;140:197–207.
113. Leboeuf D, Letellier K, Alos N, Edery P, Moldovan F. Do estrogens impact adolescent idiopathic scoliosis? Trends Endocrinol Metab. 2009;20(4):147–52.
114. Rubin C, Turner AS, Bain S, Mallinckrodt C, McLeod K. Low mechanical signals strengthen long bones. Nature. 2001;412(6847):603–4.
115. Gilsanz V, Wren TA, Sanchez M, Dorey F, Judex S, Rubin C. Low-level, high-frequency mechanical signals enhance musculoskeletal development of young women with low BMD. J Bone Miner Res. 2006;21(9):1464–74.
116. Rubin C, Recker R, Cullen D, Ryaby J, McCabe J, McLeod K. Prevention of postmenopausal bone loss by a low-magnitude, high-frequency mechanical stimuli: a clinical trial assessing compliance, efficacy, and safety. J Bone Miner Res. 2004;19(3):343–51.
117. Slatkovska L, Alibhai SM, Beyene J, Cheung AM. Effect of whole-body vibration on BMD: a systematic review and meta-analysis. Osteoporos Int. 2010;21(12):1969–80.
118. Kohrt WM. Aging and the osteogenic response to mechanical loading. Int J Sport Nutr Exerc Metab. 2001;11(Suppl):S137–42.
119. Lam TP, Ng BK, Cheung LW, Lee KM, Qin L, Cheng JC. Effect of whole body vibration (WBV) therapy on bone density and bone quality in osteopenic girls with adolescent idiopathic scoliosis: a randomized, controlled trial. Osteoporos Int. 2013;24(5):1623–36.
120. Lee WT, Jiang J. The resurgence of the importance of vitamin D in bone health. Asia Pac J Clin Nutr. 2008;17(Suppl 1):138–42.
121. Grivas TB, Vasiliadis E, Savvidou O, Mouzakis V, Koufopoulos G. Geographic latitude and prevalence of adolescent idiopathic scoliosis. Stud Health Technol Inform. 2006;123:84–9.
122. Lam TP, Yu WS, Mak WY, Cheung TF, Lee KM, BKW N, et al., editors. Vitamin D insufficiency and its association with low bone mass in girls with adolescent idiopathic scoliosis (AIS). 48th Scoliosis Research Society (SRS) annual meeting, Sep 2013. Lyon: Scoliosis Research Society (SRS); 2013.
123. Hung VWY, Qin L, Cheung CSK, Lam TP, Ng BKW, Tse YK, et al. Osteopenia: a new prognostic factor of curve progression in adolescent idiopathic scoliosis. J Bone Joint Surg Am. 2005;87:2709–16.
124. Schneider P, Meier M, Wepf R, Muller R. Towards quantitative 3D imaging of the osteocyte lacuno-canalicular network. Bone. 2010;47(5):848–58.
125. Ruchon AF, Tenenhouse HS, Marcinkiewicz M, Siegfried G, Aubin JE, DesGroseillers L, et al. Developmental expression and tissue distribution of Phex protein: effect of the Hyp mutation and relationship to bone markers. J Bone Miner Res. 2000;15(8):1440–50.
126. Zhao CQ, Liu D, Li H, Jiang LS, Dai LY. Expression of leptin and its functional receptor on disc cells: contribution to cell proliferation. Spine (Phila Pa 1976). 2008;33(23):E858–64.
127. Jones SJ, Glorieux FH, Travers R, Boyde A. The microscopic structure of bone in normal children and patients with osteogenesis imperfecta: a survey using backscattered electron imaging. Calcif Tissue Int. 1999;64(1):8–17.
128. Knothe Tate ML, Adamson JR, Tami AE, Bauer TW. The osteocyte. Int J Biochem Cell Biol. 2004;36(1):1–8.
129. Cheng JC, Tang SP, Guo X, Chan CW, Qin L. Osteopenia in adolescent idiopathic scoliosis: a histomorphometric study. Spine (Phila Pa 1976). 2001;26(3):E19–23.
130. Ren Y, Lin S, Jing Y, Dechow PC, Feng JQ. A novel way to statistically analyze morphologic changes in Dmp1-null osteocytes. Connect Tissue Res. 2014;55(Suppl 1):129–33.
131. Cejka D, Jager-Lansky A, Kieweg H, Weber M, Bieglmayer C, Haider DG, et al. Sclerostin serum levels correlate positively with bone mineral density and microarchitecture in haemodialysis patients. Nephrol Dial Transplant. 2012;27(1):226–30.
132. Christen P, Ito K, Ellouz R, Boutroy S, Sornay-Rendu E, Chapurlat RD, et al. Bone remodelling in humans is load-driven but not lazy. Nat Commun. 2014;5:4855.

Chapter 7
Neurological Research in Idiopathic Scoliosis

Masafumi Machida

7.1 Introduction

Idiopathic scoliosis (IS) is a three-dimensional deformity of the spine with lateral curvature combined with vertebral rotation. The primary lesion, however, lies in the sagittal plane, taking the form of lordosis. It was first described by Hippocrates, and the term "scoliosis" was first coined by Galen (AD 131–201). IS, therefore, refers to a structural scoliosis with lordosis and vertebral rotation. This is the most common and clincally important type of idiopathic scoliosis, which affects more offen in girls. The spine curvature progresses during the growing years, particularly during the preadolescent and adolescent growth spurt, and halts as growth ceases. Although the clinical manifestations of scoliosis have been well described, its etiology and pathogenesis of IS have not been clearly elucidated.

IS is a multifactorial disease which involves intrinsic factors such as the growth of vertebral bodies, abnormal morphometry of the posterior elements, and asymmetrical growth of the neurocentral cartilage. Other multiple factors have been proposed such as genetics, extra-spinal left-right asymmetrical body growth and development, imbalance of muscle structures, dysfunction of the nervous, somatosensory and vestibular functions, length discrepancy between spine and spinal cord, abnormal platelet calmodulin, and abnormality in melatonin metabolism [1]. Recently, research of IS etiology has focused on the structural elements of the spine such as musculature and collagenous structures, systemic factors such as endocrine and central nervous system, and also genetics [2] (Fig. 7.1), but none has shown convincing evidence for the cause of IS. Results of various animal

M. Machida, M.D., D.Med.Sci
Department of Spine and Spinal Cord Surgery,
Yokohama Brain and Spine Center, Yokohama, Kanagawa, Japan
e-mail: m.m.spine@gmail.com

M. Machida et al. (eds.), *Pathogenesis of Idiopathic Scoliosis*,
https://doi.org/10.1007/978-4-431-56541-3_7

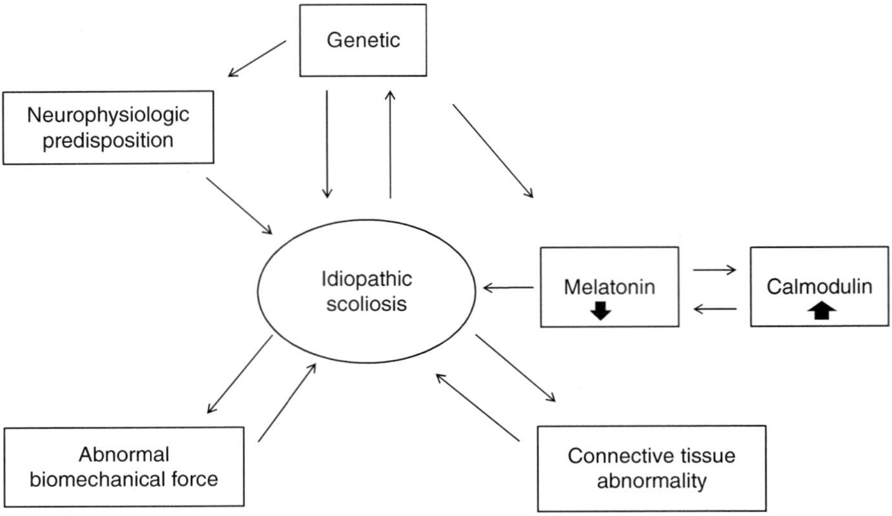

Fig. 7.1 Interrelationships among various factors that have a potential role in the etiology of idiopathic scoliosis

experimental models and clinical studies have indicated possible anatomical or functional components as a cause of IS, but many of these may be epiphenomena rather than the cause.

This chapter is a review of the neurological causative factors thus far proposed for IS and a discussion of where the research is heading in order to find the etiology of IS.

7.2 Erect Posture and Paravertebral Muscles

Bipedalism with an upright posture predisposed humans to a series of three-dimensional changes in the spine and trunk, affecting the sagittal shape pelvic-spine rotation/counter-rotation in the horizontal plane, and trunk broadening in the coronary plane. The fully erect posture, which is unique to humans, seems to be a prerequisite for the development of IS. From a biomechanical standpoint of view, this transformation could be economical and functional, but it tends to weaken the spinal column resulting in a form of "backward shear stress (dorsal shear force)" to which the vertebrae are not accustomed. The effects of dorsal shear force can be further enhanced by the rotational instability associated with the hypokyphosis or lordosis caused by the relative anterior spinal overgrowth (RASO) and the axial spinal movements unique to humans. Consequently, the upright bipedal posture may contribute to the rotator instability from which scoliosis originates. This has been confirmed by the experimental rat studies of Machida et al., in which experimental scoliosis developed only in pinealectomized bipedal, but not in quadrupedal, rats

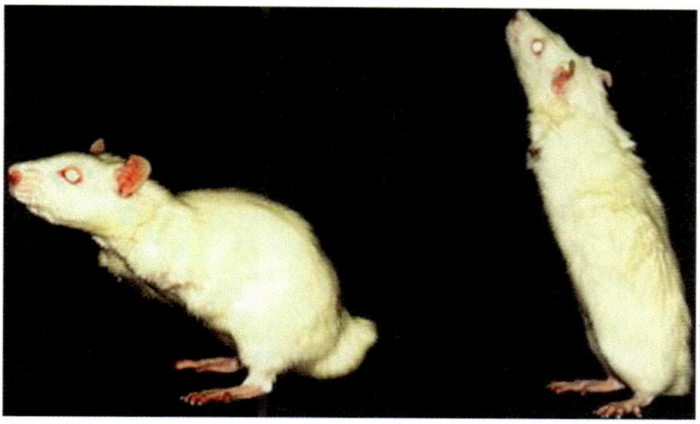

Fig. 7.2 Resection of the forelimbs and tail produced bipedal rats. The standing position induces experimental scoliosis

[3, 4]. These results support the notion that the bipedal posture may play an important role in the development of scoliosis (Fig. 7.2).

The idea that erector spine asymmetry might be the source of scoliosis is by no means new; tenotomy of the multifidus muscle had been suggested as far back as the nineteenth century a treatment for scoliosis [5]. The idea is evidently related to the high frequency of scoliosis in childhood neuromuscular disease. A few decades later another connection between scoliosis and muscle function was proposed by Eulenberg, in which asymmetrical muscle action between the concave and convex sides contributes to the deformity formation. Objecting to this idea, Adams thought that the role of the musculature in scoliosis was secondary by the overreaction of the convex paraspinal muscles attempting to stabilize the spine and prevent aggravation of the curvature [6]. He described fatty degeneration in the paraspinal muscle of the concave side of the curve, but focused on a similar pathology in the convex side of musculature at later stages with advanced deformity. Malgaigne had already suggested that scoliotic deformity was due to weakness of the muscle on the convex side in association with weak ligaments. Trontelj et al. also demonstrated asymmetrical muscle tone in the rotators of the spine on the two sides of the curve [7]. Conceivably this could be either due to an altered descending control of the spinal neurons or to a segmental neurogenic lesion involving one or a few segments that lead to asymmetric muscle weakness.

During the last century, research was focused on the role of neuromuscular factors in the causation and progression of IS. Spencer and Eccles were the first to describe the presence of two types of muscle fibers in the paraspinal muscles of AIS patients [8]. They differentiated between type-I (slow-twitch) and type-II (fast-twitch) fibers and noted that the number of type-II fibers was lower in AIS patients, suggesting a myopathic etiology for IS. Bylund et al. described a normal distribution of type-I and type-II fibers on the convexity of the curve but a lower frequency of type-I fibers on the concave side [9]. By studying biopsy samples of the paraspinal muscles in AIS patients, Slager and Hsu confirmed a decrease in the number and size of type-II fibers with no preference for either the convex or the concave [10]. In an effort to support a global myopathy, Yarom et al. found similar findings in muscle from distant sites and concluded that this represented a myopathic process [11, 12].

The myopathy differs from the known forms of congenital myopathies by its lack of specific morphology, asymmetry, and mildness.

The first studies using the electromyography (EMG) were reported by Riddles and Roaf [13]. Surface electrodes overlying the paraspinal muscles at the apex of the scoliotic curve were studied, although some of their studies including the deeper layers of the spinal muscles using needle electrodes were performed. They surmised that the unopposed activity of the deep spinal muscles would give rise to vertebral rotation as the first stage of developing scoliosis and suggested that weakening the muscle on the convex side might have stopped curve progression. Henssge studied the needle EMG potentials of paraspinal muscles in IS patients and concluded that there was evidence of muscle denervation in the deep layers in certain types of curvature [14]. In contrast, Badger found no evidence of increased EMG activity at the convex side and suggested the presence of a primary myopathic process [15]. However, Walfe reported that the EMG findings revealed variable degrees of myopathy in the deltoids of the concave side [16].

Trontelj et al. studied segmental spinal reflexes (stretch reflex) in patients with scoliosis [7]. The proprioceptive responses to the phasic stretch of the paraspinal muscles were asymmetric in all patients and were higher in the convex side. The increase in reflex response of the superficial muscles on the convex side can be attributed to diminished reciprocal inhibition from the weak and deep muscles. They concluded that a segmental neurogenic disorder predominantly involving the deep paraspinal muscles of the convex side may be the primary lesion responsible for the development of scoliosis.

Trontelj later reported the results of evaluation of single-fiber EMG (SFEMG) studies in IS patients [17]. He found an increase in fiber density, correlating with the fiber type grouping noted on histomorphometric examinations. There was increased "jitter" which was defined as abnormal conduction across the terminal axon and end plate, which is observed in both neurogenic and myopathic muscle pathologies. He also reported changes in conduction time, which correlate with changes in fiber size. Fernandez also studied the SFEMG in 51 patients with moderate idiopathic juvenile scoliosis [18]. A mild but significant neuromuscular transmission abnormality and a moderate prolonged mean of interspike latency were observed in extensor digitorum communis (EDC) musculus. The paraspinal and intercostal muscles at the apex of the scoliosis curvature in the same patients showed similar abnormalities. The study suggested the existence of a subclinical and systemic neuromuscular disorder in patients with IS, which might have a pathogenic significance. These studies suggested the presence of a systemic neuromuscular conduction defect may be the cause, rather than the effect, of the deformity. This theory was further supported in patients with a strong family history of IS who showed unilateral EMG abnormalities as early as 6 months before any radiological signs of scoliosis became evident [19]. Based on these studies, there appears to be little doubt that asymmetric EMG abnormalities exist in the paraspinal muscles of IS patients, especially in the erect posture.

Whether the EMG asymmetry results from hyperactivity on the convex side or from reduced activity on the concave side remains elusive, and there is little evidence to confirm or deny the primary importance of this EMG asymmetry contributing for the pathogenesis of IS. Although the abnormality of the paraspinal muscles has long been considered as a cause of IS, Yarom and Robin found myofilament disarray, central core formation, fiber splitting, and a marked increase in muscle calcium not only in spinal muscles but also in distal muscles like the gluteus maximus [20]. High calcium concentration was also found in the tongue muscles of IS patients with mild curvature. They attributed this to a generalized membrane defect—namely, an impaired calcium pump. Following this line of thought, low bone quality has been observed in IS patients, with changes in bone density at sites remote from the spine.

Biochemical analyses of the muscles in IS patients have found on tissue enzyme actovity and protein synthesis. Gibson et al. analyzed protein synthesis in paraspinal muscle biopsy specimens obtained bilaterally from the top, bottom, and apex of the curve in IS patients using the stable isotope-labeled L-leucine [21] and found no difference between the two sides of the spine. However, at the apex of the curve, protein synthesis was higher on the convexity than on the concavity, and muscle ribonucleic acid activity was lower on the concavity than on the convexity. They believed that these results were consistent with the effects on muscle protein turnover secondary to increased muscle contraction and functional immobilization that occurs on the concave aspect of the curve.

Although the idea that an abnormality of the paraspinal muscles might be the cause of IS has been proposed many times throughout the years, there is insufficient data to back this claim. Morphological changes were most pronounced in the concave paraspinal muscles, but similar changes were found in other muscles such as the gluteus and deltoid muscles. Whatever the etiology of the myopathy and its asymmetry, these muscle changes may be more effectual than the causal in the pathogenesis of IS; most of the abnormalities that have been noted in the muscles may be more likely secondary to the deformity itself than the cause.

7.3 Calmodulin and Melatonin

There is a close relationship between calcium and muscle contraction with the binding of calcium to troponin on contractile protein structure being the initiating factor for contraction. Troponin found by Ebashi and Endo in 1968 inhibits the interaction of myosin and actin, and the inhibition is removed by Ca^{++} [22]. Since elevated calcium stimulates ATPase function and leads to contraction, the presence of an increased sarcoplasmic calcium concentration in IS patients has suggested a possible true role of calcium-related myopathy in IS pathogenesis.

Calmodulin, another calcium-binding receptor protein, is a critical mediator of eukaryotic cellular calcium function and a regulator of many important enzymatic systems. Calmodulin regulates the contractile properties of muscles and platelets through its interaction with actin and myosin and regulates calcium fluxes from the sarcoplasmic reticulum. Several studies on platelet abnormalities in IS were reported in the 1980s based on the similarity between the cytoskeleton of skeletal muscle cells and platelet cells. An abnormal platelet aggregation in IS patients with a large Cobb angle has been confirmed, and increased platelet calmodulin levels have been shown to be associated with the progression of AIS. Cohen et al. found a 2.5- to 3-fold increase in the calmodulin activity in platelets of AIS patients [23] and suggested that the platelet calmodulin levels may be a better predictor for scoliosis progression than the Risser sign. Kindsfater et al. showed that platelet calmodulin levels were significantly higher in patients with a progressive curve than in patients with stable curvature [24]. Using calmodulin as a systemic mediator of contracting tissue, the relationship between platelet calmodulin level changes and Cobb angle changes in AIS patients suggested that altered paraspinal muscle activity may be a cause of scoliosis. Asymmetric distribution of calmodulin reported in another study further supports this hypothesis [25]. Lowe et al. noted that AIS through bracing or spinal fusion resulted in a decrease of the platelet calmodulin levels in many patients with AIS [26, 27], but the cause of this decrease in platelet calmodulin is unknown.

Recent evidence suggests that melatonin which binds to calmodulin with high affinity and acts as a calmodulin antagonist may modulate calcium-activated calmodulin. Since melatonin is to be tightly associated with the sleep-wake cycle, it may diurnally modulate many cellular functions involving calcium transport [28, 29]. Although there were some reports that platelet calmodulin may be related to muscle disorders, the high levels of calmodulin in the brain suggests that the role of calmodulin in IS may more likely be related to an abnormality in the central nervous system rather than abnormal skeletal muscles.

Thillard was the first to report the development of scoliosis in pinealectomized chickens [30], and her findings were confirmed by Dubousset and Machida [31–35] (Fig. 7.3). As melatonin is a neuromodulator which is present in the pineal gland, we put forward the hypothesis that the pathogenic mechanism is associated with a postural equilibrium induced by melatonin deficiency. We also investigated the effect of pinealectomy in rats. We performed pinealectomy not only in quadrupedal rats but also in bipedal rats created by resection of the forearms and tails. It was found that scoliosis developed in all bipedal rats (Fig. 7.4) but not in quadrupedal rats. Based upon these results, we postulated that the scoliotic deformity of the fibroelastic and bony structures of the spine in humans was associated with the bipedal condition [3]. An inherited disorder of neuromodulators and/or neurohormones affecting melatonin synthesis produces a systemic imbalance that generates an abnormal force leading to scoliosis. Furthermore, bipedal C57BL/6J mice, which have in a reduced plasma and pineal melatonin levels due to a natural knockout in a major enzyme required for melatonin synthesis (NAT gene), developed scoliosis without resection of the pineal gland [36] (Fig. 7.5). Supplementation of melatonin or pineal gland transplantation in melatonin-deficient chickens, rats, and mice prevented the development of scoliosis [3, 33, 36]. Later, Chung et al., investigating the effects of pinealectomy in monkeys, which are much closer to human beings, demonstrated that melatonin deficiency in nonhuman primates did not induce scoliosis [37]. They concluded that the factors producing scoliosis in lower animals, such as

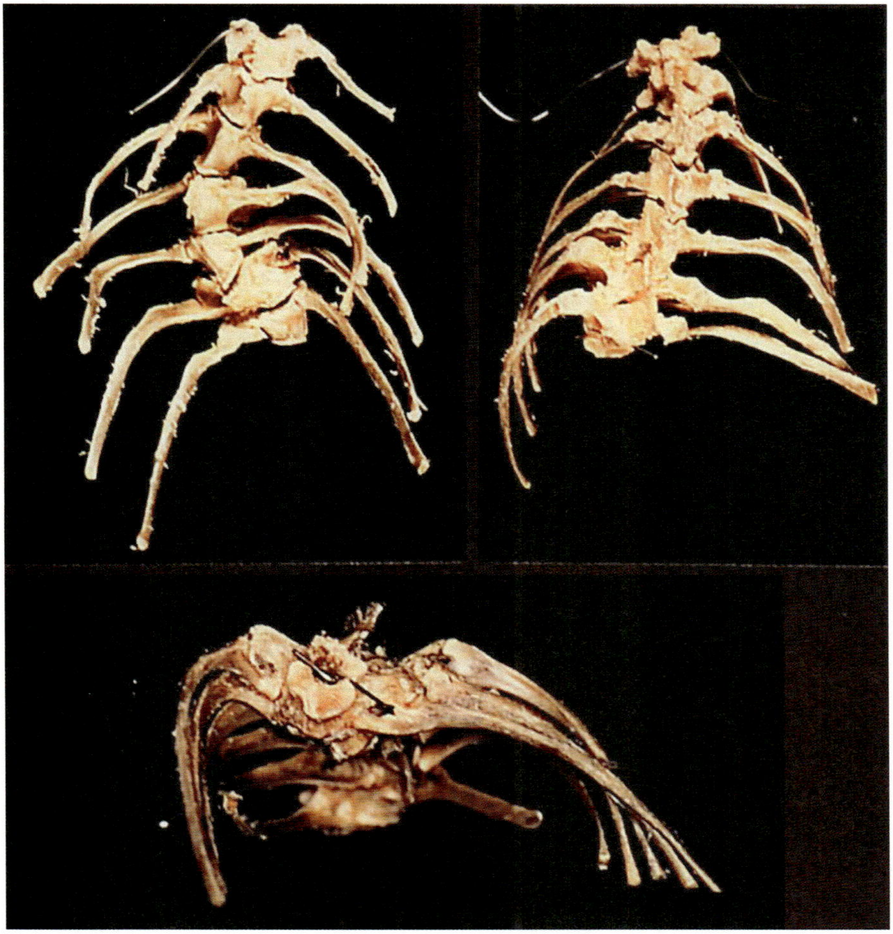

Fig. 7.3 The pictures of the thoracic spine in a pinealectomized chicken. The scoliotic deformity is lordoscoliosis with vertebral rotation. The vertebral body is compressed downward on the concave side leading to a wedge-shaped deformity. The posterior elements of a scoliotic vertebra show much more complicated deformity

chickens and rats, are different from the etiological factors in nonhuman and human primates, but we strongly disagree with their conclusion, because monkeys are mostly of quadrupedal gait, though they are capable of bipedal standing.

Utilizing a [^{125}I]iodomelatonin-binding assay in the experimental scoliosis model of melatonin-deficient C57BL/6J mice, we recently found that the responsible site for scoliosis development was likely to be the melatonin receptor in the paraventricular thalamic nucleus [38] (Fig. 7.6). There are melatonin receptors at the cerebral cortex, striatum, hippocampus, thalamus, paraventricular thalamic nucleus, hypothalamus, midbrain, and cerebellum in the brain. Mice treated with melatonin had uniformly lower total binding of [^{125}I]iodomelatonin, but mice that did not

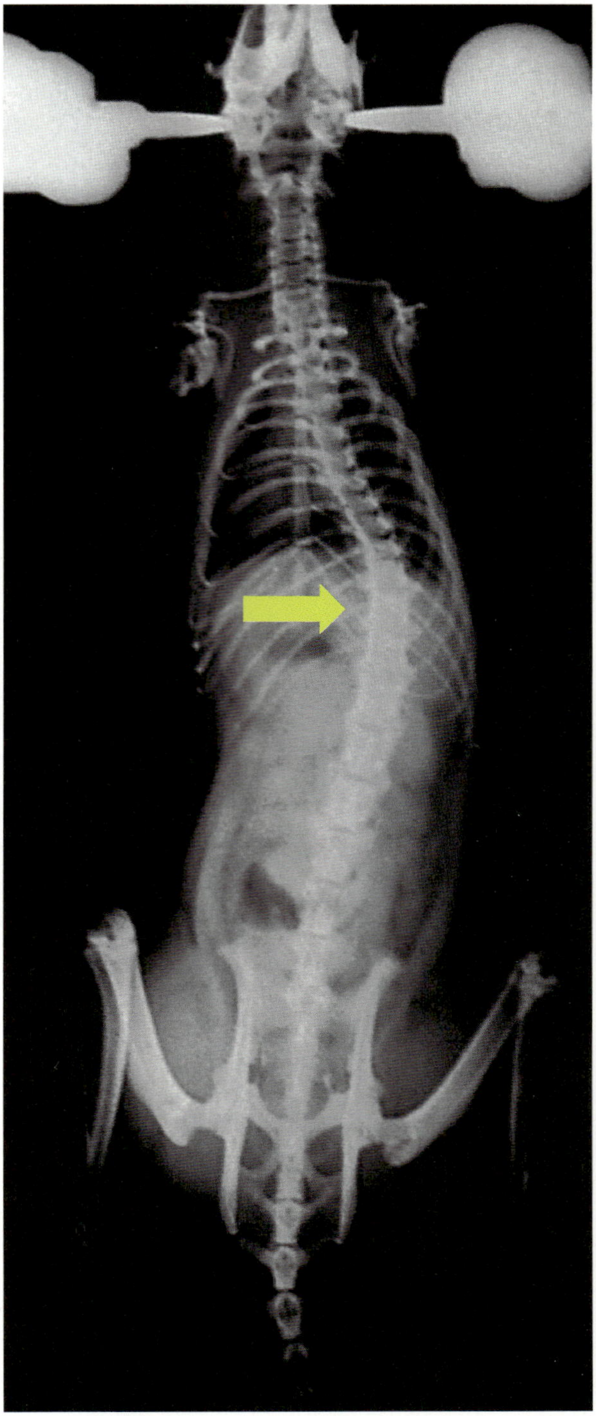

Fig. 7.4 Radiograph of the scoliotic deformity with vertebral rotation in a pinealectomized bipedal rat

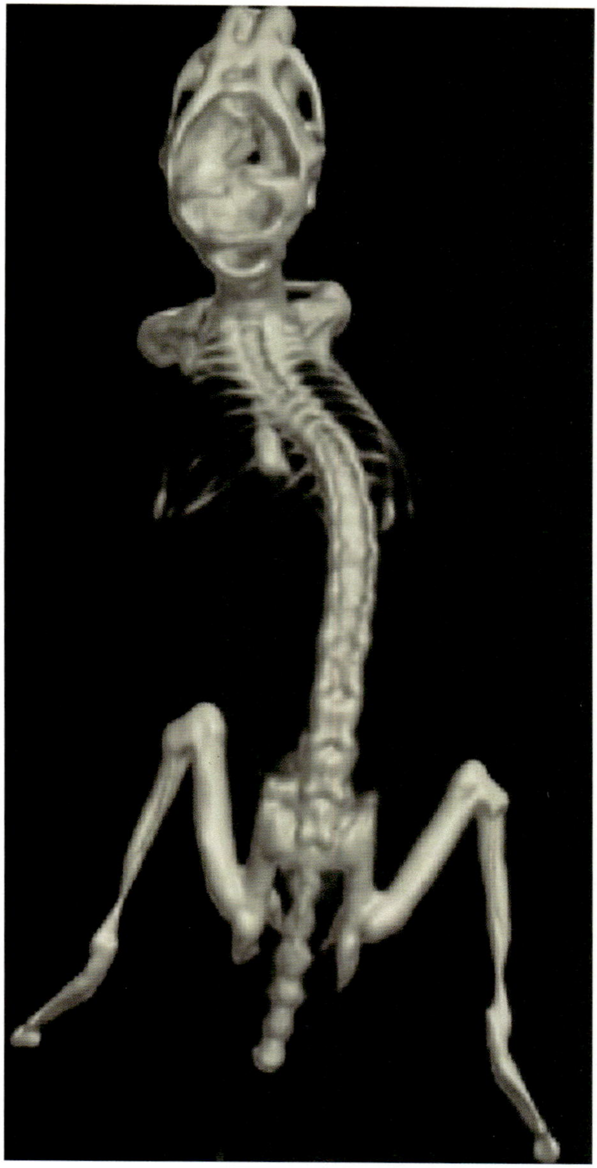

Fig. 7.5 Helical 3D-CT image clearly shows a scoliosis with right convexity and asymmetry of the thoracic cage in a bipedal mouse. There is rotation of the apical vertebra toward the convexity of the curve

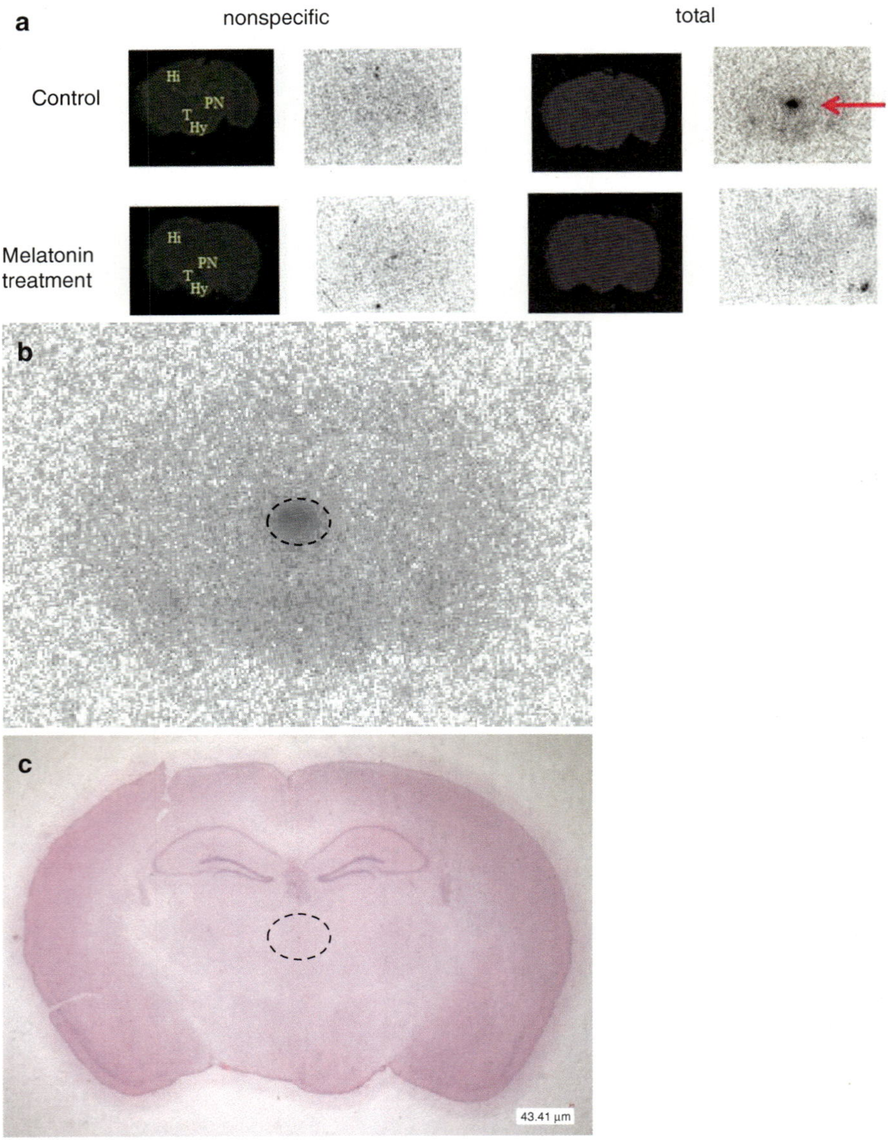

Fig. 7.6 (**a**, **b**) Distribution of [^{125}I]iodomelatonin binding sites in the bipedal C57BL/6J mouse with and without melatonin treatment. The binding density at the paraventricular thalamic nucleus (PTN) which was extremely high without melatonin treatment is uniformly lower in mice treated with melatonin. (**c**) An HE stain of the brain level in which the PTN is located. (**d**) Brain map

d

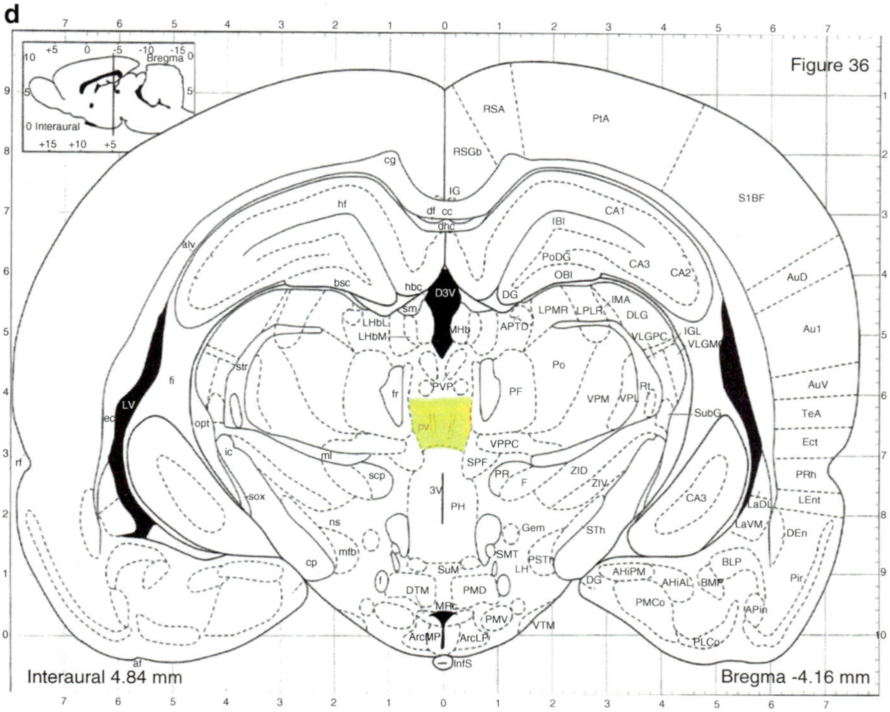

Fig. 7.6 (continued)

receive melatonin treatment had an unproportionately high density of melatonin receptors in the paraventricular thalamic nucleus compared to other sites of the brain. In contrast, mice treated with melatonin had a comparable density of melatonin receptors throughout the brain.

In agreement with the view that melatonin is deficient in IS patients, decreased melatonin levels have been observed in adolescent carriers of scoliosis [39–41]. We also reported that the melatonin concentration throughout a 24-h period was significantly lower in patients with progressive scoliosis than in patients with stable curves and normal controls (Fig. 7.7). Changes in melatonin receptor binding have also been mentioned as a possible factor in the development of IS [42, 43]. Along with this line of thought, we studied a group of 40 AIS patients with moderate to severe scoliosis, and we investigated the correlation between serum melatonin levels and curve progression and studied the effects of melatonin therapy in patients with reduced levels of endogenous melatonin. Our findings suggested that transient melatonin deficiency may be associated with deterioration of scoliosis and that melatonin levels may serve as a useful predictor for progression of spine curvature in patients with IS. Our results also suggested that melatonin treatment may provide some benefit in preventing the progression of scoliosis in melatonin-deficient patients, if the curves do not exceed 35° [41] (Fig. 7.8). Moreau et al. reported that

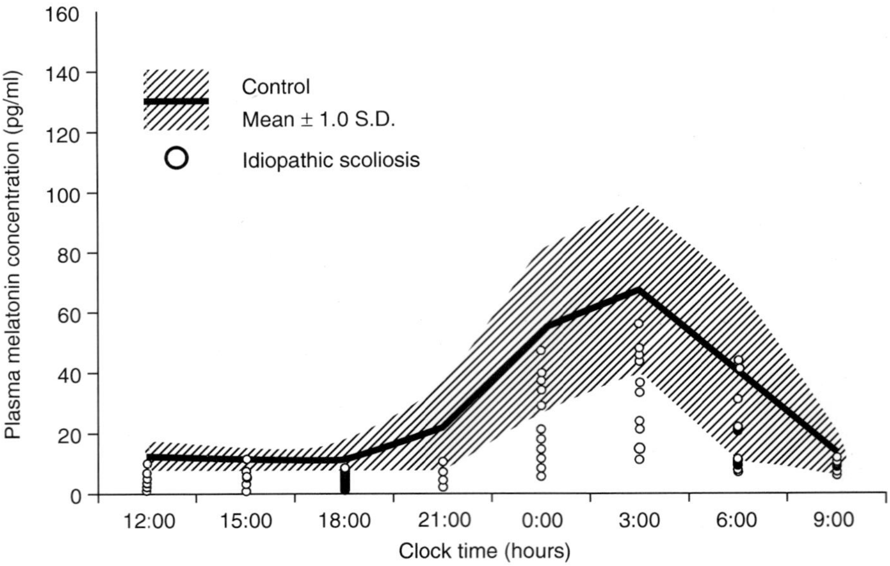

Fig. 7.7 Circadian cycle of plasma melatonin concentration in 12 patients with progressive spinal curves reveals low melatonin concentration

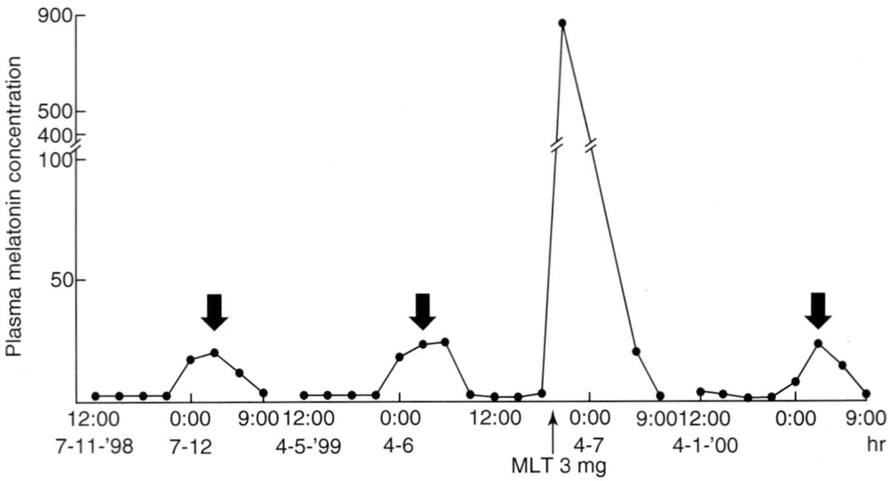

Fig. 7.8 Plasma melatonin levels before and after melatonin administration. This case that received melatonin administration for a year showed no progression in the scoliosis until maturity

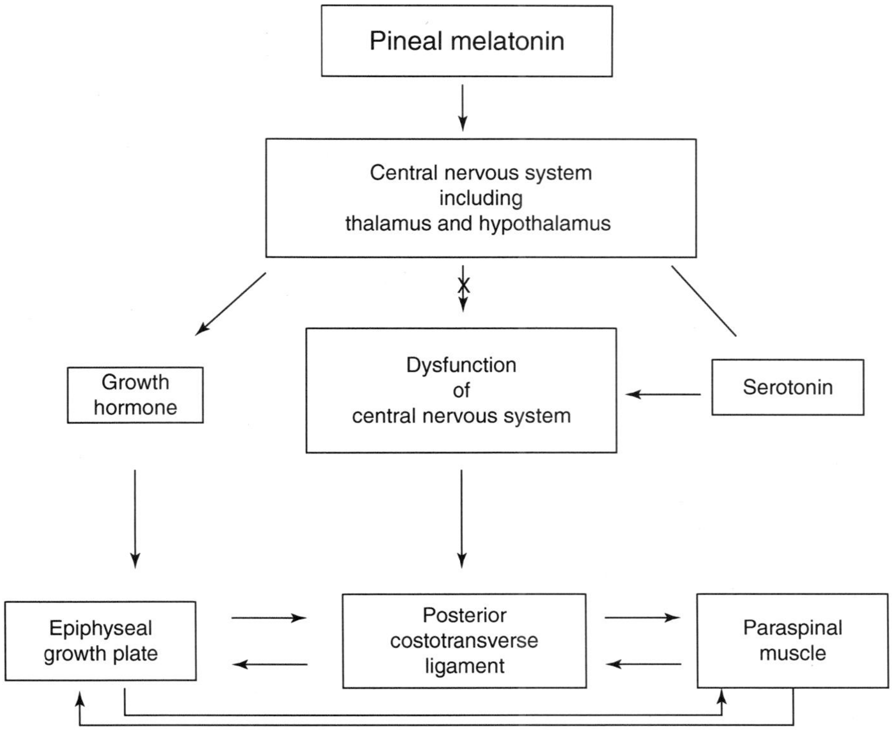

Fig. 7.9 A diagram depicting the potential sites of pineal melatonin action in a model of experimental site

the progression character of scoliosis is associated with a membrane anomaly in the melatonin receptor [44, 45]. However, recent studies in patients with AIS have shown that no evidence of mutations in the melatonin gene receptor [42, 43]. Asymmetric expression of melatonin receptor mRNA in the paraspinal muscles and melatonin signaling dysfunction in osteoblasts have been demonstrated in AIS, but it is not clear whether these findings are causative or secondary changes [44, 46]. Lowe et al. concluded that IS does not result from a simple absence of melatonin but rather an alteration in the system of melatonin production with direct or indirect consequences upon growth mechanisms [2] (Fig. 7.9).

7.4 Nervous System

Scoliosis is seen in various neurological disorders at different levels of the nervous system, from the peripheral nerves up to the central nervous system, but the abnormalities in the central nervous system have long been thought to play a role in the pathogenesis of AIS. The studies carried out at Tokushima University in

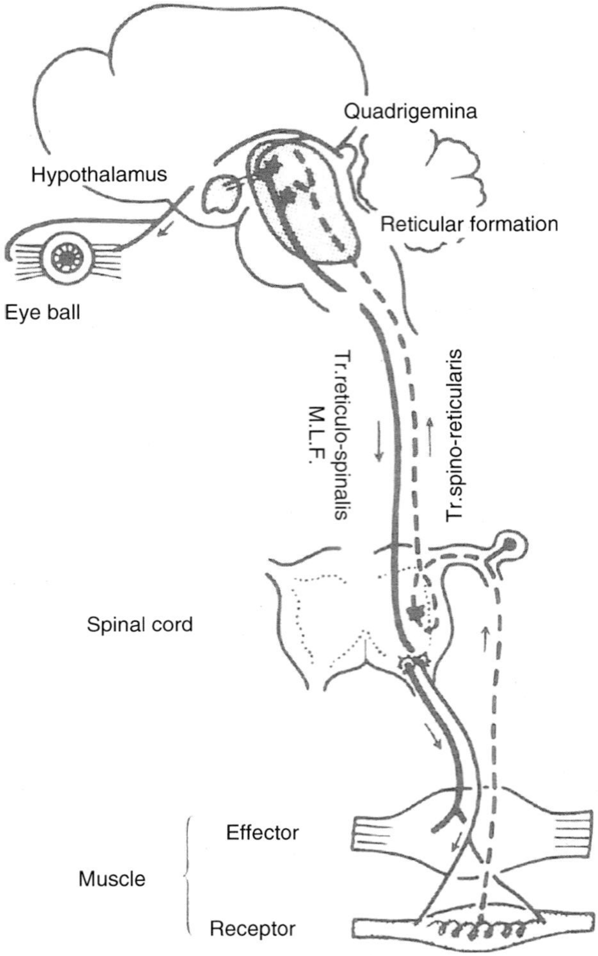

Fig. 7.10 Postural reflex pathway. Reprinted from Yamamoto H. A postural disequilibrium as an etiological factor in idiopathic scoliosis. Pathogenesis of Idiopathic Scoliosis. Edit by Jacobs RR. Published Scoliosis Research Society 1984. Courtesy from Professor Hiroshi Yamamoto (Kochi University)

Japan since 1965 were primarily designed to investigate the effect of scoliosis on postural tone, i.e., a reflex function depending on afferent stimuli from somatic proprioceptive organs onto the vestibular mechanism of the inner ears and the visual input from the eyes [47–51] (Fig. 7.10). At the 2000 Scoliosis Research Society Symposium, Lowe et al. concluded that there is a defect of central control or processing in the central nervous system affecting the growth of spine; the most consistent clinical studies point to the pontine and hindbrain regions as the most likely sites of primary pathology [2].

Relevant studies can be divided into two major groups: neuromorphologic studies and neurophysiologic studies. Utilizing the high resolution of magnetic resonance imaging (MRI) and advanced computer-aided images to compare the central nervous system of AIS patients and normal adolescents, the studies were concluded in regional brain volumes, the white matter in the corpus callosum and internal capsule [52], and the vestibular system morphology, particularly in the alignment of the semicircular canals [53–55]. Apart from the investigation of neuromorphology, functional studies in AIS subjects have shown varieties of abnormalities in the multiple systems/functions as follows: postural balance, somatosensory function, equilibrium [56–59], proprioceptive function [60], oculovestibular function [61], lateral gaze palsy [62], electromyography [63], somatosensory evoked potentials [64–67], and even electroencephalography [68]. There were also contradictory findings regarding vibratory responses [60, 69], transcranial magnetic stimulation [70, 71] and motor cortex hyperexcitability [72], and gait studies [73–76].

7.4.1 *Spinal Cord*

Experimentally induced spinal cord scoliosis has been produced in mammals through microsurgical dorsal rhizotomies [77–79]. All animals in which three or more roots were transected developed a progressive scoliosis. Histological examination of the spinal cord in the scoliosis animals showed no evidence of anterior horn damage, infarct, or ischemic change. Dorsal rhizotomies were believed to lead to spinal deformity due to the proprioceptive deficit that followed the transection of the nerve roots. Pincott et al. also reported the development of scoliosis after transection of the dorsal roots in a series of primate animals. They found that the frequency of scoliosis was higher when more roots were transected and that the addition of transecting a ventral root showed no effect on the production of a spinal deformity. In all animals, the spinal deformity convexity was on the side of the experimental lesions [80]. This supported the hypothesis that the scoliosis could be created by asymmetrical spinal muscle weakness due to loss of proprioception.

In another series of animal experiments, experimental scoliosis was produced in animals by both anterior and posterior spinal rhizotomies over several levels [81]. Scoliosis also occurred when the posterior horn cells along with the central posterior gray matter and adjacent Clarke columns were damaged on the convex side of the spinal cord. Injection of attenuated polio virus into the spinal cords of monkeys also produced scoliosis [82]. Although there was obvious spinal cord damage, scoliosis was thought not to be due to poliomyelitis because the anterior horn was not involved. This experiment provided a useful animal model, but the scoliosis that developed was similar to a paralytic or neuropathic deformity than IS, since rotation deformity was not detected.

Segmental destruction of the vascular supply in the spinal cord of rabbits gave rise to a progressive scoliotic deformity, radiologically similar to IS. In these experiments, the nerve damage was seen mainly in the posterior and lateral columns along with anterior horn, suggesting that segmental damage to the proprioceptive control of spinal musculature could have occurred [83]. Barrios et al. also produced scoliotic deformity in rabbits by using laser or electrocoagulation to induce focal damage to the posterior horn of the spinal cord [84]. This preparation produced scoliotic deformity. The areas of neuronal necrosis and/or gliosis were limited entirely to the posterior horn and the contiguous parts of the posterior and lateral columns. The scoliosis created was always convex on the side of the cord lesion. In a clinical study, Dubousset et al. reported spinal deformities in all 30 cases that received excision of spinal cord neuroblastomas, with the spinal curvature always on the convex side. The ligation or coagulation of the intercostal neurovascular bundle within foramen might have resulted in posterior horn damage of the spinal cord [85].

Scoliosis has been induced in animals through selective destruction of the posterior column at the spinal cord level, the brainstem, and the posterior hypothalamus. Clinical studies assessing posterior column function have consistently shown significant differences between scoliotic subjects and controls, and numerous studies have shown that AIS patients display abnormal postural equilibrium. Proprioceptive input, a prominent component of postural equilibrium, has been hypothesized to play a significant role in the etiology of AIS, and multiple clinical studies have supported this theory. Since proprioceptive and vibratory inputs are conducted through the posterior column system, reports of significant differences in somatosensory evoked potentials (SEPs) between AIS and normal controls imply posterior column dysfunction [86]. However, whether abnormal postural equilibrium is the primary etiologic factor or whether it is secondary to spinal deformity cannot be determined. Whitecloud et al. showed deceased sensitivity to vibration in the lower but not the upper extremities in patients with congenital scoliosis, demonstrating the presence of a sensory deficit that is secondary to the congenital curve itself or an associated subclinical spinal cord lesion; they argued that the sensory deficit is secondary to the spinal deformity rather than a primary etiologic factor. Furthermore, equilibrium dysfunction was shown to be correlated with the progression of scoliosis, regardless of whether the curve was idiopathic or congenital in origin [87] and suggested that equilibrium dysfunction was secondary to the curve but not the primary etiological factor. Since no significant asymmetry in vibration response was found between the concave and convex sides in the IS patients or the right and left sides in the control subjects, it is unlikely that a lesion of the posterior column is the primary cause for IS.

The advent of MRI has led to renewed interest in abnormal neuroanatomy seen in condition such as Chiari malformation or tethered spinal cord, both of which have been linked to scoliosis. In patients with IS, there is a substantially higher prevalence of cervicothoracic syrinxes associated with Chiari type I malformations at the foramen magnum particularly in those who exhibit a juvenile onset of this disorder [88–90]. A review of the literature revealed that the prevalence of a syrinx in a comparable series of patients with scoliosis ranged from 10% to 47% [90] [91]. The site and extent of the curve showed no differences from those found in IS without a syrinx, but there was a greater prevalence of left-sided thoracic deformity in patients with a syrinx. Neurologic function was normal in most patients, although some patients showed asymmetrical superficial abdominal reflexes. It is not yet known whether this is secondary to the syrinx formation as the first sign of syringomyelia or whether this asymmetrical reflex might reflect a more proximal hindbrain or midbrain lesion. A brain lesion could be linked to or even cause the syrinx, the tonsillar prolapse, and the scoliosis. Alternatively, the Chiari malformation and the syrinx could be the result of traction acting upon the medulla distally through the foramen magnum. It is also possible that growth of the spinal cord is slower in patients with IS, resulting in a cord that is shorter than the more rapidly growing spinal canal [92]. Reduced growth of the cord may also be due to pineal dysfunction, perhaps involving a melatonin deficiency, leading to a discrepancy between the lengths of the spinal column and the spinal cord in the normal spine [93].

In 1968, Roth proposed that shortening of the spinal cord can lead to IS. He explained the patho-mechanism of IS by a spring-string model and believed that the disturbed symmetry of nerve tension causes lateral flexion of the spine toward the side of increased tension [92]. Later, Porter, analyzing the axial lengths of the spinal column and the spinal canal in normal and IS spines, found no significant difference between the two groups in the lengths of the spine [94]. He hypothesized that a short spinal canal could tether the posterior elements, and the continuing growth of the vertebral bodies would result in buckling and rotation of the spine around the axis of the spinal cord; he called this the theory of "uncoupled neuro-osseous growth" [95]. Recently, Chu et al. reported on relative overgrowth of the spinal column in AIS without a corresponding increase in the length of the spinal cord, postulating that the fixed spinal cord could act as a functional tether [96]. The role of the spinal cord itself in the development of AIS, however, remains controversial.

7.4.2 Brainstem

It is conceivable that lateral displacement of the vertebrae requires an altered postural tone to maintain the balance of the body, which is regulated by a postural reflex mechanism: this mechanism originates from the proprioceptors, the vestibules of the internal ears, and the optic organs, ending at the equilibrium center of the brainstem. If disturbances occur at any level of the postural reflex circuit system, the stability of the axis skeleton and spine is at risk and may contribute to development of scoliosis (Yamamoto [47]) (Fig. 7.11). The imbalance may be in the primary or secondary afferent systems, but there are also clinical and experimental evidences that brainstem dysfunction may contribute to the etiology of IS [97].

The spinal column, the main axis of posture, is maintained and dynamically regulated by a postural reflex mechanism in the gamma system which operates between the peripheral proprioceptive organs and the brainstem center. Much of the input concerning postural equilibrium is coordinated with proper motor commands at the supraspinal center through a continuous integration of the impulses from a different receptor system.

Magnus performed a series of experiments in which he excised one labyrinth in dogs and found not only that a spinal deviation ensued but also that this deviation could be corrected by excising the contralateral labyrinth at a later stage [98]. These

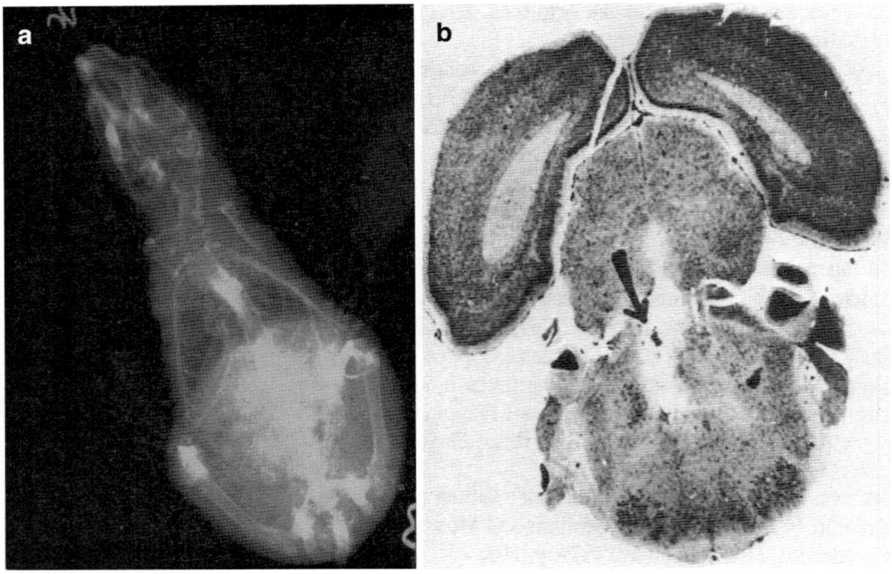

Fig. 7.11 (**a**) Experimental scoliosis produced by stereotaxic destruction of the brainstem in a young bipedal rat. (**b**) Site of lesion (arrow) in the brainstem. Reprinted from Yamamoto H. A postural disequilibrium as an etiological factor in idiopathic scoliosis. 213. Pathogenesis of Idiopathic Scoliosis. Edit by Jacobs RR. Published Scoliosis Research Society 1984. Courtesy from Professor Hiroshi Yamamoto (Kochi University)

experiments were in fact the first demonstration of the effects of conduction disturbances between the inner ear and spinal posture, although no evidence was presented as to whether true structural curvatures of the spine were produced or whether they were only postural deformities. The latter possibility was substantiated by the findings in *Xenopus laevis*, an amphibian species established previously as a model for developmental and lesion-induced plasticity of the vestibular reflex [99, 100]. After unilateral labyrinthectomy at the larval stages, adult Xenopus frogs exhibited a postural asymmetry and skeletal deformation with many characteristics reminiscent of human AIS [101]. However, this model resulted in kyphoscoliosis and not lordoscoliosis, which would cause an asymmetric and tonic contraction of the bilateral axial muscles and a continuous pull on the mostly cartilaginous skeletal elements during early ontogeny.

The vestibular system is essential for postural control and intimately interacts with the visual and proprioceptive systems. Integration of impulses from those different systems takes place mainly at the brainstem level. When vestibular function is unbalanced, skeletal muscle tone can be influenced reflexively through afferent tracts, resulting in a deviation and rotation of the body toward the side with lower muscle tone. The abnormal asymmetric posture demonstrated by the spine in these circumstances resembles the characteristics of a scoliotic deformity.

Rousie et al. found an abnormal connection between the lymphatic lateral and posterior semicircular canals (LPCC) in 52/95 (55%) of IS patients. They evaluated the functional impact of LPCC by testing the vestibule-ocular reflex (VOR) in the horizontal and vertical planes and found reproducible abnormal responses. They found that ampullofugal displacement of the fluid in the posterior canal unexpectedly produced an upbeat nystagmus and suggested that it could be due to an abnormal congenital process of ossification of the canal [53].

Shi et al. examined vestibular deficits in AIS. Geometric morphological differences were detected by vestibular analysis on the left semicircular canals in AIS patients with a right thoracic curve but not in healthy controls [52]. These morphological changes are likely to cause subclinical postural, vestibular, and proprioceptive dysfunctions. Further longitudinal studies could help to define the link between morphological and functional dysfunctions, which may have important predictive and prognostic values on curvature development and progression.

It is difficult to distinguish the cause from effect when a neurological abnormality is associated with IS. For example, an abnormal sway pattern is one area of proprioception that can be measured with a "stabilimeter," which has force transducers placed at the center of the four sides of a square platform on which the subject stands. Although sway was originally thought to be a primary abnormality that causes scoliosis [102], it is now considered to be secondary to scoliosis, i.e., a result of the spinal deformity [103]. It tends to be more marked when the central nervous system is still immature [104] and apparently reverts to normal as growth ceases, despite the residual scoliosis [103]. Therefore, the observed abnormality in equilibrium believed to be secondary to scoliosis may actually be a compensatory phenomenon of an immature neurologic system.

Sahlstrand et al. found significantly poorer postural control in 57 patients with AIS compared with normal children [105]. The difference was most pronounced in tests in which the proprioceptive functions were most important for maintaining the postural equilibriums, and the greatest abnormality was observed in the subgroup with small curvatures. They concluded that their results indirectly indicated that postural disequilibrium is a contributory causative factor for AIS. On the other hand, Gregoric et al. reported that IS patients showed no significant difference in postural equilibrium from the control group, although there was a tendency toward increased oscillations in some patients, especially when recorded with the eyes closed. With the mean oscillation frequency practically identical to the control subjects, this study did not support the theory that the pathogenesis of scoliosis is triggered by an impairment of descending postural control [106]. It is worth noting that visual input is important for IS patients to improve their postural stability.

Sahlstrand et al. studied the effects of Barany caloric stimulation on postural sway by comparing IS children and normal controls. They found that stimulation of the labyrinth on the convex side increased the area of sway, as measured on the "stabilimeter," while concave stimulation had much less effect [105]. In general, the effects of caloric stimulation in the children with scoliosis were much more pronounced than in the normal controls, and the two sides tended to be asymmetric in IS cases, which is usually symmetric in most control cases. Sahlstrand et al. also combined caloric stimulation with electronystagmographic examination with various positions of the trunk [107]. It was noted that the increase in the degree of the spinal curvature was limited to a change from an erect posture that did not affect the increased caloric response on the convex side of the curvature. This suggested that the degree of spinal curvature was not the primary reason for the abnormal vestibular response but rather that the labyrinthine asymmetry might be a basic factor of the condition. It was difficult, however, to draw a definite conclusion as to whether the vestibular imbalance was a contributory factor to AIS or whether the vestibular findings were a feedback effect from the deformed spine.

Equilibrium function should develop in pace with the growth of the body and reach maturity around the time of prepuberty. The developmental retardation of the postural reflex during the rapid growth of the body induces a risky situation for stabilizing the juvenile spine. Yamada et al. performed a series of clinical and experimental investigations of postural equilibrium dysfunction in the proprioceptive and/or the ocular reflex. 119 of 150 patients with IS (79%) showed marked equilibrium dysfunction in at least one of the equilibrium function tests while only one of 20 control subjects showed any dysfunction [47]. After cessation of vertebral growth, the equilibrium dysfunction gradually decreases and finally disappears when the subject is about 20 years of age, irrespective of degree of the curve. As for the pattern of the ocular reflex system in IS, equilibrium dysfunction was improved by changing posture from a standing or sitting to a supine position. These results demonstrate that disequilibrium in IS is dependent upon the posture, and equilibrium disorder may be a dysfunction of the reflex system which operates between the peripheral proprioceptive organs and the brainstem. Studies uncovered functional and organic impairments of the brainstem center for the posture equilibrium, suggesting the possibility that progressive scoliosis during the growth stages could be brought about by dysfunction of the postural reflex control that is derived from a functional or organic disorder at the brainstem [47].

Using sophisticated equipment, Herman and MacEwen detected a significant difference in the brainstem function between IS and control cases and between congenital scoliosis and healthy children [108]. Hinoki investigated the ocular motor system and found unstable foveal stabilization in the pursuit movement system which can be interpreted as a functional impairment of the brainstem [109]. Although a different anatomical location of the brainstem is implicated, many researchers agree that dysfunction of the brainstem plays a role in the development of IS. The clinical investigations mentioned previously revealed that most of the patients with IS showed equilibrium dysfunction in the proprioceptive and/or ocular reflex system during growth.

The dysfunction initially appeared to be a secondary phenomenon resulting from a positive feedback mechanism in the postural circuit system. However, the possibility that a brainstem disorder could be a primary etiological factor was implied by the following studies. In order to clarify the effect of brainstem lesions on development scoliosis, Yamamoto and Yamada et al. produced experimental scoliosis in bipedal rats by microscopic electrocoagulation to create stereotactic lesion in the brainstem. Histology of the lesions in the bipedal rats, which all developed scoliosis, revealed lesions in the periaqueductal gray matter, including Schutz's longitudinal dorsal bundle, at the level of the midbrain and/or the pons, close to the vestibular and periocular nuclei (Fig. 7.11). This experiment suggested that equilibrium dysfunction brought out by a disturbance in the interaction between proprioceptors of the trunk and equilibrium centers within the brainstem caused scoliosis. Yamada et al. explored further the role of the equilibrium center at the brainstem has on development of experimental scoliosis by the recording the optokinetic reflex through electronystagmography. The optokinetic reflex gradually develops in the rat with growth, but when scoliosis is experimentally produced with semicarbazides, the development of the optokinetic nystagmus was inhibited. From these results, they concluded that the scoliosis was caused by a functional disorder of equilibrium center at the brainstem [103] and proposed that there are two specific groups of patients with disequilibrium: one is due to functional disturbance and the other is due to an organic disorder within the brainstem centers. They also stated that the equilibrium disorders, whether induced by proprioceptor reflexes (functional) or brainstem lesions (organic), had a distinct relationship to the progress and the degree of the scoliosis curve. They emphasized that proprioceptors have a positive feedback influence to the equilibrium control centers, but no evidence was provided for this notion [103].

A number of studies have shown an abnormal nystagmus response during caloric testing in patients with IS, suggesting an oculovestibular abnormality. Herman et al. proposed that a dysfunction of the motor cortex that controls disturbing the axial posture due to a sensory input deficiency concerning spatial orientation and concluded that this effect probably results from central proprioceptive sources involving visual and vestibular function [110]. The clinical syndrome of symmetrical horizontal or lateral gaze palsy is often seen in patients with IS [111]. The site of neurological abnormality in this condition is thought to reside in the paramedian pontine reticular formation, which links the periocular motor nuclei and the vestibular nuclei [112].

It has been suggested that brainstem dysfunction may be a cause of IS, but whether the disturbances are indeed primary or whether they develop secondary to the existence of a scoliosis remains to be further elucidated. Equilibrium dysfunction is characteristic in patients with progressive curves, regardless of etiology, implying that it is secondary to the curve rather than a primary event [113]. Equilibrium dysfunction has been previously reported in numerous scoliosis groups reporting multifactorial abnormalities such as impaired postural control [47, 105, 106], spontaneous and positional nystagmus [47, 104, 105], abnormal smooth pursuit [97, 108], and changes in vestibular-induced nystagmus [104, 108]. The idiopathic progressive and congenital progressive patients performed the worst, with abnormal results on all of the above tests [113]. While the idiopathic nonprogressive group also demonstrated abnormalities in postural control, spontaneous and positional nystagmus episodes, and disorders in smooth visual pursuit, the equilibrium and oculovestibular functions were almost uniformly normal. The message from these studies is that equilibrium dysfunction correlates with progression of scoliosis, irrespective of the curve being either idiopathic or congenital in origin. This in turn suggests that the dysfunction is secondary to the curve rather than being a primary event.

Changes in vestibular-induced nystagmus including impaired quality, decreased duration of nystagmus, and asymmetric labyrinthine sensitivity have also been associated with IS, and such equilibrium dysfunction has been shown to be characteristic of patients with progressive curves. It is also possible that some of the abnormalities found in IS are related to a delay in maturation of the central nervous system.

7.4.3 Cerebellum

Recent research supports that the theory that scoliosis is a multifactorial disease involving abnormalities in postural disequilibrium [114, 115], vestibular dysfunction [101], and communication between the cerebellum and the vestibular system [116]. Since the posterior cerebellum and floplease cculonodular lobe have extensive afferent and efferent connections with vestibular nuclei [117, 118], the function and morphology of the cerebellum should be examined in AIS research studies.

Previous studies mainly looking into the abnormal morphology of the cerebellum in IS patients have suggested that the cerebellar dysfunction may play a role in AIS development. Shi et al. measured and compared the volume of the cerebellum between AIS patients and normal controls [119] and reported that the volumes of four regions, namely, the right VIIa, right VIIb, left X, and right X, were significantly increased by approximately 7.43–8.25% in the AIS group when compared to the control group. The increase in AIS cerebellar volume is mainly observed in the regions of the prepyramidal/prebiventer and intrabiventer fissures, the intrabiventer and secondary fissures, and the flocculonodular (X)-posterolateral fissures to the inferior hemispheric margin. They concluded that the volume differences could be compensatory consequences of the central nervous system brought out by the patient's efforts to maintain body balance an asymmetric spine [119].

Further research is required to better understand the role of anatomic changes in the cerebellum of AIS cases, and functional imaging studies to examine the correlation between the structural and functional abnormalities are anticipated. There are a small number of AIS cases reporting the cross-sectional studies, but longitudinal studies are required to further understand the role of anatomic changes in the cerebellum from onset to progression of AIS.

7.4.4 Brain

The brain or cerebrum has been one of the major factors examined in the pathogenesis of AIS. To ascertain the relationship between organic brain lesions and the development of scoliosis, stereotaxic destruction of the hypothalamus using minute electrical charges was performed in the bipedal rats [50, 103]. Marked scoliosis developed in 16 of 103 bipedal rats, and they showed equilibrium dysfunction more frequently than the rats without scoliosis. Histologic examination of the brain in the rats with scoliosis revealed lesions in the posterior hypothalamus, leading Kawata to postulate that a lesion in posterior hypothalamus may disturb the reticular formation of the brainstem and lead to scoliosis in bipedal rats [50]. Machida et al. produced experimental scoliosis in melatonin-deficient C57BL/6J mice and investigated the action sites of melatonin in the brain utilizing morphological analyses with [^{125}I]iodomelatonin. Our results suggest that the site in the brain most responsible for the etiology of scoliosis is likely to be the paraventricular thalamic nucleus (Fig. 7.6) [50].

Recently, various neuroanatomical studies of the brain have been proposed to explore the relationship between brain dysfunction and pathogenesis of AIS. Structural brain MRI analyses, such as region volume [120], cortical thickness [121], comprehensive morphometry of corpus callosum [122], vestibular morphoanatomy [56], and volume-based morphometry [52], have been used to investigate the morphological changes in the brain of AIS patients. Preliminary analyses of regional brain volume have indicated an anatomical asymmetry in brain regions functionally related to somatic motor control and coordination, and Wang et al. recently reported the thinning of the cerebral cortex in AIS patients and demonstrated that the "small-world" architecture (Walls and Strongatz 1998) and organization of the cortical networks in AIS patients was fully preserved, but there is hemispheric asymmetry in AIS brains. Their results suggested an increased central role of temporal and occipital cortexes and a decreased central role of limbic cortex in AIS patients when compared to normal controls. Furthermore, decreased structural connectivity between the two hemispheres and increased connectivity in several cortical regions within one hemisphere demonstrate an alteration of cortical network in the AIS brain [111].

Shi et al. applied MRI volume-based morphometry to test their hypothesis that there are neuroanatomic changes in patients with AIS [52]. It has been reported that patients with left thoracic curves have a slightly higher prevalence of neuroanatomic brain abnormalities than those with right thoracic curves. White matter attenuation in the corpus callosum and left internal capsule, which are responsible for interhemispheric communication and acts a conduit for corticothalamic projectional fibers, respectively, were found to be slightly lower in left thoracic AIS cases when compared to control subjects; however, this was not evident in right thoracic AIS cases. Lee et al. found no significant difference between left thoracic AIS and controls [123]. Joly et al. investigated the in vivo microstructures of the white matter within the corpus callosum in AIS patients using diffusion magnetic imaging and found that the corpus callosum had significantly lower fractional anisotropy in patients with right thoracic AIS than in controls. In particular, the anterior part of the corpus callosum (region II) revealed significantly lower value in both the voxel- and ROI-based analyses. He hypothesized that defective sensorimotor integration at the cortical level plays a role in AIS [124]. Confirmation of these findings is required in future research to evaluate the relationship of white matter abnormality with curve laterality, pathogenesis, and prognosis in patients with AIS.

To better understand the role of neuroanatomic changes in AIS, functional imaging studies that correlate structural changes with functional impairments are needed. In the past, electroencephalographic (EEG) studies were utilized to localize intracerebral defects in AIS patients. Peterson et al. carried out an EEG investigation in 57 patients with AIS and found that 30% exhibited "increase of low-frequency activity" only or "paroxysmal activity," compared to 17% in control cases [68]. On further examination, however, it was noted that these abnormalities tended to appear only at rest, and that there was no statistical difference between the scoliotic and the normal children if their EEG recordings included "activation procedures" such as hyperventilation, photic stimulation, or sleep. They concluded that centrally located subcortical structures are involved in the pathologic process in AIS. They also pointed out that the previously noted paroxysmal activity was like an age-dependent phenomenon, and the possibility therefore existed that the "abnormalities" found in scoliotic children were due to cerebral immaturity. However, frequency analysis of the EEG recordings, which is a quantitative measure for determining brain maturity, showed no differences between the scoliotic subjects and the controls (Peterson et al. [68]). In fact, there was an inverse relationship between the degree of curvature and the presence of abnormal paroxysmal EEG waves. This inversed activity in the patients with less advanced deformity was not an age-related phenomenon, since there was no statistical difference between the age of the patients and degree of curvatures. They also noted that there was no correlation between the direction of the curve and any asymmetry of EEG activity.

Data indicating the presence of EEG changes in IS was presented by Lukeschitsch et al. who compared 115 children with IS with 35 children suffering from congenital scoliosis. Fifty of the children with IS showed abnormalities in their EEGs, while the incidence was even greater in the congenital scoliosis group with 20 out of 35. No relationship was found between EEG abnormalities and the degree of curvature or the presence of other neurological changes [125]. In contrast, the study by Peterson showed that only a small number of the IS cases (seven out of 50) were associated with paroxysmal activity. Leonard also carried out an EEG examination in 57 patients with IS and found that 22 patients (38%) were considered to have abnormal EEGs. He postulated that the abnormality was emanating from the midline subcortical structures in the brainstem region [126]. Dretakis et al. also showed an increased frequency of EEG changes in IS patients when compared to normal controls. The EEG changes were even more evident after "activation" by sleep, hyperventilation, or photic stimulation. There were no specific EEG changes in IS, but the data raised the possibility of minor brain trauma during birth both in the children with IS and those with congenital spinal deformity. They also reported that the EEG abnormalities were related to the location of curve with focal EEG changes observed in the brain hemisphere opposite the curve direction in the case with lumbar curves, while EEG changes were observed in the ipsilateral brain hemisphere in cases with thoracolumbar curves. In cases with thoracic curves, EEG abnormalities suggestive of subcortical changes were found in 50% of the patients with abnormal EEGs. Bilateral synchronous abnormalities were predominant in children with

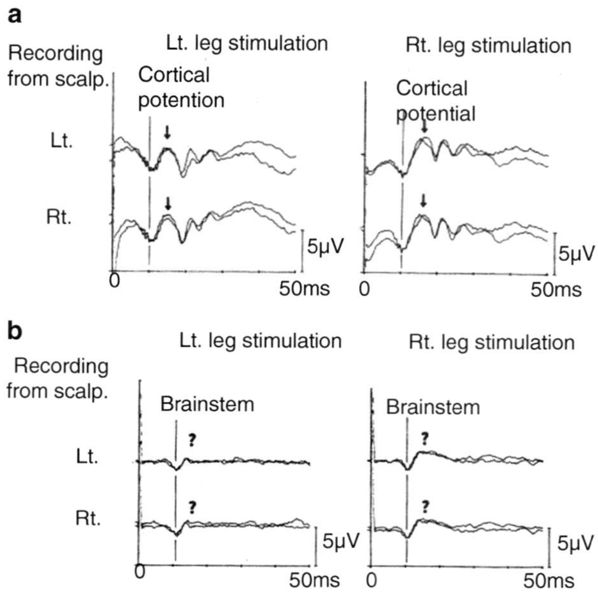

Fig. 7.12 (**a**) Waveform somatosensory evoked potentials (SEPs) in control chicken after stimulation of the leg consists of an initial positive peak followed by subsequent negative and positive peaks. The initial positive peak originates in the brainstem, and negative peak arises from the cortex. Note that identical SEP latencies are observed bilaterally. (**b**) Waveform SEPs in pinealectomized chicken reveal a normal initial positive potential but lacks subsequent negative peak

thoracic scoliosis, whereas focal EEG changes were more frequently seen in children with other locations of scoliosis. However, there are studies that contradict the presence of EEG abnormalities [127]. Robb et al. performed EEG examinations in 25 children with IS and compared the results with those achieved in 25 age- and sex-matched normal children. All of the IS cases and 24 out of 25 controls had normal EEGs resulting to the view that IS has a central neurologic that can be assessed by EEG [128]. Although there are numerous studies using EEG to evaluate IS pathology, it is important to remember that EEG cannot detect subcortical abnormalities.

Identifying neurologic deficits in IS not only helps in defining possible etiologies but may also provide useful clinical information. Schneider et al. examined the spinal vertebrae and the spinal cord in eight IS patients that exhibited abnormal somatosensory evoked potentials (SEPs) and found that six children showed structural abnormalities in the spine or the spinal cord. Based on these findings, they recommend SEPs as a screening method for hidden lesions of the central nervous system [129]. We studied SEPs in 20 chickens with experimentally induced scoliosis after pinealectomy and found that SEPs after leg stimulation were significantly delayed in the scoliosis group compared to the controls (Fig. 7.12). We then compared SEPs taken from 100 patients with AIS and 20 age-matched healthy youngsters without scoliosis and found that the latency of cortical potential (N37) after

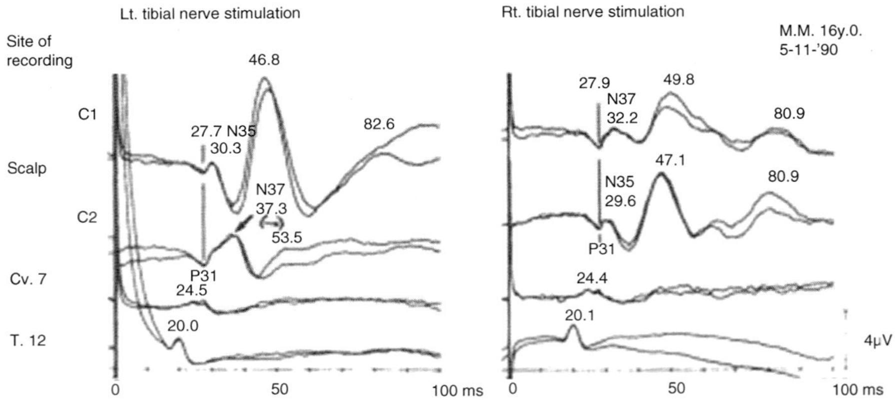

Fig. 7.13 SEPs from the scalp, neck (Cv7), and thoracic (T12) spine after stimulation of the tibial nerve. Tibial SEP showed asymmetric latencies between right and left stimulation with delayed cortical potential (N37) after stimulation of left tibial nerve side

stimulation of the tibial nerve was longer in the scoliosis group than in the control group (Fig. 7.13). Analysis of individual patients revealed SEPs abnormalities in all except for three patients. Our findings in both experimental and clinical studies strongly support the hypothesis that IS results from dysfunction, somewhere within the central nervous system related to sensory pathway [64].

Hausman et al. also reported an increase in SEPs latencies after stimulation of the tibial nerve in 68 of 100 patients with AIS [66]. Pathological SEPs are indicative of functional abnormalities with subclinical involvement of the recorded neuronal pathways. Chau et al. suggested that the site of SEP abnormalities in AIS originates from a level above the cervical spine and is likely to involve disturbances along the spinocortical pathway [130]. Other studies involving late reflexes and SEPs in patients undergoing surgery for AIS have demonstrated abnormal and asymmetrical latencies, correlating with the side and indeed the progression of the scoliosis [131]. They concluded that these findings suggested a problem of the midbrain and/or brainstem, where primary neurological pathogenesis might cause a functional asymmetry in balance and consequently result in scoliosis [131]. Whether these findings are primary etiological factors or secondary to the spinal deformity is not known.

In order to find the etiology and pathogenesis of AIS, as shown in this review, extensive studies have been conducted exploring entire neurological systems, from peripheral nerve to the brain. Although many possible findings were discovered in multiple organs and systems, none showed conclusively the true etiology of AIS. Continued researches to find the true etiology of AIS is imperative in order to provide appropriate and successful treatment for AIS.

References

1. Kouwenhoven JW, Castelein RM. The pathogenesis of adolescent idiopathic scoliosis: review of the literature. Spine. 2008;33:2898–908.
2. Low TG, Edgard M, Margulies JY, et al. Etiology of idiopathic scoliosis: current trends in research. J Bone Joint Surg. 2000;82A:1157–68.
3. Machida M, Murai I, Miyashita Y, et al. Pathogenesis of idiopathic scoliosis: experimental study in rats. Spine. 1999;24:1985–9.
4. Machida M, Saito M, Dubousset J, et al. Pathological mechanism of idiopathic scoliosis: experimental scoliosis in pinealectomized rats. Eur Spine J. 2005;14:843–8.
5. Guerin J. Letter sur le traitement des deviations laterals de l'epine par la section sous-cutanee des muscles de dos et de la colonne vertebrale. Gaz Med Paris. 1839;7:403–4.
6. Adams W. Lectures on the pathology and treatment of lateral and other forms of curvature of the spine. London: Churchill & Sons; 1865.
7. Trontelj JV, Pecak F, Dimitrijevic MR. Segmental neurophysiological mechanisms in scoliosis. J Bone Joint Surg. 1979;61B:310–3.
8. Spencer GSG, Eccles MJ. Spinal muscle in scoliosis. Part 2. The proportion and size of type I and type II skeletal muscle fibers measured using a computer controlled microscope. J Neurol Sci. 1976;30:143–54.
9. Bylund P, Jansson E, Dahlberg E, et al. Muscle fiber types in thoracic erector spinae muscles. Fiber types in idiopathic and other forms of scoliosis. Clin Orthop. 1987;214:222–8.
10. Slager UT, Hsu JD. Morphometry and pathology of the paraspinous muscles in idiopathic scoliosis. Dev Med Child Neurol. 1986;28:749–56.
11. Yarom R, Robin GC, Gorodetsky R. X-Ray fluorescence analysis of muscle in scoliosis. Spine. 1978;3:142–5.
12. Yarom R, Robin GC. Studies on spinal and peripheral muscles from patients with scoliosis. Spine. 1979;4:12–21.
13. Riddle HVF, Roaf R. Muscle imbalance in the causation of scoliosis. Lancet. 1955;1:1245–7.
14. Henssge J. Are signs of denervation of muscles of the spine primary or secondary findings in cases of scoliosis? J Bone Joint Surg. 1968;50B:882.
15. Badger VM. Correlation studies on muscle in scoliosis: histochemistry, EMG, EM and quantitative enzyme estimation. J Bone Joint Surg. 1969;51A:204.
16. Walf E, Robin GC, Yarom R, et al. Myopathy of deltoid muscle in patients with idiopathic scoliosis. Electromyogr Clin Neurophysiol. 1982;22:357–69.
17. Trontelj JV. The motor unit in idiopathic scoliosis. Acta Orth Jugosl. 1984;15:7–14.
18. Fernandez JM. Single fiber EMG in juvenile idiopathic scoliosis. Muscle Nerve. 1988;11:297–300.
19. Valentino B, Maccauro L, Mango G. Electromyography in the investigation and early diagnosis of scoliosis. Anat Clin. 1985;7:55–9.
20. Yarom R, Robin GC. Muscle pathology in idiopathic scoliosis. Isr J Med Sci. 1979;15:917–24.
21. Gibson JN, McMaster MJ, Scrimgeour CM, et al. Rates of muscle protein synthesis in paraspinal muscle: lateral disparity in children with idiopathic scoliosis. Clin Sci. 1988;75:79–83.
22. Ebashi S, Endo M. Calcium and muscle contraction. Prog Biophys Mol Biol. 1968;18:123–83.
23. Cohen DS, Solomons CS, Lowe TG. Altered platelet calmodulin activity in AIS. Orthop Trans. 1985;9:106.
24. Kindsfater K, Lowe T, Lawellin D, et al. Levels of platelet calmodulin for the prediction of progression and severity of adolescent idiopathic scoliosis. J Bone Joint Surg. 1994;76A:1186–92.

25. Acaroglu RE, Akel I, Alanay A, et al. Comparison of the melatonin and calmodulin in paraventral muscle and platelets of patients with or without adolescent idiopathic scoliosis. Spine J. 2009;34:E659–63.
26. Lowe TG, Lawellin D, Smith D, et al. Platelet calmodulin levels in adolescent idiopathic scoliosis: do the levels correlate with curve progression and severity? Spine. 2002;27:768–75.
27. Lowe TG, Buewell RG, Dangerfield PH. Platelet calmodulin levels in adolescent idiopathic scoliosis (AIS): can they predict curve progression and severity? Summary of an electronic focus group debate of the IBSE. Eur Spine J. 2004;13:257–65.
28. Benitex-King G, Anton-Tay F. Calmodulin mediates melatonin cytoskeletal effects. Experientia. 1993;49:635–41.
29. Brezeniski AA. melatonin in humans. New Engl J Med. 1997;336:186–9.
30. Thillard MJ. Deformation de la colonne vertebrale consecutives a l'epiphysectomie chez le poussin. Extrait Compt Rendus Assoc Anat. 1959;XLVI:22–6.
31. Dubousset J, Queneau P, Thillard MJ. Experimental scoliosis induced by pineal and dicephalic lesions in young chickens: its relation with clinical findings in idiopathic scoliosis. Orthop Trans. 1983;7:7.
32. Machida M, Dubousset J, Imamura Y, et al. An experimental study in chickens for the pathogenesis of idiopathic scoliosis. Spine. 1993;18:1609–15.
33. Machida M, Dubousset J, Imamura Y, et al. Role of melatonin deficiency in the development of scoliosis in pinealectomised chickens. J Bone Joint Surg. 1995;77B:134–8.
34. Dubousset J, Machida M. Possible role of the pineal gland in the pathogenesis of idiopathic scoliosis. Experimental and clinical studies. Bull Acad Natl Med. 2001;185:593–602.
35. Machida M, Dubousset J, Sato T, et al. Pathological mechanism of experimental scoliosis in pinealectomized chickens. Spine. 2001;26:E385–91.
36. Machida M, Dubousset J, Yamada T, et al. Experimental scoliosis in melatonin-deficient C57BL/6J mice without pinealectomy. J Pineal Res. 2006;41:1–7.
37. Cheung KM, Wang T, Poon AM, et al. The effect of pinealectomy in scoliosis development in young nonhuman primates. Spine. 2005;30:2009–13.
38. Machida M, Dubousset J, Miyake A, et al. The possible pathogenesis in adolescent idiopathic scoliosis based on experimental model of melatonin-deficient C57BL/65J mice. Presented at 51st annual meeting of Scoliosis Research Society in Prague, Sep 2016. Prague: Scoliosis Research Society; 2016. p. 22.
39. Machida M, Dubousset J, Imamura Y, et al. Melatonin. A possible role in pathogenesis of adolescent idiopathic scoliosis. Spine. 1996;21:1147–52.
40. Machida M. Cause of idiopathic scoliosis. Spine. 1999;24:2576–83.
41. Machida M, Dubousset J, Yamada T, et al. Serum melatonin levels in adolescent idiopathic scoliosis prediction and prevention for curve progression – a prospective study. J Pineal Res. 2009;46:344–8.
42. Morcuende JA, Minhas R, Dolan L, et al. Allelic variants of human melatonin 1A receptor in patients with familial adolescent idiopathic scoliosis. Spine. 2003;28:2025–8.
43. Qiu XS, Tang NL, Yeung HY, et al. The role of melatonin receptor 1B gene (MTNR1B) in adolescent idiopathic scoliosis – a genetic association study. Stud Health Technol Inform. 2006;123:3–8.
44. Moreau A, Wang DS, Forget S, et al. Melatonin signaling dysfunction in adolescent idiopathic scoliosis. Spine. 2004;29:1772–81.
45. Akoume MY, Azeddine B, Turgeon I, et al. Cell-based screening test for idiopathic scoliosis using cellular dielectric spectroscopy. Spine. 2010;35:E601–8.
46. Wu J, Qiu Y, Zhang L, et al. Association of estrogen receptor gene polymorphisms with susceptibility to adolescent idiopathic scoliosis. Spine. 2006;31:1131–6.
47. Yamada K, Ikata T, Yamamoto H, et al. Equilibrium function in scoliosis and active corrective plaster jacket for the treatment. Tokushima J Med. 1969;16:1–7.
48. Tezuka A. Development of scoliosis in cases with congenital organic abnormalities of the brain stem. A report of seven cases. Tokushima J Exp Med. 1971;18:49–62.

49. Yamamoto H, Yamada K. Equilibrium approach to scoliotic posture. Agressologie. 1976;17:61–6.
50. Kawata S. Experimental scoliosis produced by stereotaxic destruction of the posterior part of the hypothalamus in bipedal rats. Shikoku Acta Med. 1976;32:125–31.
51. Yamada K, Yamamoto H. Neuromuscular and neurohormonal approaches to the etiology of idiopathic scoliosis. Orth Trans. 1978;2:277.
52. Shi L, Wang D, Chu WCW, et al. Volume-based morphometry of brain MR images in adolescent idiopathic scoliosis and healthy control subjects. Am J Neuroradiol. 2009;30:1302–7.
53. Rousie DL, Hache JC, Pellerin P, et al. Oculomotor, postural, and perceptual asymmetries and asymmetries in vestibular organ anatomy. Ann N Y Acad Sci. 1999;871:439–46.
54. Chu WC, Shi L, Wang D, et al. Variations of semicircular canals orientation and left-right asymmetry in adolescent idiopathic scoliosis (AIS) comparing with normal controls: MR morphometry study using advanced image computation techniques. Stud Health Technol Inform. 2008;140:333.
55. Shi L, Wang D, Chu WC, et al. Automatic MRI segmentation and morphoanatomy analysis of the vestibular system in adolescent idiopathic scoliosis. NeuroImage. 2011;54:S180–8.
56. Guo X, Chau W, Hui-Chan CWY, et al. Balance control in adolescents with idiopathic scoliosis and disturbed somatosensory function. Spine. 2006;31:E437–40.
57. Lao ML, Chow DH, Guo X, et al. Impaired dynamic balance control in adolescents with idiopathic scoliosis and abnormal somatosensory evoked potentials. J Pediatr Orthop. 2006;28:846–9.
58. Beaulieu M, Toulotte C, Gatto L, et al. Postural imbalance in nontreated adolescent idiopathic scoliosis at different periods of progression. Eur Spine J. 2009;18:38–44.
59. Simoneau M, Richer N, Mercier P, et al. Sensory deprivation and balance control in idiopathic scoliosis adolescent. Exp Brain Res. 2006;170:576–82.
60. Barrack RL, Wyatt MP, Whitecloud TSIII, et al. Vibratory hypersensitivity in idiopathic scoliosis. J Pediatr Orthop. 1988;8:389–95.
61. Wiener-Vacher SR, Mazda K. Asymmetric otolith vestibule-ocular responses in children with idiopathic scoliosis. J Pediatr. 1998;132:1028–32.
62. Jen J, Coulin CJ, Bosley TM, et al. Familial horizontal gaze palsy with progressive scoliosis maps to chromosome 11q23-25. Neurology. 2002;59:432–5.
63. Cheung J, Veldhuizen AG, Jp H, et al. Geometric and myographic assessments in the evaluation of curve progression in idiopathic scoliosis. Spine. 2006;31:322–9.
64. Machida M, Dubousset J, Imamura Y, et al. Pathogenesis of idiopathic scoliosis: SEPs in chickens with experimentally induced scoliosis and in patients with idiopathic scoliosis. J Pediatr Orthop. 1994;14:329–35.
65. Cheng JC, Guo X, Sher AH, et al. Correlation between curve severity, somatosensory evoked potentials, and magnetic resonance imaging in adolescents idiopathic scoliosis. Spine. 1999;23:332–7.
66. Hausmann ON, Boni T, Pfirrmann CW, et al. Preoperative radiological and electrophysiological evaluation in 100 adolescent idiopathic scoliosis patients. Eur Spine J. 2003;12:501–6.
67. Lao ML, Chow DH, Guo X, et al. Impaired dynamic balance control in adolescents with idiopathic scoliosis and abnormal somatosensory evoked potentials. J Pediatr Orthop. 2008;28:846–9.
68. Peterson I, Sahlstrand T, Sellden U. EEG investigation of patients with adolescent idiopathic scoliosis. Acta Orth Scand. 1979;50:283–93.
69. McInnes E, Hill DL, Raso VJ, et al. Vibratory response in adolescents who have idiopathic scoliosis. J Bone Joint Surg. 1991;73A:1208–12.
70. Kimiskidis VK, Potoupnis M, Papagiannopoulos SK, et al. Idiopathic scoliosis: a transcranial magnetic stimulation study. J Musculoskelet Neuronal Interact. 2007;7:155–60.
71. Mihailia D, Calancie B. Is corticospinal tract organization different in idiopathic scoliosis? Stud Health Technol Inform. 2008;140:350.
72. Domenech J, Torms JM, Barrios C, et al. Motor cortical hyperexcitability in idiopathic scoliosis: could focal dystonia be a subclinical etiological factor? Eur Spine J. 2010;19:223–30.

73. Chockalingam N, Dangerfield PH, Rahmatalla A, et al. Assessment of ground reaction force during scoliotic gait. Eur Spine J. 2004;13:750–4.
74. Chow DH, Kwok ML, Cheng JC, et al. The effect of backpack weight on the standing posture and balance of schoolgirls with adolescent idiopathic scoliosis and normal controls. Gait Posture. 2006;24:173–81.
75. Bruyneel AV, Chavet P, Bollini G, et al. Dynamical asymmetries in idiopathic scoliosis during forward and lateral initiation step. Eur Spine J. 2009;18:188–95.
76. Mahaudens P, Banse X, Mousny M, et al. Gait in adolescent idiopathic scoliosis: kinematic electromyographic analysis. Eur Spine J. 2009;18:512–21.
77. Liszka O. Spinal cord mechanisms leading to scoliosis in animal experiments. Acta Med Pol. 1961;2:45–63.
78. MacEwen GD. Experimental scoliosis. In: Zorab PA, editor. Proceedings of the 2nd symposium on scoliosis: causation. Livigstone: Edinburgh; 1968. p. 14–8.
79. Alexander MA, Bunch WH, Ebbesson SOE. Can experimental dorsal rhizotomy produce scoliosis? J Bone Joint Surg. 1972;54A:1509–13.
80. Pincott JR, Davies JS, Taffs LF. Scoliosis caused by section of dorsal spinal nerve roots. J Bone Joint Surg. 1984;66B:27–9.
81. Suk SI, Song HS, Lee CK. Scoliosis induced anterior and posterior rhizotomy. Spine. 1989;14:692–7.
82. Pincott JR, Taffs LF. Experimental scoliosis in primates. A neurological cause. J Bone Joint Surg. 1982;64B:503–7.
83. deSalis J, Beguiristain JL, Canadell J. The production of experimental scoliosis by selective arterial ablation. Int Orthop. 1980;3:311–5.
84. Barrios C, Tunon MT, deSalis JA, et al. Scoliosis induced by medullary damage: an experimental study in rabbits. Spine. 1987;12:433–9.
85. Dubousset J, Bancel PH, Missenard G. Spinal deformities secondary to the treatment of neuroblastomas in children. Presented at 15th annual meeting of scoliosis research society in Chicago, Sep 1980. Prague: Scoliosis Research Society; 1980. p. 17.
86. Cheng JC, Guo X, Shea AH. Posterior tibial nerve somatosensory cortical evoked potentials in idiopathic scoliosis. Spine. 1998;23:332–7.
87. Whitecloud TS III, Brinker MR, Barrack RL, et al. Vibratory response in congenital scoliosis. J Pediatr Orthop. 1989;9:422–6.
88. Isu T, Chono Y, Iwasaki Y, et al. Scoliosis associated with syringomyelia presenting in children. Childs Nerv Syst. 1992;8:97–100.
89. Arai S, Ohtsuka Y, Moriya H, et al. Scoliosis associated with syringomyelia. Spine. 1993;18:1591–2.
90. Gupta P, Lenke LG, Bridwell KH. Incidence of neural axis abnormalities in infantile and juvenile patients with spinal deformity. Is a magnetic resonance image screening necessary? Spine. 1998;23:206–10.
91. Singhal R, Perry DC, Prasad S, et al. The use of routine preoperative magnetic resonance imaging in identifying intraspinal anomalies in patients with idiopathic scoliosis: a 10-year review. Eur Spine J. 2013;22:355–9.
92. Roth M. Idiopathic scoliosis caused by a short spinal cord. Acta Radiol Diagn (Stockh). 1968;7:257–2571.
93. Porter RW. Can a short spinal cord produce scoliosis? Eur Spine J. 2001;10:2–9.
94. Porter RW. Idiopathic scoliosis: the relation between the vertebral canal and the vertebral bodies. Spine. 2000;25:1360–6.
95. Porter RW. The pathogenesis of idiopathic scoliosis: uncoupled neuro-osseous growth? Eur Spine J. 2001;10:473–81.
96. Chu WC, Lam WW, Chan YL, et al. Relative shortening and functional tethering of spinal cord in adolescent idiopathic scoliosis?: study with multiplanar reformat magnetic resonance imaging and somatosensory evoked potential. Spine. 2001;10:482–7.
97. Yamamoto H. A postural disequilibrium as an etiological factor in idiopathic scoliosis. In: Jacobs RR, editor. Pathogenesis of idiopathic scoliosis: proceeding of an international conference. Prague: Scoliosis Research Society; 1983.

98. Magnus R. Korperstellung. Berlin: Springer; 1925. (cited by Stilwell DL, 1962)
99. Horn E, Rayer B. Compensation of vestibular lesions in relation to development. Naturwissenscaften. 1978;65:441.
100. Rayer B, Horn E. The development of the static vestibule-ocular reflex in the Southern Clawed Toad, Xenopus laevis. III Chronic hemilabyrinthectomized tadpoles. J Com Physiol A. 1986;159:887–95.
101. Lambert FM, Malinvaud D, Glaunes J, et al. Vestibular asymmetry as the cause of idiopathic scoliosis: a possible answer from Xenopus. J Neurosci. 2009;29:12477–83.
102. Nachemson A, Sahlstrand F. Etiologic factors in adolescent idiopathic scoliosis. Spine. 1977;3:176–82.
103. Yamada K, Yamamoto H, Nakagawa Y, et al. Etiology of idiopathic scoliosis. Clin Orthop. 1984;184:50–7.
104. Sahlstrand T, Petrusson B. A study of labyrinthine function in patients with adolescent idiopathic scoliosis. (i) An electronystagmographic study. Acta Orth Scan. 1979;50:759–69.
105. Sahlstrand T, Ortengren R, Nachemson A. Postural equilibrium in idiopathic scoliosis. Acta Orth Scand. 1978;49:354–65.
106. Gregoric M, Pecak F, Trontelj JV, et al. Postural control in scoliosis: a statokinesimetric study in patients with scoliosis due to neuromuscular disorders and in patients with idiopathic scoliosis. Acta Orthop Scand. 1981;52:59–63.
107. Sahlstrand T, Petrusson B. Postural effects on nystagmus response during caloric stimulation in patients with adolescent idiopathic scoliosis. (ii) an electronystagmographic study. Acta Orth Scan. 1979;50:771–5.
108. Herman R, MacEwen GD. Idiopathic scoliosis: a visio-vesticular disorder of the central nervous system. In: Zorab PA, editor. Scoliosis. Preceeding of the sixth symposium. London: Academic; 1978. p. 61–9.
109. Hinoki M. Measurement of the slow phase of optokinetic nystagmus in patients with scoliosis. Agressologie. 1979;2D–C:223–4.
110. Herman R, Mixon J, Fisher A, et al. Idiopathic scoliosis and the central nervous system: a motor control problem. Spine. 1985;10:1–14.
111. Hamanishi C, Tanaka S, Kasahara Y, et al. Progressive scoliosis associated with lateral gaze palsy. Spine. 1993;18:2545–8.
112. Herman R, Maulucci R, Stuyck J, et al. Vestibular functioning in idiopathic scoliosis. Orth Trans. 1979;3:218–9.
113. O'Beirne J, Goldberg C, Dowling E, et al. Equilibrium dysfunction in scoliosis – cause or effect? J Spinal Dis. 1989;2:184–9.
114. Byl NH, Hollands S, Jurek A, et al. Postural imbalance and vibratory sensitivity in patients with idiopathic scoliosis: implications for treatment. J Orthop Sports Phys Ther. 1997;26:60–8.
115. Mirovsky Y, Blankstei A, Shlamkovitch N. Postural control in patients with severe idiopathic scoliosis: a prospective study. J Pediatr Orthop. 2006;15B:168–71.
116. Simoneuau M, Lamothe V, Hutin T, et al. Evidence for cognitive vestibular integration impairment in idiopathic scoliosis patients. BMC Neurosci. 2009;10:102.
117. Ghez C, Farn S. The cerebellum. In: Kandel ER, Schwartz JH, editors. Principle of neural science. 2nd ed. New York, NY: Elsevier; 1985. p. 502–22.
118. Barmack NH. Central vestibular system: vestibular nuclei and posterior cerebellum. Brain Res Bull. 2003;60:511–41.
119. Shi L, Wang D, Hui SCN, et al. Volumetric changes in cerebellar regions in adolescent idiopathic scoliosis compared with healthy controls. Spine J. 2013;
120. Liu T, Chu WC Yeung G, et al. MR analysis of regional brain volume in adolescent idiopathic scoliosis: neurological manifestation of a systemic disease. J Magn Reson Imaging. 2008;27:732–6.
121. Wang D, Shi L, Chu WC, et al. Abnormal cerebral cortical thinning pattern in adolescent idiopathic scoliosis. NeuroImage. 2012;59:935–42.

122. Wang D, Shi L, Chu WCW, et al. A comparison of morphometric techniques for studying the shape of corpus callosum in adolescent idiopathic scoliosis. NeuroImage. 2009;45:738–48.
123. Lee JS, Kim S-J, Suh KT, et al. Adolescent idiopathic scoliosis may not be associated with brain anomalies. Acta Radiol. 2009;50:941–6.
124. Joly O, Rousie D, Jissendi P, et al. A new approach to corpus callosum anomalies in idiopathic scoliosis using diffusion tensor magnetic resonance imaging. Eur Spine J. 2014;22:2643–9.
125. Lukeschitsch G, Meznik F, Feldner-Bustin H. Zerebrale dysfunction bei patenten mit idiopatische skoliose. Ztsch Orth. 1980;118:372–5.
126. Leonard MA. An investigation into the EEG findings in patients with idiopathic scoliosis. J Bone Joint Surg. 1981;63B:632.
127. Dretakins EK, Parskevaidis H, Zarkadoulas V, et al. Electroencephalographic study of school children with adolescent idiopathic scoliosis. Spine. 1988;13:143–5.
128. Robb JE, Conner AN, Stephenson JBT. Normal electroencephalograms in idiopathic scoliosis. Act Orth Scand. 1985;57:220–1.
129. Schneider E, Niethard FU, Schiek H, et al. Wie idioppathisch ist die idiopathische Skoliose? Ergebnisse neurologischer Untersuchungen mit somatosensorisch evozierten Potentialen bei Kindern und Jugendlichen. Z Orthop. 1991;129:355–61.
130. Chau WW, Guo X, Fu LL, et al. Abnormal sensory evoked potential (SSEP) in adolescents with idiopathic scoliosis – the site of abnormality. In: Sawatzky BJ, editor. International Research Society of spinal deformities symposium. Vancouver, BC: International Research Society; 2004. p. 279–81.
131. Maguire J, Madigan R, Wallance S, et al. Intraoperative long-latency reflex activity in adolescent idiopathic scoliosis demonstrates abnormal central processing. A possible cause of adolescent idiopathic scoliosis. Spine. 1993;18:1621–6.

Printed by Printforce, the Netherlands